Social Housing in Transition Countries

Routledge Studies in Health and Social Welfare

1 **Researching Trust and Health**
Edited by Julie Brownlie, Alexandra Greene and Alexandra Howson

2 **Health, Illness and Culture**
Broken Narratives
Edited by Lars-Christer Hydén and Jens Brockmeier

3 **Biopolitics and the 'Obesity Epidemic'**
Governing Bodies
Edited by Jan Wright and Valerie Harwood

4 **Globalization and Health**
Pathways, Evidence and Policy
Edited by Ronald Labonté, Ted Schrecker, Corinne Packer, and Vivien Runnels

5 **Gender Equity in Health**
The Shifting Frontiers of Evidence and Action
Edited by Gita Sen and Piroska Östlin

6 **Perspectives on Care at Home for Older People**
Edited by Christine Ceci, Kristín Björnsdóttir and Mary Ellen Purkis

7 **Transnational Social Support**
Edited by Adrienne Chambon, Wolfgang Schröer and Cornelia Schweppe

8 **The Transformation of Contemporary Health Care**
The Market, the Laboratory, and the Forum
Tiago Moreira

9 **Children with Gender Identity Disorder**
A Clinical, Ethical, and Legal Analysis
Simona Giordano

10 **Social Housing in Transition Countries**
Edited by József Hegedüs, Martin Lux and Nóra Teller

Social Housing in Transition Countries

Edited by József Hegedüs, Martin Lux and Nóra Teller

Routledge
Taylor & Francis Group
NEW YORK LONDON

First published 2013
by Routledge
711 Third Avenue, New York, NY 10017

Simultaneously published in the UK
by Routledge
2 Park Square, Milton Park, Abingdon, Oxfordshire OX14 4RN

First issued in paperback 2014

Routledge is an imprint of the Taylor & Francis Group, an informa business

Library of Congress Cataloging-in-Publication Data

Social housing in transition countries / edited by József Hegedüs, Martin Lux, and Nóra Teller. — 1st ed.
p. cm. — (Routledge studies in health and social welfare ; 10)
Includes bibliographical references and index.
1. Public housing—Europe, Eastern. 2. Housing policy—Europe, Eastern. 3. Former communist countries—Social policy—Case studies. I. Hegedus, Jozsef, 1951– II. Lux, Martin. III. Teller, Nóra.
HD7288.78.E86S63 2012
363.50947—dc23
2012011133

ISBN 978-0-415-89014-4 (hbk)
ISBN 978-1-138-80956-7 (pbk)
ISBN 978-0-203-09590-4 (ebk)

Typeset in Sabon
by IBT Global.

Contents

Figures

Tables

Preface

This volume intends to fill the gap in the range of publications on post-transitional social housing policy developments in Central and Eastern Europe, delivering a critical evaluation of the developments in selected countries' social housing sectors.

The first part of the volume provides a conceptual framework for understanding the process of transition, with particular emphasis on the question of convergence and divergence within the region. The second part focuses on housing policy issues such as privatization, housing finance and management, rent regulation, and the situation of the Roma, which have had a major effect on the development of the housing system. The case studies making up the third part of the volume focus on the specific aspect of social housing that was most relevant to each country. The final part summarizes the current problems facing the social housing systems in the region.

The entire book concludes that social housing policy developments are still trapped by the legacy of privatization, the paradox of decentralization, and the informal economy, all of which lead to inefficient allocation practices. The systems remain without an adequate response to basic social housing needs and are continuously destabilized by general economic and fiscal policy changes in the broader European context.

Acknowledgments

The idea of this book emerged from an international workshop on social housing in Central and Eastern Europe held in Budapest in autumn 2008 with the generous support of the Council of Europe and Habitat for Humanity International. Some of the chapters were developed based on the papers presented and discussed during this event and in the following years in the thematic working group on Central and Eastern Europe of the European Network of Housing Research.

The work on this book was also supported by the Grant Agency of the Czech Republic, grant "Social Inequalities and the Market Risks Following from Housing Consumption. The Real and Desirable Response of State Fiscal and Monetary Policies" no. 403/09/1915, as well as the Metropolitan Research Institute.

We are deeply indebted to our editorial assistants, Agnes Bezeczky, Robin Cassling, and Andrea Judit Tóth, whose patient and thorough work made the publication of these texts possible. We would also like to acknowledge the support of Ildikó Horváth throughout the process of editing.

Part I

1 The Transformation of the Social Housing Sector in Eastern Europe

A Conceptual Framework

József Hegedüs

HOUSING IN THE NEW ECONOMIC AND SOCIAL SYSTEM

The tradition of social housing in Europe goes back to the social conflicts related to urbanization in the nineteenth century, and it became a determining factor in the housing system after World War I, largely because of the introduction of rent control regulations. Social housing in different European countries developed independently for the most part, following the political and historical traditions of individual countries. The creation of the EU made the question of divergence and convergence highly relevant, despite the fact that housing is not an EU-level competency (Priemus 2004; Doling 1997; Gibb 2002; Oxley 2000; Priemus and Dieleman 2002; Scalon and Whithead 2007). The European social housing sector is undergoing changes that point towards both convergence and divergence (Harloe 1995; Kemeny 1995, 2006). However, convergence tends to dominate: "we would expect all advanced capitalist countries to be experiencing the same sorts of pressures and to be responding in similar ways and we might expect to find superficial evidence of similarity and a vulnerability to the advancing hegemony of the neo-liberal economic model" (Malpass 2008, 24).

Post-socialist countries went through a radical transition process that has led to the dissolution of the original Eastern European Housing Model (EEHM) and the creation of a new housing system. Our goal is to describe the housing system that emerged and, more particularly, the role of social housing within the new system. We start out by summarizing the main elements of the EEHM, and argue that it constitutes one model with several submodels (Hegedüs and Tosics 1996; Hegedüs 2011) rather than different models with no common core element (Kemeny and Lowe 1998). Our next step is to develop a conceptual framework for the analysis inspired by a special reading of the Varieties of Capitalism literature (Hall and Soskice 2001) and the Welfare Regime (Esping-Andersen 1990) literature. This will help us to describe housing in its interconnectedness with economic institutions (such as the finance system, construction industry, etc.) and with the social welfare system (housing subsidies, social programs, etc.). We describe those factors of the political and economic transition that we consider to have had an effect on the formation of the new social housing system. This was not an easy task, because the transition process in these countries is not over.

The second section of the chapter deals with the transformation of the housing system in the region, focusing on the changing role of social housing. Although the countries differed in terms of economic development and housing conditions, large-scale privatization of the state-owned housing stock took place across the region. Affordability emerged as a central problem for all of the new housing systems, which is why our discussion of the social housing programs focuses on the ability to pay the cost of housing and the cost of access to housing.

In our conclusion, we return to the question of convergence and divergence. We do not support ready-made typologies of the transitional countries; we believe that the differences are the result of conflicts between different interest groups and organizations that reach a consensus and stabilize the institutions from time to time, which then again leads to new conflicts and a new consensus. Social housing policy is a result of these conflicts and their solutions or, as we will show, the lack of a solution. Just as "cracks" in the EEHM distorted the existing institutional structures, new social "cracks" have emerged in the process of transformation from state socialism to a market society, and the responses to these new "cracks" shape the social housing system.[1] Consequently, we cannot promise to offer a clean picture or describe well-defined models; we will instead concentrate on trends, problems, and alternative solutions in different countries, which can sometimes be contradictory.

INTRODUCTION: A BROAD DEFINITION OF SOCIAL HOUSING

In this volume, we will try to adopt a broad concept of social housing. According to mainstream approaches, social housing is generally defined as housing provided on a not-for-profit basis, managed either by the state or by various permutations of not-for-profit or community agencies that range from housing associations to cooperatives (Burke 2004). This focus hinders mainstream approaches from accounting for the effects of income distribution, the tax system, and other income support programs on the housing system. John Hills is one of the theorists to suggest that the concept must include all benefit programs that have a bearing on housing: "in designing social housing finance and housing benefit systems, potential reforms should be judged in terms of the fundamental aim of the system—to support those who would not otherwise be able to afford an acceptable standard of housing" (2000, 1).[2] Economics-based theories also use a broader concept of social housing; they generally consider its definitive feature to be the combination of a lower-than-market price or rent with a need-based allocation system. For instance, Maclennan and More (1997) describe social housing policy as a field that may include "provision in owner occupation as well as private and non-private rental units and the term relates to the purpose of policy rather than the means" (535).

Kemeny's (1981) highly influential housing theory also implicitly identifies the social sector with the public rental sector. Kemeny's typology distinguishes between the residual and unitary rental regimes as the two basic options of the social housing model. The analyses involve explicit and implicit judgments that imply that the unitary model is superior to the residual model because the latter results in the stigmatization and territorial concentration of the poor, and thus contributes to the poverty trap. Kemeny claims that the size of the social rental sector (whether residual or unitary) is itself an important symptom of existing social structures and social values. For instance, in *The Myth of Home Ownership* (1981), Kemeny describes Australia as a society that does not take responsibility for providing its poor with housing, as the size of the sector was only 5 percent. However, if we want to use a truly broad concept of social housing, then categories such as the size of the public rental sector are not an adequate gauge of a social housing regime. Instead, we need to take the effects of income distribution, income benefit programs, and the tax system into account to establish whether the private rental sector is affordable for a broad swath of the population, particularly low-income households.

The weakness of mainstream approaches is that they necessarily omit two important issues that influence the housing situation of low-income groups, particularly in less-developed countries. The first of these is the question of income inequality if we factor in income benefit programs. Certain income benefit programs enable low-income households to find housing in the private sector. However, benefit programs that effectively achieve the same goals as social housing do not show up in analyses of the social housing sector. The second issue concerns homeownership programs for low-income households (so-called social homeownership; see Oxley 2009). Although such programs have a significant effect on housing provision in countries that do not have a highly developed rental sector (such as Spain, Greece, Portugal, and the Eastern European countries discussed in this volume), they are seldom discussed in the context of social housing because of the lack of a public ownership component. We will attempt to take the influence of these two issues on social housing into consideration in the course of our analyses.

SOCIAL HOUSING IN THE EASTERN EUROPEAN HOUSING MODEL

The main characteristics of the EEHM (Hegedüs and Tosics 1996) were single-party political control over the housing sector, the subordinate role of market mechanisms, a lack of market competition among housing agencies (bureaucratic coordination), and broad control over the allocation of housing services (huge, nontransparent subsidies). However, several versions of this model emerged as individual countries responded differently to problems within the socialist economy (Turner, Hegedüs, and Tosics 1992). Thus, structural explanations form the main features of the model, whereas the divergences can be characterized as "policy options" taken by individual governments.[3]

From an economic point of view, the housing system was part of the shortage economy (Kornai 1992). In this system, bureaucratic coordination rather than market mechanisms integrated the various parts of the economy. Resource allocation to the housing sector (investments, loans, etc.) was controlled by the state,[4] decoupled from supply and demand factors. The vast majority of services were provided "in kind" or below the market price, allocated according to "merit". The artificially low, subsidized housing prices resulted in constant shortages, which led to the development of a dual housing market. This meant that an informal economy existed side by side with the state-controlled housing sector, consisting of self-help buildings, private transactions in the rental sector, private real estate market transactions, a market for subtenancy, and a small entirely private rental sector (Alexeev 1988, 1990; Hegedüs and Tosics 1996).

In sociological terms, the problems in the socialist housing system were caused by the disparity between housing policy aims and reality. The rapid process of industrialization and urbanization confronted the socialist housing system with insurmountable difficulties. This resulted in "cracks" (Hegedüs 1992) in the housing model: in order to circumvent the problems with the system, the behavior of the agents in the housing system no longer corresponded to centrally planned state policy, and the institutional and legal framework could not easily hinder this process. Countries responded differently to the appearance of these "cracks": they could either implement strict control mechanisms (Bulgaria, Russia, East Germany) or allow quasi-market processes (Yugoslavia, Hungary). Thus, Yugoslavian guest workers brought home their earnings from Western Europe and invested them in private housing. Similarly, in Hungary, income from the informal economy, mainly from agricultural production, was used to improve housing conditions. As there was a shortage in construction materials, the state could have attempted to intervene in both cases, but it chose not to. Uncontrolled private transactions in the public sector, such as apartment exchanges, provide another example: they also forced the system to either allow these transactions in a controlled framework or use tough sanctions in order to minimize the scope of the private sector.

It is difficult to establish a concept of social housing for the EEHM, because it was clearly not identical to public rental housing. State housing included housing provision of different tenure types (rental, cooperative, and owner-occupied), which were all under strict state control in terms of investment, housing standards, costs, and prices. There was no special subsector or sphere that could be called "social housing". Thus, there was no need for housing assistance in the formal housing market because of the heavily subsidized housing services, and as the informal market was not officially acknowledged, no income support was applied.

The "public rental" sector was a comprehensive category that included various types of public housing: enterprise housing, council housing, and the rental stock under the shared control of the councils and the enterprises. "Enterprise housing" meant that, in an economic and political structure dominated by the sectoral ministries, the large state-owned enterprises developed and managed their own housing stock. Working hostels were a special type of enterprise housing that served to provide shelter to the first generation of industrial workers who migrated from rural areas. Enterprise housing was very significant in the Soviet Union, but it also made up 13 percent of the housing stock in Poland and 6 percent in Slovakia (Hajduk 1996). In the council housing system, the local governments (as deconcentrated agents of the central government) had the right to develop, manage, and allocate the public housing stock. This was typical in Poland, Hungary, the Czech Republic, and so on. There was a third type of public housing in the former Yugoslavia, where, according to the model of socialist self-management, public housing was under the shared control of the local enterprises and the councils. Finally, there were other special forms of tenure that fall into the category of public rental. Various kinds of "tied accommodation" meant that rental tenure was connected to certain jobs, such as army or police officer or national railway company employee. In Hungary, public housing management companies provided the caretakers of the buildings with apartments. Tenants typically had strong tenancy rights in all of these tenure forms: they often had the right to exchange, inherit, and "sell" a tenancy (Alexeev 1988; Hegedüs and Tosics 1996). Only the tenants in tied accommodation sometimes had more limited tenancy rights.

This overview of the EEHM shows that social housing policy is part of the broader welfare system and should be analyzed within this wider context. However, comparative studies have had difficulties in conceptualizing the Soviet "welfare system". A classification as the "Industrial Achievement–Performance model" (Wilensky 1975) or "authoritarian welfare state" (Aidukaite 2009) do not bring us closer to understanding the welfare regimes of the socialist countries. According to the ideology (constitution, laws, and policy guidelines), these societies ought to have been quite egalitarian, but detailed analyses show that in reality, the individual's long-term prospects were determined by his/her political and economic position (Szelényi 1983; Szelényi and Manchin 1987). According to research on the pre-transition housing systems, state housing subsidies increased rather than decreased inequality, favoring higher income and more influential groups (Szelényi 1983; Hegedüs and Tosics 1986; Alexeev 1988).

VARIETIES OF TRANSFORMATION ANALYSIS

The events of 1989–1990 brought about the establishment of a democratic political system that removed political constraints on the introduction of market mechanisms. The introduction of a multiparty political system, radical privatization, and rapid decentralization characterized the transition from a 'planned' to a 'market' economy. Liberal economic approaches (promoted, for instance, by technical assistance agencies) have dominated the transition literature (Mykhnenko 2004; Kornai 1998, 2000). They focused on the process of overcoming the economic and institutional constraints that hindered the development of the market economy.

There were several attempts to classify Eastern European countries according to differences in the transition process. One mode of analysis was based on the *Varieties of Capitalism* approach (Hall and Soskice 2001); it produced some interesting results that provide a background for understanding the housing system transition. There is widespread agreement that countries followed different developmental paths in terms of the institutional setting. Greskovits (2008) defined four variants of Eastern European capitalism based on the role of leading sectors in macroeconomic stabilization, the formation of the social welfare system, and industrial restructuring.

A recent study by M. Myant and J. Drahokoupil (2010) tries to develop a more sophisticated typology of transition economies. They define five important aspects of institutional development that influence the way in which a national economy can be integrated into the global economy. Analyzing these five dimensions (relationship between politics and business, the rule of law, the role of the state in the economy, the structure of business, and the finance system) they define six forms of international integration that "do not provide 'pure' varieties of capitalism, partly because every country combined more than one form of international integration and partly because different institutional forms were often compatible with the same kind of international integration" (14).[5] The authors conclude that there are five types of post-socialist economies, but they emphasize that there are no unique causal links between the form of integration and the institutional preconditions: "by combining forms of integration with internal economic, political and institutional forms, an approximate classification into five types can be made. In some cases there is overlap between them and none is fixed. All are, to varying extents, in a process of change" (21).

Mitra (2001) used a political science approach and defined four types of transitional economies: competitive democracies that guarantee civil liberties and political rights through a free democratic election system (CEB countries); concentrated political regimes that provide the legal framework of free elections but in practice limit "political competition through constraints on civil liberties" (Romania, Bulgaria, the Ukraine, etc.); noncompetitive political regimes that constrain the political opposition through the control of political freedoms and civil rights (Belarus,

Kazakhstan, Turkmenistan, Uzbekistan, and Kazakhstan); and war-torn political regimes that still suffered from the effects of civil war (Albania, Armenia, Azerbaijan, Bosnia and Herzegovina, Georgia, and Tajikistan). This typology reflected the situation around 2000, but as the author noted, the political system of a country is subject to change: "political systems are still evolving, so countries have been shifting over time across different ideal types" (Mitra 2001, 99). The countries can thus fall into different categories at different times, as recent developments in Romania, Bulgaria, or Hungary show.

Analyses of the social housing sector in transitional countries also have accounted for changes in the welfare regimes. Esping-Andersen (1990) originally identified three basic types: the liberal, the social-democratic, and the conservative/corporatist welfare regimes, which was later supplemented by the Mediterranean (Ferrera 1996) type. After 1990, the challenge was to find a separate heading for the transitional countries. Deacon (1998, 2000) created a separate post-socialist category, whereas Bohle and Greskovits (2007) divided them up among the already existing headings, with the Baltic states classified as liberal, the Visegrad countries as social-democratic, and Slovenia as a corporatist welfare regime. There is no agreement among researchers whether any general conclusions can be drawn concerning the development of welfare systems in transition countries. The main obstacle to research is that public sector reforms (education, health care system, etc.) are incomplete, policy and institutions in different welfare sectors follow different principles even within a single country, and there is a big gap between the rhetoric of programs and their actual implementation. Most of the research is nonconclusive, which is a clear sign of the ongoing conflicting processes in welfare politics (Tomka 2005; Ferge 2001; Cerami 2005; Tausz 2009).

Kasza (2002) questioned the validity of regime typologies. He could not find consistency among different spheres of the welfare system because "(1) each welfare policy tends to change incrementally over many years; (2) different welfare policies in the same country typically have different histories; (3) discrete sets of policy actors are involved in the various fields of welfare policy; (4) variations in the policymaking process affect the substance of policy; and (5) borrowing from foreign models introduces diverse practical and normative elements into each country's welfare package" (2002, 282).[6]

The development of welfare policy in the region did not originate from a consistent ideological model; the policymakers followed no grand plan. Instead, welfare policies evolved in direct reaction to specific societal problems. The various areas of welfare policy (income benefit programs, education, the pension system, etc.) were generally modified with loosely coordinated measures (Hegedüs and Szemző 2010). This type of "trial and error" or "scrambling through" approach was more or less a general phenomenon in the region (Tsenkova 2009).

Three Conflicting Factors of Housing Sector Development

The mainstream approach in housing policy proposed that all aspects of the housing sector (legal, financial, etc.) should undergo systematic reform, thus freeing the housing market from the control of the socialist state. This normative approach dominated housing research in the early 1990s, based on the enabling housing policy of the World Bank (1993). It aimed to identify and describe well-defined legal institutions (property rights, building regulations, flexible planning structure, etc.) and market institutions (housing finance systems, property management, etc.) and to introduce targeted social programs. The ideal housing model was a housing system in which market mechanisms dominate the production, allocation, and consumption of housing; there is sufficient competition among agents and institutions in the interrelated markets for housing finance, resources, and services; and governments provide subsidies that are relatively transparent, progressively targeted, and budgeted in sustainable ways (see, for example, Hegedüs, Mayo, and Tosics 1996; Pichler-Milanovich 2001; Buckley and Tsenkova 2001; Tsenkova 2009).

However, subsequent studies have shown that the transformation was not such a clear-cut, linear process. In order to better describe what actually happened, we distinguish three main factors that are significant for the analysis of the transition: (a) market creation strategies, which help establish new market mechanisms; (b) market correction strategies, which actively alleviate the negative social effects of the new market mechanisms; and (c) the "political stasis factor", which makes it difficult to alter popular elements of the existing system, such as across-the-board subsidies or even regressive tax policy.

The market creation strategy could be implemented without difficulty in sectors where there were no basic social barriers to major change (the construction industry, production of and trade in building materials). However, in the area of housing services (water, heating, etc.) and housing finance, the introduction of market mechanisms created social conflicts arising from price liberalization, enforcement of foreclosures, evictions due to nonpayment, and unaffordable user charges.

The most important market correction strategy was the creation of social benefit programs that help households facing economic hardship. However, it is very difficult to run these programs efficiently because the low public administration capacity and the significance of the informal economy make it hard to gather reliable information on households' incomes. Social housing programs as a market correction mechanism had a low priority until the end of the 1990s.

The "political stasis factors" play an important role in decreasing and postponing the social conflicts of the transition. In the field of housing, which is particularly liable to social conflict, there has been a temptation to retain the popular elements of the socialist housing system: across-the-board subsidies that maintain rent levels below the actual cost of rent; public management companies; price control of energy costs; and a lack of retribution for nonpayment (eviction evasions). Furthermore, these factors do not only contribute to the conservation of the status quo; they often have a regressive redistributive effect, as in, for instance, the reluctance to develop means-tested benefit programs or the massive support for homeownership in the form of mortgage subsidies and contract savings schemes.

How will these three factors enable us to describe the transition process in all its complexity? Let us now turn to their effect on households. During the transition, households had to adapt to the way in which these factors shaped political and economic life by taking them into account in their coping strategies. The transitional recession meant that many households had to struggle to keep a balanced budget, relying on extended family networks and the informal economy to do so (Smith 2000; Pavlovskaya 2004). However, this process of adaptation was not passive: the households' strategies influenced political and economic development, and social policy was also necessarily sensitive to changes in the behavior of the households (Hegedüs and Szemző 2010). Furthermore, households do not only have an individual effect; they are also enmeshed in a political environment where trade unions, political parties, and so on, are constantly competing for political power. Such political entities also play a role in modifying both the policy options and the behavior of the households. Thus, we need to understand the dynamics of this two-way interaction between households and policy if we are to provide an adequate description of the transition.

THE HOUSING SYSTEM TRANSITION AND SOCIAL HOUSING

The new Central and Eastern European (CEE) social housing regimes are still undergoing a process of transition. They have three important elements in common: the limited role of the social landlords due to privatization, an affordability problem due to the divergence in incomes and housing costs in both the public rental and the homeownership sector, and an accessibility problem in both rental and owner-occupied housing for low-income groups. We will argue that the institutional answers to these structural problems may differ from country to country, but they nevertheless form subspecies of the same theoretical model.

Housing Conditions after the Transition

The transitional countries analyzed in this volume differ greatly in terms of population and land area, with Slovenia and Russia at the two extremes. They are at significantly different levels of economic development and recovered from the transitional recession at varying speeds. Slovenia's GDP is more than triple that of the Ukraine (measured in purchasing power parity per capity in 2003). The Baltic states and Central European countries went through a successful economic recovery after the transition and reached 1.5–3.1 percent annual GDP growth between 1990 and 2003, whereas Southeastern European countries, which suffered from the Balkan War and thus implemented reforms later, experienced much slower development. By 2008, the Visegrad and the Baltic countries had reached 130–170 percent of their 1989 GDP, whereas the real GDP of the two new Balkan member states is around the same level as in 1989. The other Balkan countries have yet to reach 1989 levels again.

However, despite the huge differences in the economic recovery and in the institutional response to the transition, similar processes took place in the housing sector: the state-owned construction and building materials industry and the banking sector were privatized and social housing management was decentralized. Institutional solutions continue to vary from country to country.

Comparisons of key housing statistics at the beginning of the transition period suggested that the Eastern European model performed quite well in comparison with countries at the same level of GDP (Hegedüs, Mayo, and Tosics 1996). Expectations that the introduction of market mechanisms would lead to an increase in housing investment proved to be false: housing

Table 1.1 Housing Condition in New Member States of Europe, 2010

	Population in 2009 (thousand people)	Dwelling per 1,000 inhabitants (in 2000)	m²/ person	Bath/ shower (%)	N of rooms	Housing cost level (EU-27 = 100)	GDP in PPP (EU-27 = 100)
Slovenia	2,032	358	30.9	92.3	2.8	69.3	87.0
Czech Republic	10,468	427	28.7	95.5	2.9	58.0	78.0
Hungary	10,031	399	31.2	91.3	2.6	46.5	63.0
Poland	38,136	307	24.2	86.9	3.7	47.6	49.0
Slovak Republic	5,412	310	26.0	92.8	3.2	52.4	72.0
Estonia	1,340	454	29.7	67.1	3.3	74.7	63.0
Latvia	2,261	398	27.0	60.3	2.5	62.9	61.0
Lithuania	3,350	375	24.9	71.1	2.5	45.3	53.0
Bulgaria	7,607	450	25.2	n.a.	n.a.	32.4	43.0
Romania	21,499	352	15.0	58.9	2.6	55.1	42.0
EU-10	102,136	356	23.9	80.6	3.1	50.1	54.0
EU-17*	397,588	462	39.9	97.4	4.4	108.9	109.0

Source: EU Housing Statistics (2010). * European Union except the 10 new member states.

investment declined in the 1990s as a reaction to the transitional recession. After twenty years of transition, there is a large gap between old and new EU member states in terms of housing quality and quantity. There was a 22 percent gap in dwellings per one thousand inhabitants, a 17 percent gap in the share of housing units with a bathroom, and a 30 percent gap in the number of rooms between the EU17 and the EU10 in 2010. However, the housing stock in the new member states is, on average, far better than what might be expected on the basis of the difference in income levels, as the gap in per capita GDP (in PPP) was 50 percent.

It is worth highlighting some of the differences among the new member states. The housing stock in Romania tends to be the worst in terms of size (floor space per capita and the share of flats with a bathroom), which can probably be explained by extreme industrialization in the pre-transition period. Housing policy papers in Poland—both official government documents and research studies—argue that the housing shortage is a huge impediment to development. Recent housing statistics do not fully support this hypothesis, as Poland has the highest average number of rooms per housing units. The relatively good conditions in the Baltic states are due to migration in the last two decades. The proportion of empty housing is increasing in the region. It is at 11 percent in Estonia and 6 percent in Hungary.

Social Housing and the New Tenure Structure

The processes of privatization and restitution had a huge impact on housing systems in the region (for a detailed analysis of the privatization process, see Chapter 2 in this volume). Privatization could not have been avoided, because all social forces were in favor of it at the time; in fact, it is in all actors' short-term interests even today. The public rental sector virtually disappeared in most of the transitional countries as a result. Some countries initially seemed to be exceptions to this trend (e.g., Czech Republic, Poland, Latvia, and Russia), but today, we consider these differences to simply be due to a slower pace of privatization. Privatization had a regressive social effect: financial gains were proportional to the households' wealth, which meant that low-income households were trapped in the social rental sector and were unable to buy their homes at a discount price. The social rental sector has thus become a residualized sector, which houses the most vulnerable social groups.

There was an interesting attempt to categorize housing systems according to privatization strategy, but this method proved insufficient to explain the sociologically important differences between the countries. Lux (2003) followed this approach in his privatization policy-based typology (first used by Hegedüs and Tosics 1998). He differentiated three "models": 'fast privatizers' (Hungary, Slovenia, Estonia, etc.) and 'slow privatizers' (Poland, Latvia, and the Czech Republic), with one strong outlier: Bulgaria—a country that had low levels of public housing even at the beginning of transition. The case of Bulgaria highlights the limitations of the tenure-oriented approach; the typology does not help us understand how Bulgaria went through the transition or how Bulgarian social housing policy managed affordability problems. Indeed, a typology based on privatization strategies could not succeed, as the privatization process is not yet over. It is predicted that, as in other countries, more than 80 percent of the stock will be privatized in both Latvia and the Czech Republic, and privatization continues to take place in Russia (see Chapter 2, this volume).

Beyond the institutional development discussed by the mainstream economic literature (property rights, rule of law, etc.), decentralization also played an important role in the development of housing regimes. This process took on various different forms throughout the region (Bird, Ebel, and Wallich 1995; Dabla-Norris 2006; Rodríguez-Pose and Krøijer 2008). It is very difficult for housing theory to establish a causal connection between decentralization and different social housing models. It is difficult to generalize the impact of local governments on social housing, because different degrees of fiscal decentralization characterize the different countries.

The municipalities became the most important new social landlords. In the new, decentralized system, the framework set up by new housing legislation gave them substantial autonomy to set policy in the social rental sector. There are major differences between countries in terms of the municipalities' scope of autonomy and their financial incentives. For example, municipalities were free to choose among different forms of housing management in several countries (Hungary, Czech Republic, Poland, etc.), whereas the surviving communal enterprises kept their management monopoly over the municipal housing stock (and, for a while, even over privatized apartments in multistory buildings) in others (Russia, the Ukraine, etc.). The structural factors in the changed environment (relatively deteriorated stock, dominance of socially vulnerable and low-income people among the tenants, permanent fiscal pressure on local governments, the lack of efficient monitoring, and enforcement of central government policies and laws) were common to all the countries in the region.

The social housing sector is changing in terms of tenure rights, rent regulation, and allocation rules. As the case studies in this volume show, the new social landlords are implementing different solutions that can fit into the legal framework. However these changes have yet to create a transparent and sustainable system. No professional social landlord has emerged that could undertake the capital investments necessary for the renewal and maintenance of the remaining housing stock or for the expansion of the sector based on future rent revenues and predictable central government grants.

Social housing programs in the region are generally too small to meet demand and depend on grants from the central government. Private financial institutions seldom participate in these projects. The rents paid by the tenants and the subsidies paid by the governments do not provide a stable

Table 1.2 Change of the Tenure Structure in Selected Transitional Countries, 1990, 2001

	Year	public rental	co-oper-ative	private rental	owner occu-pied	other	total
Albania	1990	35.5			64.5		100
	2001	1		5	94		100
Bulgaria	1990	6.6	1.5		91.7	0.2	100
	2001	3		0	96.5	0.5	100
Croatia	1990	24		3.5	67.5	5	100
	2001	2.9		10.8	82.9	3.4	100
Czech Republic	1990	39.1	20.4		40.5		100
	2001	29	17.4	6.7	46.9		100
	2008	14	12.4	13	60.6		100
Estonia	1990	61	4		35		100
	2001	5.2			94.8		100
Hungary	1990	23		3	74		100
	2001	4		4	91	1	100
Latvia	1990	59	5		36		100
	2001	16	2		82		100
Lithuania	1990	60.8			39.2		100
	2001	2.4			94.5	3.1	100
Poland	1990	31.6	25.4		43		100
	2001	16.1	28.6		55.3		100
	2009	10	19.4		70.4	0.2	100
Romania	1990	32.7			67.3		100
	2001	2.7		1.1	96.2	0	100
Russian Federation	1990	67	4		26	3	100
	2001	29			66	5	100
Serbia	1990	23		3	64	10	100
	2001	2.6		4.4	81.6	11.4	100
Slovakia	1990	27.7	22.1		50.2		100
	2001	6.5	15.6	4.1	73.8		100
Slovenia	1990	31		1	68		100
	2001	3		7	82	8	100
Ukraine	1991	47.3			52.7		100
	2001	20			80		100

Source: Own estimates based on Turner, Hegedüs, and Tosics (1992), Hegedüs, Lux, and Sunega (2011), Lux (2003), Bežovan (case study in this volume), Petrovic (case study in this volume), and Muzioł-Węcławowicz (case study in this volume).

and predictable revenue that could reassure private investors about the profitability of such programs.

In almost every country in the region, politics (and housing policy) recognized the need for social housing after mass privatization and the economic recovery had already taken place. A number of programs aimed to increase the size of the social rental sector, but none of them seem to have led to a breakthrough. Realizing that municipalities are under political and financial pressure that limits the development of the social housing, both governments and donor agencies looked for other solutions in the field of nonprofit housing schemes. Some examples are municipal housing funds in Slovenia, nonprofit housing cooperatives in Slovakia, TBSs (social building associations) in Poland, or the Serbian municipal housing agencies. The TBSs in Poland are the most frequently quoted example, but as the case study on Polish social housing in this volume shows, their dependence on the central budget and the pressure from the tenants to have the apartments privatized makes the long-term sustainability of this model uncertain.

Thus, although governments implemented social housing programs across the region, the sector has only experienced limited expansion. Furthermore, the social and financial sustainability of the new social housing system could not be guaranteed: the operation of the sector requires huge subsidies to bridge the gap between market rents and "social" rents; tenants retained extensive tenancy rights; allocation principles remained nontransparent; the down-payment requirement as a precondition to enter the sector led to an indirect regressive selection among possible tenants; and a number of negative factors (e.g., nonpayment, deterioration of the stock, etc.) emerged. These problems and uncertainties explain why both tenants and landlords continue to press for further privatization.

Homeownership became the dominant tenure form. Cooperatives kept their legal status, but in practice, the property rights of the members are hardly different from that of homeowners in condominiums. Housing policies in the region have a bias towards homeownership. The subsidies (mortgage subsidies, contract saving schemes, capital grants for private construction, etc.) and tax regulations make homeownership much more favorable than any options in the rental sector. This bias remains even if we take the "economic subsidies" (hidden subsidies that are equal to the difference between the regulated rent and market rent) into consideration (Lux 2009). This means that the tenants in the rental sector are those who cannot afford to enter owner-occupation. Moreover, legal uncertainty constrains the development of the rental sector.

Private rentals become a crucial area for housing policy, although we have very limited information on it because it belongs mostly to the informal sector. As a consequence of restitution, a new private rental sector emerged, which has become an area of conflict between the private tenants and landlords. The new owners were generally successful in putting the burden of increased rents on the tenants and the governments in the form of rent subsidies (e.g., in Slovenia, Slovakia, Poland, and, to a smaller extent, in the Czech Republic). Another possible consequence of restitution was that the restituted housing units remained part of the formal economy, in contrast to the housing let by individual owners (not professional landlords) typically without registration or taxes. Those low-income tenants who are forced to rent apartments in the informal rental market are extremely vulnerable, as they are not eligible for social programs if they cannot register with the authorities.

The future role of the private rental sector is a key issue. This sector can contribute to the efficiency of the housing system by making higher mobility possible, providing a more flexible housing supply and helping to eliminate distortions in the system, etc. (Lowe 2003; Erdősi, Hegedüs, and Somogyi 2000; Dübel, Hamilton, and Brzeski 2006; Belniak 2007). Moreover, the private sector can be used for social purposes, as in the case of social rental agencies in countries like Holland, Belgium, Italy, and so on, which can be especially important at a time when there is no demographic pressure for new construction. However, we have to emphasize again that there is little reliable information concerning this part of the informal economy. The official data are much lower than expert estimates: for instance, research has showed that 12.2 percent of the Lithuanian and 16.8 percent of the Polish housing stock is made up of private rentals (Dübel, Hamilton, and Brzeski 2006).

Housing Cost and Income Distribution—Affordability

After more than twenty years of transition, Eastern and Central European societies have become nonegalitarian: income inequality has increased (see Table 1.3), unemployment (including hidden unemployment) is high, and insecurity is part of everyday life (arrears, homelessness). The dramatic growth in income inequality took place during the 1990s, when average incomes decreased during the first half of the decade and then stagnated. Real incomes finally started to increase in 2000 and continued to grow until the economic crisis in 2008. Poverty became a huge problem that affects 10 percent of the households even in the new EU member states (Leitner and Holzner 2008). Although the data clearly demonstrate the growth in inequality throughout the region, they provide a less clear picture of the differences between the countries. The new EU member states are generally considered to have less income inequality than other countries formerly part of the Soviet Union, as measured by key factors like wage distribution, employment, entrepreneurial incomes, social safety nets, and other public policy measures (Mitra and Yemtsov 2006). The economic recession associated with the transition also increased regional inequalities within countries. In Hungary the net income per capita is 50 percent higher in the most developed region than in the two least developed regions.

Increases in social inequality were caused by regressive public policy decisions as well as by "market creation" strategies (see Chapter 2, this volume). Social exclusion also played a role, as the Roma population had much fewer opportunities to adjust to the new situation. Five million Roma people live in the Czech Republic, Hungary, Slovakia, Romania, and Bulgaria in very difficult conditions (see Chapter 6, this volume).

There have been several analyses of housing affordability in the region (World Bank 2000; EBRD 2001; Fankhauser and Tepic 2005; Buzar 2007). All of the studies agreed that the data are unreliable, which makes comparison across different countries very difficult. However, some general trends can be identified despite the imprecision of the data. Housing costs (especially utility costs such as water and sewage fees or heating costs) have increased throughout the region at such a rapid pace that household incomes could not keep up.[7] By 1994 utility costs relative to incomes had risen on average from 5.8 percent to 11.4 percent in ten post-socialist countries (Hegedüs, Mayo, and Tosics 1996). Utility companies have generally not reached full cost recovery yet, but the share of utility costs in the households' budgets had increased again significantly by the middle of the 2000s. Fankhauser and Tepic's (2005) study shows variation among the different countries, with households' electricity costs varying between 1.6 percent of household income in Russia and 5.5 percent in Serbia, whereas water fees move between 0.7 percent in Serbia and 4.1 percent in Hungary. However,

Table 1.3 The Gini Coefficients of Income per Capita

Country	Gini Coefficient of Income per Capita		
	1987–1990	1996–1998	2007–2008
Bosnia and Herzegovina	n.a	n.a	0.36
Bulgaria	0.23	0.41	0.45
Croatia	0.36	0.35	0.34
Czech Republic	0.19	0.25	0.26
Estonia	0.23	0.37	0.36
Hungary	0.21	0.25	0.31
Latvia	0.24	0.32	0.36
Lithuania	0.23	0.34	0.38
Poland	0.28	0.33	0.34
Romania	0.23	0.3	0.31
Russia	0.22	0.3	0.42
Serbia	n.a	n.a	0.28
Slovakia	0.22	0.3	0.26
Slovenia	0.22	0.3	0.31
Ukraine	0.24	0.47	0.28

Source: Mitra (2001, 9); Wikipedia (Gini coefficients by country).

Table 1.4 Housing Affordability around 2002–2004 in Selected Transitional Countries (Utility Cost as a Percentage of Household Budget)

	Utility Cost Affordability					
	Across All Income Groups			Of Lowest Income Decile		
Countries	Electricity	Water	Total	Electricity	Water	Total
Bosnia and Herzegovina	5.4	1.1	6.5	8.4	0.7	9.1
Croatia	3.9	1.3	5.2	10.9	2.3	13.2
Czech Republic	4.2	1.2	5.4	5.5	1.5	7
Estonia	3.2	1	4.2	8.2	2.4	10.6
Hungary	5.3	4.1	9.4	6.3	4	10.3
Poland	4.5	2	6.5	5.7	1.8	7.5
Romania	4.8	3.1	7.9	4.1	0.7	4.8
Russia	1.6	3.5	5.1	2.1	4.5	6.6
Serbia	5.5	0.7	6.2	7.2	2.1	9.3
Slovakia	3.5	1.3	4.8	11.4	4.3	15.7
Slovenia	4.5	1.3	5.8	9.4	2.6	12
Ukraine	2.1	1.2	3.3	2.5	0.6	3.2

Source: Fankhauser and Tepic. (2005).

the lowest-income group spent a much bigger share of its income (over 10 percent) on utilities in Hungary, Slovakia, Croatia, and Estonia. Buzar describes the phenomenon of "energy poverty", when households cannot afford to keep adequately warm at a reasonable share of their income, which "arises out of the inadequate co-ordination of energy, social welfare and housing policies" (2007, 224).

The basic economic reason for this problem is that the production costs of energy, heating, water, and other utilities are increasing. Although there are differences between resource-rich and resource-poor countries, the global market sets energy prices for both groups. However, a country can choose the extent to which it liberalizes energy prices. Complete price liberalization would make a large group of vulnerable consumers unable to pay for energy, which leaves governments with two options. They can either offer an across-the-board subsidy to the service providers, which lowers costs for all consumers (but may require higher taxes or slow down economic growth), or they can develop programs targeted only at vulnerable consumers.

The affordability problem can be handled in two ways: either by increasing household incomes or by decreasing housing expenditures. Struggling households can reduce their housing costs through social migration, by moving to a smaller housing unit with lower expenses. This tendency can lead to unintended negative consequences if, as a consequence of downward mobility, the household ends up in an underdeveloped region and its members lose their chance to enter the labor market, education system, and health system, and do not have access to other welfare benefits. Alternatively, households can try to decrease their energy costs. Although a number of energy-efficiency programs were initiated in the 2000s, they did not systematically create an adequate incentive for households to rationalize their energy consumption.

The second way to handle the affordability problem is to increase household incomes. Most countries introduced a range of different income benefit programs, including housing allowance programs, to help low-income households. However, these programs could not bridge the increasing gap between housing costs and incomes because of limited resources and a lack of institutional capacity. As a consequence, the number of households that had difficulties in paying the housing costs increased. Households' coping strategies include applying for additional, non-housing-related income benefits such as childcare benefits, medicine grant, and so on;[8] taking jobs in the informal economy; or getting help from the wider family. However, those who are not able or willing to take these options accumulate debt.

Accumulated arrears can force households to move to a less valuable home and use their equity to pay back their debts to the utility companies. It is becoming more and more frequent for utility companies to start foreclosure procedures. This type of "downward mobility" was a fairly new phenomenon in transitional countries; it contributed to the development of slums in remote villages and urban areas. In Slovakia, the poor housing allowance system led to the mass disconnection of vulnerable consumers. As no rules "on disconnection (termination is left to the contract), the protection of vulnerable consumers, and an appropriate dispute resolution mechanism" (Bartl 2010, 237) were implemented, the number of disconnected households made up 3 percent of the population in 2008.

In Hungary, a new type of crime appeared that profited from the arrears issue. Households with high utility debts (typically also struggling with other social problems) were cheated by the so-called 'real estate mafia', which offered an inhabitable home (typically in a dead-end village or slum area of a city) in exchange for the apartment with debt. Over four hundred such cases were registered between 2001 and 2003, but they were probably only the tip of the iceberg.

Housing market processes contribute to the economic segregation of all disadvantaged social groups, including low-income groups in general as well as the Roma and other ethnic minorities. Institutional segregation by the housing market agents (local governments, banks, developers, etc.) compounds the problem. This is illustrated by cases in Hungary when urban local governments have offered cash grants to Roma people in order to get them to move from their jurisdiction to rural, remote areas. In other cases, developers have used subsidy programs to build new but very poor-quality houses in segregated areas in villages.

Housing Market and Access to Housing—Affordability

As homeownership is the dominant tenure form in the region, the affordability of private homes became an important housing policy question. The state-dominated housing finance system collapsed in 1990 and it took eight to twelve years to develop a new market-based housing finance system. Mortgage products existed on a small scale in most of the countries, but the size of the market was very small because of their high price and the lack

Table 1.5 New Housing Construction 1990–2009 (Number of Units/1.000 Inhabitants)

	1990	1993	1997	2001	2002	2006	2007	2008	2009
Croatia	4.1	1.9	2.8	2.8	4.0	5.0	5.8	5.7	4.2
Czech Republic	4.4	3.1	1.7	2.4	2.7	2.9	4.0	3.7	3.7
Estonia	4.8	1.6	0.7	0.4	0.8	3.8	5.3	4.0	2.3
Hungary	4.2	2.0	2.7	2.8	3.1	3.4	3.6	3.6	3.2
Poland	3.5	2.5	1.9	2.7	2.5	3.0	3.5	4.3	4.2
Romania	2.1	1.3	1.4	1.3	1.2	1.8	2.2	3.1	2.9
Slovakia	3.9	2.6	1.3	1.9	2.6	2.7	3.1	3.2	3.5
Slovenia	3.9	4.0	3.0	3.2	3.6	3.8	4.2	4.9	4.2
Country average	3.4	2.2	1.9	2.3	2.4	2.9	3.4	3.9	3.7

Source: UNECE, National Statistical Institutes, and EU Housing Statistics (2010) (country average is weighted by the population in 2002).

Table 1.6 Outstanding Mortgage as a Percent of the GDP

	2002	2004	2006	2008
Bulgaria	0.7%	2.6%	7.0%	12.2%
Croatia	6.9%	10.3%	12.7%	15.1%
Czech	4.6%	7.6%	14.5%	18.0%
Estonia	7.9%	16.6%	32.3%	38.6%
Hungary	4.8%	10.4%	15.0%	23.2%
Latvia	4.2%	11.5%	29.1%	31.0%
Lithuania	2.3%	7.0%	28.0%	36.4%
Poland	3.5%	5.5%	10.7%	12.8%
Romania	1.0%	1.4%	1.8%	3.7%
Slovenia	0.8%	1.5%	5.1%	7.2%
Slovakia	4.0%	6.1%	10.3%	17.8%

Source: European Mortgage Federation (Hypostat), European Banking Statistics, 2009, for Hungary Hungarian National Bank.

of a legal framework (especially foreclosure regulations). This was demonstrated by the low mortgage loan/GDP ratio.

As Table 1.5 shows, housing output decreased drastically in all the countries at the beginning of the transition. However, the slump was less severe in countries with a higher GDP and a faster recovery: Slovenia and Croatia only suffered a 20–30 percent decrease, whereas Estonian output had decreased by 80 percent in 1997. The overall average was 45 percent.

The development of the mortgage finance system became possible throughout the region around 2000, after macroeconomic stabilization (improvements in GDP growth, inflation, interest rates, the banking system, and the legal framework of foreclosure). There was an extreme increase in outstanding loans in the Baltic states, especially Latvia and Estonia, where the loan to GDP ratio surpassed 30 percent. In fact, outstanding mortgage loans to GDP increased all over the region, but continued to lag behind EU levels. However, mortgage repayment costs much the same as in developed countries because of the higher interest rates and spread in transitional countries (Table 1.6).

In some countries, mortgage finance development was influenced by speculative demand due to an increase in house prices (Estonia, Latvia, and to a certain extent in Lithuania), to generous homeownership subsidies (Hungary, until 2004), or to the cheap interest rate of foreign currency loans (Hungary, after 2004). In other countries, the mortgage market grew rapidly, but became more balanced (e.g., in the Czech Republic, Poland, Slovakia, and Slovenia). In yet other countries, the development of the mortgage market only started around 2004 (Romania and Bulgaria).

Foreign currency (euro and Swiss franc denominated) loans were popular throughout the region (for instance, in Croatia, Poland, Romania, and Hungary). These loans had lower interest rates than the loans offered in the national currencies, but the exchange rate risk and interest rate risk remained with the households (the related affordability issues only became obvious with the 2008–2009 recession, e.g., in Hungary). The share of FX-denominated loans was typically about 40 percent in 2006, but there were some important exceptions (e.g., Czech Republic).

As a consequence of the emerging new housing finance system, housing affordability improved despite the fact that house prices increased more quickly than household income. Decreasing interest rates after 2000 made mortgages affordable for the upper 40 percent of the households, thus relaxing the pressure on social housing. A number of countries subsidized the home buyers through tax exemptions, interest rate subsidies, mortgage guarantees, and contract savings premiums, but these subsidies were typically not unmanageable. Hungary was an exception: it introduced substantial support for home buyers, which resulted in an unsustainably high fiscal commitment for the budget; the subsidy program had to be discontinued in 2004.

After the collapse of the centrally planned economy, reported house price to income (P/I) ratios were initially very high and then tended to decrease. Possible reasons for this were decreasing demographic pressure, the increased housing supply due to privatization, decreases in real income, macroeconomic insecurity, and similar factors. The reported P/I ratio improved greatly in the second half of the 1990s, reaching 4–6, although this was still high compared with some market housing systems in developed countries (Hegedüs, Mayo, and Tosics 1996). The number of transactions started to increase around this time—a sign of a healthy housing market—but reported mobility rates remained quite low in comparison with Western countries. In 2007, well under 10 percent of households in the new EU member states bought/sold their homes, whereas the same indicator was well over 15 percent in the old member states (EU-SILC, 2007).

At the end of the 1990s, housing prices started to increase again as a consequence of economic stabilization. As the increase in average income did not keep pace with the price increases, the increased P/I ratio pointed to an affordability problem. However, it is not easy to demonstrate this trend, as price information is quite unreliable in transition countries; the housing market worked on a cash basis with family transfers and loans playing an important role.

The existence of the informal economy may help explain the relatively high P/I ratios. The informal economy was estimated to be as large as 25–33 percent of GDP between 1990 and 1999, and informal transactions are still widely accepted today by consumers (VAT tax evasion), employees (wages are often paid directly into the "pocket" of 25 percent of all employees), service providers (tax evasion), and so on (Schneider 2002; Buehn and Schneider 2009). According to Glovackas's (2007) estimate, the size of the shadow economy may reach 20 percent of GDP in the new EU member states.

Intergenerational transfers (transfers of family savings and inheritance) played an increasingly important role in how households solved the problem of accessing the owner-occupied market. This, together with the role of the informal economy, can explain how the housing market could exist with such a high P/I ratio and low housing affordability index.

The crisis of 2008 has slowed down the development of the mortgage market. The crisis also led to the development of a new problem, mass evictions, particularly in the worst hit countries, such as the Baltic states, Romania, and Hungary. A large number of households are in danger of losing their homes, and the social housing sector is not prepared to house them all. The share of nonperforming loans increased to 35 percent in Romania, 17–18 percent in the Baltic states, and 14 percent in Hungary in 2011 (Kubik, Predescu, and Rodado 2011). In Hungary, 140,000 borrowers have arrears of more than ninety days, a huge number in comparison with the 120,000 units in the municipal housing stock in 2010.

CONCLUSION: TOWARDS A NEW MODEL?

Our description of how the EEHM changed as a result of the transition process fits into the framework of "soft globalization" theories. We established that, on the one hand, post-socialist countries underwent highly similar structural changes; on the other hand, their policy responses showed major variation. The end of the one-party system, privatization and price liberalization, the development of a new financial sector, growing integration into the world economy, public sector restructuring, and decentralization all show a certain extent of convergence. However, these countries responded to the challenges of the transition process in very different ways in areas such as the structure of the political system, the role of the state in the economy, and the institutional structure of the financial sector, as discussed with differing degrees of success in the "varieties of capitalism" literature. Partly as a consequence of these factors, economic development in terms of GDP growth varies. We are persuaded that the evidence for divergence is not insignificant, but we did not find any typology in the political science, sociology, or political economy literature that could provide a solid basis for an analysis of the changes in housing sector.

We saw that some trends hold true across all of the housing systems in the region, thus strengthening the convergence theory. The social rental sector was largely privatized; it became a residual sector that concentrates the most vulnerable social groups. In most countries, politics (and housing policy) only recognized the need for social housing after mass privatization and economic recovery had already taken place. Programs to expand the social rental sector did not lead to a breakthrough, and its social and financial sustainability remains very weak. Although there have been a number of attempts to modernize the sector, powerful new social landlords have yet to emerge. Two factors hinder the active participation of local governments in such programs: high costs and social conflicts generated by the social rental sector.

The development of the private rental sector has brought about the expansion of a tenure form that is new to the region. However, private rentals are still part of the informal economy in most of the countries, which makes it very difficult to integrate this sector into social housing.

Donor assistance programs had a great deal of influence on the development of the nongovernmental sector in the region, and EU housing policy may have a large impact in the future. UN-Habitat, NGOs from Austria and Holland, and other organizations devised projects to expand the social rental sector. The Council of Europe Development Bank also ran programs in the region (although these were not limited to social rental housing). However, the NGOs did not have much success in the field of social housing. They might gain in significance once a neutral grant allocation system is in place that will enable them to participate in housing management and provision. Furthermore, international organizations should cooperate more extensively; at the moment, every organization focuses only on meeting its own criteria for success (like in the EU structural programs for the new member states).

Housing policy is the result of an interaction between the stakeholders, who all have a very distinct set of political and economic interests. Housing programs are lobbied by local governments, building companies, mortgage banks, financial institutions (such as contract saving banks), and other interest groups, but the details of the decision-making process remain hidden. Governments have frequently made changes to housing policy over the last twenty years, but these changes were generally guided by short-term political and economic interests rather than by political (socialist versus conservative) ideology. There was always a large gap between the rhetoric and the actual effects of a program. A housing policy white paper can promise anything, but implementation and enforcement are another matter altogether.

The region is characterized by "weak government", which is also a factor to explain the lack of efficient housing policy. This means, firstly, that governments are under the influence of private interests interlocked with banks and entrepreneurs; they have little capacity to balance between the different social groups. Secondly, trade unions are more or less powerless in the private sector; they have more power in the public sector and tend to protest reforms. Thirdly, the capacity of governments to introduce and monitor reforms is limited because of the fiscal pressure on the budget and competition with the private sector. Fourthly, decentralization has led to the creation of a public administration that is quite responsive to local interests but has made the public sector as a whole fragmented and inefficient. Finally, the integrity of the public sector has been damaged; corruption cases (especially unrevealed and pardoned cases) make the governments too weak to be a champion of reforms.

The social and economic problems caused by the transition forced governments to introduce changes in the welfare system. The variation in the institutional answers to these cracks (social/political tensions in the self-governing market integration mechanism) may explain the differences between the new welfare regimes. However, it is unclear what kind of welfare regime transitional countries are moving towards, whether it will become a new model that combines the elements of modern European welfare regimes with the 'socialist tradition'. One main trend seems to be that the state plays a smaller and smaller role in the housing and welfare systems. However, welfare policies develop through loosely coordinated measures across different areas (income benefit programs, education, pension system, etc.) in reaction to emerging societal problems—policymakers have no consistent model to be implemented in mind.

Social institutions do not have the capacity and resources to operate an efficient safety net in the new environment (high unemployment, large informal economy, etc.). Poverty is not only due to the income disparity–generating effect of the market economy; it can be also considered as the failure of the welfare system. As incomes from the informal economy remain untaxed, scarce resources are split up among programs that cannot guarantee the affordability of housing costs. Several housing programs contributed to the reproduction of social inequality caused by the labor market and the education system both through market processes and institutional mechanisms (deficiencies in the legal framework and the discriminatory behavior of the housing market agents). Further research is needed to understand the behavior of the different actors in the housing system with respect to the welfare system and to explore in greater detail what social mechanisms lead to the strengthening or weakening of inequity and conflicts among different social groups. The challenge for housing policy in transition countries is to provide institutional assistance to the social groups who have ended up in vulnerable situations because of the structural changes in the economy (privatization and commodification of public services).

NOTES

1. These "cracks" can best be understood in the context of Polanyi's (1957) integration mechanism theory. He distinguished three ideal types of integration mechanisms: redistribution (dominant in the EEHM); market exchange (dominant in post-transition societies); and reciprocity. The "cracks" are those social and political conflicts that are at variance with a society's integration mechanisms. The institutional solutions used to manage these conflicts lead to the emergence of different welfare regimes.
2. Further on, Hills does narrow his definition somewhat, to housing that includes "council housing and that owned by non-profit housing associations now officially known as Registered Social Landlords, RSLs" (2000, 6).
3. This approach could be conceived as a "soft structuralist" approach, which combines a "rational choice" (policy choice or agency choice) type of explanation with structural elements. In an earlier work, Hegedüs followed (1992) this argumentation, for example, in the explanation of "self-help" housing in Hungary.
4. The state meant not only the central government and the councils, but the state-owned enterprises as well, which constituted the majority of the economy and were integrated into the economy through the Communist Party.
5. These forms are: export-oriented FDI in complex sectors, export-oriented complex sectors without FDI, simple manufacturing subcontracting to MNC (multinational corporation), commodity exports, dependence on remittances and aid, and dependence on "financialized" growth.
6. O'Sullivan (2004, 327–29) arrived at the same conclusion in analyzing the Irish welfare system, which he claims could not be classified as a "liberal" welfare regime, because of the exceptional role of the family and the Catholic Church in different welfare areas.
7. Because of privatization, rents make up a negligible share of the housing costs.
8. Income benefit programs typically form a fragmented system across the region: the central government, the local governments, and nonprofit foundations may cooperate, compete, or (as is most common) simply ignore each others' programs. Affected families can become disoriented and even more defenseless due to the lack of information in this chaotic system.

REFERENCES

Aidukaite, J. 2009. "Old Welfare State Theories and New Welfare Regimes in Eastern Europe: Challenges and Implications." *Communist and Post-Communist Studies* 42:23–39.

Alexeev, M. 1988. "The Effect of Housing Allocation on Social Inequality: A Soviet Perspective." *Journal of Comparative Economics* 12:228–34.

———. 1990. "Distribution of Housing Subsidies in the USSR, with Some Soviet-Hungarian, Comparisons." *Comparative Economic Studies* 32 (3): 138–57.

Bartl, M. 2010. "The Affordability of Energy: How Much Protection for the Vulnerable Consumers?" *Journal of Consumer Policy* 33:225–45.

Belniak, S. 2007. "Housing Market Supply and Demand in Poland: The Role of Fundamentals." Paper prepared for a workshop at the Technical University of Bratislava. http://www.disparity.cz/data/USR_048_DEFAULT/Zbornik1_tlac_ISBN.pdf accessed January 12, 2011.

Bird, R. M., Ebel, R. D., and Wallich, C., eds. 1995. *Decentralization of the Socialist State. Intergovernmental Finance in Transition Economies.* Washington, DC: World Bank.

Bohle, D. and Greskovits, B. 2007, "Neoliberalism, embedded neoliberalism and neocorporatism: towards transnational capitalism in Central-Eastern Europe." *West European Politics,* 30:4, 443–446.

Buckley, R. and Tsenkova, S. 2001. "Housing Market Systems in Reforming Socialist Economies: Comparative Indicators of Performance and Policy." *European Housing Policy* 2:1–34.

Buehn, A. and Schneider, F. 2009. *Corruption and the Shadow Economy: A Structural Equation Model Approach, IZA Discussion Papers, 4182.* Institute for the Study of Labor (IZA). http://ftp.iza.org/dp4182.pdf accessed January 20, 2011.

Burke, T. 2004. *Governance and Social Housing: Can Good Governance Be Bad Practice?* Institute for Social Research, Swinburne University of Technology, Australia. http://www.sisr.net/publications/0402burke.pdf accessed February 2011.

Buzar, S. 2007. "The 'Hidden' Geographies of Energy Poverty in Post-Socialism: Between Institutions and Households." *Geoforum* 38:224–240.

Cerami, A. 2005. "Social Policy in Central and Eastern Europe: the Emergence of a New European Model of Solidarity?" Unpublished PhD Dissertation, University of Erfurt.

Dabla-Norris, E. 2006. "The Challenge of Fiscal Decentralization in Transition Countries." *Comparative Economic Studies* 48:100–131.

Deacon, B. 1998. "Global and Regional Agencies and the Making of Post-Communist Social Policy in Eastern Europe." *The Future of European Welfare. A New Social Contract?* London: Macmillan Press.

———. 2000. "Eastern European Welfare States: The Impact of the Politics of Globalization." *Journal of European Social Policy* 10 (2): 146–61.

Doling, J. 1997. *Comparative Housing Policy.* Basingstoke: Macmillan.

Dübel, J., Hamilton E., and Brzeski, J. 2006. *Rental Choice and Housing Policy Realignment in Transition: Post-Privatization Challenges in the Europe and Central Asia Region.* Policy Research Working Paper Series 3884, World Bank. http://ideas.repec.org/p/wbk/wbrwps/3884.html accessed January 20, 2011.

EBRD. 2001. Transition Report. http://www.ebrd.com/pages/research/publications/flagships/transition/archive.shtml accessed January 17 2011.

Erdősi, S., Hegedüs, J., and Somogyi, E. 2000. "Is Private Rental an Option for Urban Housing Provision in Hungary?" *Journal of Housing and Built Environment* 15 (3): 267–91.

Esping-Andersen, G. 1990. *The Three Worlds of Welfare Capitalism*. Princeton, NJ: Princeton University Press.

EU Housing Statistics, 2010. The Hague: Ministry of the Interior and Kingdom Relations Edited by Kees Dol and Marietta Haffner, OTB Research Institute for the Built Environment, Delft University of Technology September 2010.

EU-SILC, 2007. European Union statistics on income and living conditions (EU-SILC). Brussels, Eurostat, 2007.

Fankhauser, S. and Tepic, S. 2005. *Can Poor Consumers Pay for Energy and Water? An Affordability Analysis for Transition Countries, European Bank Reconstruction and Development*. Working Paper No. 92, May. http://www.ebrd.com/downloads/research/economics/workingpapers/wp0092.pdf accessed 1 March 2011.

Ferge, Zs. 2001. "European Integration and the Reform of Social Security in the Accession Countries." *Journal of Social Quality* 3 (1–2): 9–25.

Ferrera, M. 1996. "The 'Southern Model' of Welfare in Social Europe." *Journal of European Social Policy* 6 (1): 17–37.

Gibb, K. 2002. "Trends and Change in Social Housing Finance and Provision within the European Union." *Housing Studies* 17 (2): 325–36.

Glovackas, S. 2007. *The Informal Economy in Central and Eastern Europe*. www.wiego.org/papers/2005/Glovackas.doc accessed 21 March 2010.

Greskovits, B. 2008. "Leading Sectors and the Variety of Capitalism in Eastern Europe." *State and Society in Post-Socialist Economies*. Basingstoke: Palgrave Macmillan.

Hajduk, H. 1996. "Poland." *Housing Policy in Europe*.

Hall, P. A. and Soskice, D., eds. 2001. *Varieties of Capitalism: The Institutional Foundations of Comparative Advantage*. New York: Oxford University Press.

Harloe, M. 1995. The People's Home? *Social Rented Housing in Europe and America*. Oxford: Blackwell.

Hegedüs, J. 1992. "Self Help Housing in Hungary." *Beyond Self-Help Housing*, Profil Verlag, 217–3.

———. 2011. "Social Safety Nets, the Informal Economy and Housing Poverty-Experiences in Transitional Countries." *European Journal of Homelessness* 5 (1): 15–26.

Hegedüs, J., Lux, M., and Sunega, P. 2011. "Decline and Depression: The Impact of the Global Economic Crisis on Housing Markets in Two Post-Socialist States." *Journal of Housing and the Built Environment* 26 (June): 315–33.

Hegedüs, J., Mayo, E. S., and Tosics, I. 1996. "Transition of the Housing Sector in the East Central European Countries." *Review of Urban and Regional Development Studies* 8:101–36.

Hegedüs, J. and Szemző, H. 2010. *Shaping the New Welfare Regime in Transition Countries: The Interplay of Public Policies and Households' Strategies (Case of Hungary) Comparative Housing Research: Approaches and Policy Challenges in a New International Era, 24/25 March 2010, OTB Research Institute and the Faculty of Architecture*. Delft University of Technology, the Netherlands, Delft.

Hegedüs, J. and Tosics, I. 1996. "Disintegration of East-European Housing Model." *Housing Privatization in Eastern Europe*. Greenwood. Westport, Connectucut,London.

———. 1998. "Rent Reform—Issues for the Countries of Eastern Europe and the Newly Independent States." *Housing Studies*13 (5): 657–78.

Hills, J. 2000. *Reinventing Social Housing Finance*. Institute for Public Policy Research, London.

Kasza, G. 2002. "The Illusion of the Welfare 'Regime.'" *Journal of Social Policy* 31 (2): 271–87.

Kemeny, J. 1981, *The Myth of Home Ownership*. London: Routledge Kegan Paul.

———. 1995. *From Public Housing to the Social Market*. London: Routledge.
———. 2006. "Corporatism and Housing Regimes." *Housing, Theory and Society* 23 (1): 1–18.
Kemeny, J. and Lowe, S. 1998. "Schools of Comparative Housing Research: From Convergence to Divergence." *Housing Studies* 13 (2): 161–76.
Kornai, J. 1992. *The Socialist System. The Political Economy of Communism*. Oxford: Clarendon Press.
———. 1998. "From Socialism to Capitalism: What Is Meant by the 'Change of System'?" Presented at the Social Market Foundation, Centre for Post-Collectivist Studies, June.
———. 2000. "What the Change of System from Socialism to Capitalism Does and Does Not Mean." *Journal of Economic Perspectives* 14 (1): 27–42.
Kubik, Z., Predescu, V., Rodado, J. C. 2011. "Which Are the Most Fragile Banking Systems within the New Member States?" *Flash Economic Research*, December 9, No. 901. http://cib.natixis.com/flushdoc.aspx?id=61383 accessed December 20, 2011.
Leitner, S. and Holzner, M. 2008. "Economic Inequality in Central, East and Southeast Europe." *The Balkan Observatory Working Papers*. The Vienna Institute for International Economic Studies. http://ideas.repec.org/p/wii/bpaper/bowp074.html accessed December 20, 2011.
Lowe, S. 2003. "The Private Rented Sector—Evidence from Budapest and Sofia." *Housing Change in East and Central Europe (Integration or Fragmentation?*
Lux, M., ed. 2003. *Housing Policy: An End or a New Beginning?* Budapest: Open Society Institute.
———. 2009. *Housing Policy and Housing Finance in the Czech Republic during Transition (An Example of the Schism between the Still-Living Past and the Need of Reform)*. Delft: Delft University Press.
Maclennan, D. and More, A. 1997. "The Future of Social Housing: Key Economic Questions." *Housing Studies* 12:531–47.
Malpass, P. 2008. "Histories of Social Housing: A Comparative Approach." *Social Housing in Europe II—A Review of Policies and Outcomes*. London: London School of Economics.
Mitra, K. P. and Yemtsov, R. 2006. *Increasing Inequality in Transition Economies: Is There More to Come?* World Bank Policy Working Paper No. 4007. http://papers.ssrn.com/sol3/papers.cfm?abstract_id=930846 accessed November 20, 2010.
Mitra, P. 2001. *Transition—The First Ten Years: Analysis and Lessons for Eastern Europe and the Former Soviet Union*. Washington, DC: World Bank.
Myant, M. and Drahokoupil, J. 2010. *Varieties of Capitalism in Transition Economies*. http://ssrn.com/abstract=1561944 accessed November 20, 2012.
Mykhnenko, V. 2004. "The Post-Communist State and Capitalism in Transition: Towards a Complementary Relationship." Presented at the Havighurst Centre for Russian and Post-Soviet Studies, November 5–6.
O'Sullivan, E. 2004. "Welfare Regimes, Housing and Homelessness in the Republic of Ireland." *European Journal of Housing Policy* 4 (3): 323–43.
Oxley, M. 2000. *The Future of Social Housing Learning from Europe*. Institute for Public Policy Research.
———. 2009. *Financing Affordable Social Housing in Europe*. UN-HABITAT.
Pavlovskaya, M. 2004. Other transitions: multiple economies of Moscow households in the 1990s, *Annals of the Association of American Geographers*, 94(2): 329–51
Pichler-Milanovich, N. 2001. "Urban Housing Markets in Central and Eastern Europe: Convergence, Divergence or Policy Collapse." *European Journal of Housing Policy* 1 (2): 145–87.

Polanyi, K. 1957. *The Great Transformation*. New York: Rinehart.
Priemus, H. 2004. "Dutch Housing Allowances: Social Housing at Risk." *International Journal of Urban and Regional Research* 28 (3) 706–712.
Priemus, H. and Dieleman, F. 2002. "Social Housing Policy in the European Union: Past, Present and Perspectives." *Urban Studies* 39 (2): 191–200.
Rodríguez-Pose, A. and Krøijer, A. 2008. *Fiscal Decentralization and Economic: Growth in Central and Eastern Europe*. Working Paper Series in Economics and Social Science, 2008/08.
Scanlon, K. and Whitehead, C. 2007. *Social Housing in Europe*. London: London School of Economics.
Schneider, F. 2002. "Size and Measurement of the Informal Economy in 110 Countries around the World." Paper presented at the Workshop of Australian National Tax Centre, ANU, Canberra, Australia, July 17. http://www.amnet.co.il/attachments/informal_economy110.pdf accessed April 15 2010.
Smith, A. 2000. "Employment restructuring and household survival in 'postcommunist transition': rethinking economic practices in Eastern Europe" *Environment and Planning A* 32 (10): 1759—80
Szelényi, I. 1983. *Urban Inequalities under State Socialism*. Oxford: Oxford University Press.
Szelényi, I. and Manchin, R. 1987. "Social Policy under State Socialism: Market Redistribution and Social Inequalities in East European Socialist Societies." *Stagnation and Renewal in Social Policy: The Rise and Fall of Policy Regimes*. Armonk, NY: M. E. Sharpe.
Tausz, K. 2009. From State Socialism to a Hybrid Welfare State: Hungary, K. Schubert, S. Hegelich and U. Bazant (Eds.) *The Handbook of European Welfare Systems*. New York: Routledge.
Tsenkova, S. 2009. *Housing Reforms in Post-Socialist Europe. Lost In Transition*. Heidelberg: Springer-Verlag.
Turner, B., Hegedüs, J., and Tosics, I., eds. 1992. *The Reform of Housing in Eastern Europe and the Soviet Union*. London: Routledge.
Wilensky, H. 1975. *The Welfare State and Equality: Structural and Ideological Roots of Public Expenditures*. Berkeley: University of California Press.
World Bank. 1993. *Housing: Enabling Markets to Work/With Technical Supplements*. Washington: World Bank.
———. 2000. *Maintaining Utility Services for the Poor Policies and Practices in Central and Eastern Europe and the Former Soviet Union*. Washington: World Bank.
UNECE, Bulletin of Housing Statistics for Europe and North America, 2000–2006 (downloaded from www.unece.org)

Part II

Critical Issues in the Transition Process

2 Housing Privatization and Restitution

József Hegedüs

INTRODUCTION—TENURE IN THE SOCIALIST HOUSING SYSTEM

Housing privatization and restitution was a definitive event in the history of post-socialist housing systems, and it has generated an enormous public debate (e.g., Turner, Hegedüs, and Tosics 1992; Clapham and Kintera 1996; Struyk 1996; Lux 2003; Mandic 2010). In the evaluation of the debate it is important to note that tenure meant something different in the socialist housing system than in Western societies (Marcuse 1996; Mandic and Clapham 1996; Hegedüs and Tosics 1996; Lowe and Tsenkova 2003). One of the aims of the chapter is to understand privatization and restitution in the context of the transition of the Eastern European Housing Model (EEHM; Hegedüs and Tosics 1996), emphasizing both the continuity and the contrast with previous systems.

The key factor in understanding the privatization and restitution process in transition countries is to abandon the Anglo-Saxon approach to tenure, because uncritical use of this approach leads to a misunderstanding of the social and economic consequences of privatization in this part of the world. The concept of tenure—in mainstream housing research—is defined by the terms used in the Western legal system (owner-occupied, public housing, cooperative, etc.). Tenures (or, more broadly, housing provision) differ from each other according to property rights tied to certain housing forms: the right to use, to transfer, to "tax", to invest. However, outside the Western world, a variety of other tenure forms exist based on customary and traditional practices that survived urbanization in the Third World. For example, one-third of the world population today lives in slums in unsecured tenure, from a Western point of view, but this form of tenure has a peculiar stability embodied in the informal social and economic system. This is an example of how a diverse set of social and economic relations can lead to special tenure forms, most of which do not fit into the Western tradition (Hoffman, Haupt, and Struyk 1992; Mandic and Clapham 1996).[1]

According to our approach, the EEHM is characterized by the dominance and control of the state; however, the actual tenure structure was a result of state intervention into the inherited legal/social system of tenures. Thus, it differs significantly from the expectations of theorists such as Peter Marcuse (1996), who describe the tenure structure as a compromise between socialist ideology and practice. The role of ideology was to legitimize the one-party system, and the social and legal structure of the housing system was thus formed according to the political needs and social aims of the ruling nomenclature. As a consequence, private ownership was typically under public control (limited right to sell, uncontrolled power of state agencies to ban construction on private property or to expropriate private housing for public investments, one private housing unit per family rule, etc.) whereas tenants enjoyed wide property rights under public ownership (Mandic 2010; Hegedüs and Tosics 1983; Alexeev 1988). This is an important factor in the evaluation of the economic consequences of privatization.

In Hungary, for example, the tenancy right was marketable informally; its asset value was approximately 50 percent of the privately owned units (Hegedüs and Tosics 1996, 246). In the former Soviet Republic of Latvia, once a tenant was "'given' an apartment—after waiting some twenty years or having advanced in the system through bribes or special merits—you could live there as long as you pleased, or change it for another. Apartments could even be 'inherited'" (Berglund 2002, 37). In Poland, members of housing cooperatives already enjoyed the same rights as owners in the owner-occupied sector (Tadeusz 1993).

Privatization and restitution thus took place in a housing system where, in practice, public ownership was closer to a quasi-private ownership. The blurry boundary between owning and renting had important consequences for the political and economic interpretation of privatization.

From a sociological point of view, privatization and restitution are very different things: privatization expands the existing property rights of tenants into full-fledged private ownership, whereas restitution deprives tenants of their (quasi-) property rights and turns them into real tenants. More specifically, restitution in the housing field meant that the housing properties nationalized by the socialist governments after World War II were given back to the original owners, whereas the sitting tenants became private renters with the new landlord. Privatization, on the other hand, meant that the sitting tenants of state-owned apartments had the right to buy the property (at a discount price), and as a consequence, the state rental unit became an owner-occupied unit. Whereas restitution had a limited effect on the market in terms of the number of the housing units, privatization typically changed the ownership of 60–90 percent of the stock. However, the political consequences of restitution were not negligible. Because of these differences, the chapter deals with the problem of restitution in a separate section.

THEORIES OF PRIVATIZATION

The literature on housing privatization in transition countries is dominated by descriptive analyses based on national statistics, but very few studies have used targeted surveys (Hegedüs et al. 1993; Székely 2001). Four theoretical explanations for privatization emerged in the literature: rational choice theory, path dependence, privatization as "shock absorber," and privatization as "agency of change". Each of these approaches provides theoretical insights that help us understand the social, economic, and political factors behind privatization. The next sections will summarize these theories.

Rational Choice Theory

According to this approach, privatization was the result of rational decisions taken by the various actors who had the right to sell and buy state-owned housing properties. The set of actors was made up of the local or national government (depending on the degree of decentralization) as owners of the stock and the sitting tenants. The choice between the options—to sell or not to sell, or to buy or not to buy—was based on their relative rewards. Perceived rewards were influenced by expectations (future rents, house prices, future changes of legislation, etc.); the "value gap" (the difference between the market price and the purchase price of the housing unit); and political factors (security of tenure, decentralization in the public sector, fiscal pressure on the government budget at both the central and local level). The dominant strategy of both the local governments and the households was the "sell and buy" combination in Hungary between 1990 and 1995 (Hegedüs et al. 1993).

The government's short-term decision was crucially influenced by fiscal considerations: the privatization of public housing brought in additional income and it allowed the government to transfer the social and economic problems associated with the public housing stock to the new private owners. However, in the macro-political environment following the transition, there were no political forces to argue for longer-term considerations. This meant that the long-term interests of the population who did not participate directly in the decision-making process (and who would stand in need of social housing in the future) were left out of consideration.

"Path Dependence" Theory

This theory goes back to the debate on the "theory of market transition" (discussed in Bodnár 1996). The "path dependence" argument developed by David Stark (1992) states that "previous and currently existing institutional settings constrain and orient the course of action taken in the process of transformation and influence the results of those actions" (Bodnár, 1996, 619). The path dependence argument in its simplest version claims that old structures survive the transformation and determine its results. Bodnár uses this argument to explain the outcome of privatization; she notes that privileged social groups transformed her advantage in the public sector into high capital value in the owner-occupied sector. Although their approach can elucidate the fact that the communist ruling class kept its position in the market system, its explanation of institutions' behavior is limited. In fact, analyses that point to the regressive effect of privatization reach similar conclusions as the path dependence theory, and are less likely to fall into the trap of following a conspiracy theory–like logic. These explanations may have had a value in light of the events immediately following the transition, but as time passed, they lost their strength. For example, the lack of restitution in Hungary was clearly due to the fact that privatization had started before the change of the regime. However, the framework of the path dependence theory cannot adequately explain the long process of housing privatization in the region, because this process was determined by new institutions and social groups looking to their short-term interests.

Privatization as a "Shock Absorber"

Raymond Struyk (1996) argued that privatization's most important function was to play the role of a "shock absorber", that is, it made it politically easier to accept the social consequences of the transformation crisis and helped households develop a coping strategy. Decision-makers aimed to manage the social tensions caused by the transformation recession through privatization, as it was expected to free up housing capital for households that saw their real income decrease and living costs increase. The efficiency of the "shock absorber" function depended on the allocation of the stock across different income groups. In Russia, because of the low correlation between housing value and income, it had a more progressive redistribution effect, helping low-income groups to manage economic hardship (Buckley and Gurenko 1997). Moreover, privatization was an efficient way to increase votes in the political arena. This had an effect in most of the post-socialist privatization programs.

There was an interesting conflict between the different levels of government with respect to the privatization decisions. In some cases, the central government made the decision to privatize; in other cases the local governments had the authority to do so. In countries where the property was transferred to the municipalities, the central government (and Parliament) introduced a right to buy policy to take credit politically for privatization.

Privatization as an Agency of Change

According to this theory, privatization in post-socialist countries was an integral part of the complex economic and social transformation of the "centrally planned command system". The theory implies that state ownership of housing constrained the development of market mechanisms in the housing sector. Privatization is accordingly described as an "agency for change", helping and forcing households to adapt their behavior (housing consumption) to the market conditions, and paving the way for a more efficient housing system "that would deal with housing shortages and would lead to a higher level of maintenance" (Clapham and Kintera 1996, 174). The privatized stock thus makes the adaptation process more efficient (Renaud 1996). Furthermore, the approach claimed that market development would provide such significant benefits to the population that rapid privatization was required, thus making the regressive effects of giveaway privatization secondary (see, for example, Daniell and Struyk 1994).

There is a general accusation that World Bank, IMF, and USAID, who were quite active in technical assistance programs, pushed the countries in transition to privatize the state housing stock (Lux 2009). Actually, some written documents contradict this thesis: some experts were in favor of "cautious privatization," and most of them criticized the giveaway privatization programs. For example, Struyk and Telgarsky (1991) argued that two objectives must be pursued simultaneously in the process of privatization: (a) selling units at or near market prices to tenants or other households willing to purchase them, and (b) integrating the remaining state-owned rentals with the nascent but expanding rental market.

Different privatization practices can best be explained with a combination of the theories outlined in the preceding. These theories serve to describe the interaction of the various actors and interest groups (new/old political elite, new entrepreneurial class, the influential middle class) that led to privatization. However, the models leave out some relevant factors, including the ethnic aspects of the transition process (particularly important for the Baltic countries). Andrew Roberts (2009) describes further special political factors that influenced the process.

In Latvia, for example, the discussion concerning housing privatization started in the late 1980s, and the first law on the privatization of state and municipal apartments was adopted in 1995. The delay depended mainly on the sensitive question of noncitizens' right to acquire property (Breitner 1998, 12). Noncitizens (Russians, etc.) were disfavored in the voucher system. This meant that citizens of other former Soviet republics were not necessarily able to privatize their apartment without having some capital (Berglund 2002, 40).

HOUSING PRIVATIZATION: SEVERAL VERSIONS, SAME MODEL

The housing privatization process in transitional countries varied significantly. A right to buy regulation was introduced in most countries. In Albania, housing privatization was rapidly implemented by the central government: sitting tenants only had to turn in a claim and pay a registration fee defined in a government decree (Lowry 1993). In Hungary, the right to buy regulation was introduced only in 1993; until then, the decision to privatize was in the hands of the local government. In the Czech Republic there was no "right to buy legislation" whatsoever.

In almost all countries, the first step was to transfer the state-owned residential properties to the municipalities and issue a law that regulated the conditions of privatization. (Albania was an exception.) Local governments as new landlords, however, were in a very different position from country to country, depending on the rights tied to the ownership of the stock (setting rent, allocation, allowances, privatization, etc.).

The public rental units owned by state-owned enterprises were handled differently. Privatization of enterprise-owned apartments was more complicated because of unpredictable rules in the enterprise privatization programs. In some cases the housing stock was not included in the privatization package, thus letting the housing privatization simply follow national rules. However, the new owners of the enterprise typically had the right to privatize the stock, which caused severe conflicts between the new landlords and the tenants.

Cooperative housing—in principle—represents a tenure form between public rental and owner-occupation, but there were only slight differences between living in a cooperative and a state rental in Eastern Europe, as the construction, allocation, and financing were managed by organizations under direct state control.[2] Cooperatives had an important role in Czechoslovakia (17 percent), Poland (24 percent), and the Soviet Union (4 percent) before 1990 (Clapham and Kintera 1996). In the Czech Republic, the transformation of the cooperatives was gradual, as most of them had loans that had to be paid back before privatization could take place. In Poland, the rental cooperatives were transformed into owner cooperatives, which is a form of owner-occupation (World Bank 2006).The same happened in Slovenia and Slovakia (Donner 2006). However, cooperative buildings in Latvia were given to those living there for free (Trapenciere 2006, 41). Overall, the cooperative sector was transformed into an owner-occupied housing form, even in the cases when it retained the formal structure of a cooperative.

Most countries implemented a kind of "give-away" privatization, which meant that sitting tenants paid a price that was typically less than 15 percent of the market price, and in some cases received property rights free of charge (e.g., in Russia, Georgia, etc.). Countries introduced different financial schemes, including the use of vouchers (Estonia, Latvia, etc.), compensation shares (Hungary), special loans, advance payment schemes, and so on.

In the beginning, experts and advisors thought that privatization would be a "one-step" intervention, finished in a limited time period, after which a new housing system could be developed. There was thus a time limit on privatization in most countries. However, the process took place at very different speeds. The deadline for privatization was extended in several countries like Hungary, Romania, Russia, Latvia, Slovenia, and others. In Russia, 'unconditional' privatization was extended to 2013. The Romanian government offered the right to buy to sitting tenants in newly built social rental units in 2007. And even after twenty years of transition, privatization is still possible according to the same procedures in countries like Romania, Russia, or the Czech Republic.

The fiscal effect of privatization was not negligible. However, privatization did not prove to be a significant source of revenue for the central or municipal budgets, as the prices were far below market rates and the process took very long. Some analysts proposed that receipts from the sales should be recycled back into housing or infrastructure, or used to reduce budget deficits until a reliable tax system could be devised and put in place (Katsura and Struyk 1991, 1251–73). In Slovenia, an institution was set up for this purpose: municipalities and firms had to earmark 20 percent of their proceeds from privatization for a newly formed National Housing Fund, which later became a financial vehicle for the mortgage market (Cirman 2005). In Estonia, privatization revenues were also used for preferential housing loans. Part of the money from the sale of public housing was supposed to be spent on social housing construction and to provide for housing or financial help for tenants who lost their quasi-property rights as a result of the restitution process. In Hungary, privatization revenue

Table 2.1 Housing Privatization (%)

	Public Rental % in 1990	Public Rental, around 2000	% Privatized
Albania	35.5	1.0	97.2
Lithuania	60.8	2.4	96.1
Romania	32.7	2.7	91.7
Serbia and Montenegro	22.2	2.8	87.4
Croatia	24.0	2.9	87.9
Bulgaria	6.6	3.0	54.5
Slovenia	31.0	3.0	90.3
Hungary	23.0	4.0	82.6
Armenia	52.5	4.0	92.4
Estonia	61.0	5.2	91.5
Republic of Moldova	21.0	5.5	73.8
Slovakia	27.7	6.5	76.5
Kazakhstan	66.1	6.8	72.9
Latvia	59.0	16.0	72.9
Poland	31.6	16.1	49.1
Czech Republic	39.1	17.0	56.7
Ukraine	47.3	20.0	57.7
Russian Federation	67.0	29.0	56.7

Source: UN-ECE (2002); Hegedüs and Struyk (2005).

was initially transferred to a Housing Fund, but it was barely used for the construction or renovation of social housing, as a fiscal austerity program caused shortfalls in local government budgets and these funds were appropriated to make up the difference.

As 75–95 percent of the public housing stock was sold to the sitting tenants, basically under the "give-away" financial scheme, the public rental sector shrank accordingly (see Table 2.1). The scale of the privatization depended on the size of the public rental sector at 1990. The low share of public rental sector in Bulgaria (6.6 percent) illustrates very well that tenure structure and the strictness of the state control do not necessary relate to each other. Moreover, there was no room for privatization in Bulgaria.

Early research aimed to describe the differences between the transition countries' models of privatization. Researchers described two distinct policy models based on the differences in the degree of privatization between two groups of countries. The first group, which included Albania, Estonia, Hungary, Romania, Serbia, and Slovenia, carried out extensive privatization and had a small residual public housing sector (less than 5 percent), which targeted low-income households. At the other extreme, there was a group of countries where the public housing sector remained significant in size, which included the Czech Republic (17 percent),[3] Poland (16 percent), Russia (29 percent), and Latvia (16 percent). The difference between the two groups was explained as the result of systematic policy decisions (Tsenkova and Turner 2004).

Alternatively, the latter group might not represent a distinct rental model; privatization may simply have taken place at a slower pace in these countries. Indeed, the rental sector in the second group of countries is under pressure to be privatized, partly because households expecting rent increases would like to buy their homes and partly because the local governments would like to reduce fiscal pressure by selling public housing. However, a number of factors have slowed down the process, such as the low ability of households to pay; an expected rise in maintenance costs when the property is transferred to a private owner (Russia); and complicated procedural rules (land registration, requirements that a minimum of 75 percent of the tenants have the intention to buy, etc.).

The Czech Republic provides a good example to prove that, despite differences in speed, privatization follows the same model across the region. Housing policy in the Czech Republic differs from that of most transition countries because there was no national "right to buy" policy, and municipal governments had authority over privatization decisions. In 2001, after almost a decade of privatization, 17 percent of the stock was still made up of public rentals. However, local governments planned to continue the privatization process, which was expected to speed up because of the recently introduced rent liberalization. In Pardubice, for example, the plan was to keep 2,500–3,000 of the 125,000 public housing units, that is, to privatize 75–80 percent of the stock.[4] In Prague, 54 percent of the stock had been sold by 2003, and the city—according to its housing policy paper—planned to continue privatization of the flats under a strict rent control policy (Housing Policy Concept, Prague, 2004). The share of the public rental sector will be below 10 percent once the city has completed its plans. Indeed, recent data show that the share of the public rental stock has decreased to 10–11 percent throughout the Czech Republic, which means that 70–75 percent of original public housing stock has already been sold (Lux 2009). Thus, slow privatization does not necessarily justify a separate model, as the larger public rental sector in countries like the Czech Republic did not go through any structural changes.

The countries in the second group are thus expected to continue the privatization process, and it is unlikely that they will be able to convert their "post-socialist" rental sector into a "unitary public rental sector". To create a social housing sector from the formerly state-owned rental sector would have required basic structural changes, including the introduction of allocation based on need, income-related (means-tested) housing allowances, cost-based user charges, and the reduction of tenants' property rights. Typically, the political cost of enacting these changes was high and the incentive structure was not in place to achieve them (Hegedüs 2007).

CONSEQUENCES OF PRIVATIZATION

Equity Issue

A general feature of housing privatization was that sitting tenants could buy their homes for a fraction of the market price—that is, they could profit from "privatization gain". Two factors should be taken into consideration in the evaluation of this transfer of wealth. Firstly, tenants had the right to exchange their rental units freely with other rental units (or even with a privately owned property, as in Hungary), which means that rental housing had a quasi-market value. This quasi-market value depended on expected future changes to the legal system and, more specifically, to tenancy rights. We can thus calculate privatization gain as the actual market value of a housing unit minus its quasi-exchange value and minus the sum paid to the state to secure the property rights. A number of analysts do not take the quasi-market value of apartments into account in calculating the privatization gain, and thus exaggerate the transfer of wealth that occurred in the privatization process (World Bank 2001). Secondly, the privatization gain depended on expectations concerning future rent subsidies (the difference between the actual rent and the market rent). Indeed, the tenants' decision to buy their homes depended largely on expected future subsidies, as well as "deferred maintenance" costs (the typical backlog of necessary investment in the rental stock), both of which were factored into the quasi-market value. The rational choice approach to privatization takes these factors into consideration: as there were different expectations concerning the survival of the subsidy system in different countries, this accounts for a difference in the pace of privatization.

Even so, giveaway privatization in Hungary generated a huge equity problem arising from the difference between the market value and the discounted selling price. Because the best public housing units were allocated according to merit in the socialist period, an estimated 40 percent of investment value went to households in the top quartile of the income distribution, whereas only 17 percent went to the lowest quartile (Hegedüs et al. 1996). Mandic and Stanovnik (1996) came to a similar conclusion in their analysis of the Slovenian data.

Buckley and Gurenko argue:

> Almost "give-away" privatization of housing that began in Russia in 1993 gave households at least some savings to help cushion the costs of the transition. This program was an important way of permitting households to exploit the distributional benefits of the old system, a step that has not been pursued nearly as aggressively in many other reforming economies. Because the distribution of housing income in Russia is so much less dispersed than is wage income, while at the same time the distribution of nonresidential wealth is almost certainly much more dispersed, housing's privatization had a strongly progressive effect on the distribution of wealth.
>
> The privatization of housing may also help address poverty concerns. For example, in 1992 the elderly in the lowest-income quartile had less than one seventh of the income of young households in the highest-income quartile. But they had five square meters more housing space per person. Because up to 30 percent of the elderly were below the poverty line, being able to liquidate this additional housing wealth could go a long way toward addressing their poverty problem. (1997, 29)

However, in countries where housing consumption was unequally allocated among different groups according to income, status, and social position, privatization reinforced the regressive effects. As Yemtsov argued: "Even more, given a relatively short time span the distribution of housing wealth in favour of the better off induced by privatization in some countries (in our study, Serbia and Russia), the regressive effects are not negligible" (2007, 26). Because of these two factors—the distribution of good-quality apartments and the low price charged for the privatized unit—the regressive equity effect was general throughout the region.

Some tenants were excluded from the privatization process, partly for legal/political reasons, partly because of their financial position. For example, in the Czech Republic and Estonia, tenants who happened to live in apartments in the stock that was nationalized after World War II were excluded from privatization because of restitution. Russian nationals in

Latvia faced disadvantages in the privatization process. The very poor, who had already accumulated high unpaid bills, did not have the resources to buy their homes, and could thus not profit from the privatization gain. Smaller, more specific groups were also affected. For instance, the caretakers of large apartment houses in Hungary typically lived in small apartments designed for the purpose on the ground floor; these apartments came to be owned by the newly founded condominiums together with the staircases, courtyards, attics, and so on, and the caretakers were thus forced to rent from the new owners of the building.

Efficiency—Housing Management

The privatization of urban multiunit buildings (typically housing estates) raised the question of how the new condominiums were to be managed. In principle, the new owners became responsible for the operation and modernization of the privatized housing stock, which had suffered from systematic undermaintenance in the socialist period. However, the legal framework of privatization and the emergence of inexperienced and—in many cases—poor homeowners led to problems. With the given backlog of repairs, financing the operation and renovation of the buildings put an unmanageable burden on the new owners.

Policymakers were of the view that the new owners would work out among themselves how to keep the building in good repair and how to collect the fees for common expenses. But these expectations were not fulfilled even in countries that developed a legal framework for the new condominiums and made this a precondition of privatization. The interaction of new owners led to conflicts that proved difficult to solve. The effectiveness of these new entities is in doubt, especially when the properties are in bad condition and the owners have little resources. In Slovenia, for example, low-income homeowners are already experiencing considerable difficulty in meeting the costs associated with homeownership (Sendi 1995, 2004).

It was not obligatory in a number of countries to set up a legal entity such as a condominium or homeowners' association during the process of privatization, and the homes in multiunit buildings were privatized, whereas the common part of the building remained in state/municipal ownership. As a consequence, the relation between the individual properties (flats) and the common areas (staircase, roof, structures) were legally unclear (Albania, Moldavia, etc.). In other cases, like in the three Baltic countries, only the buildings were privatized, and the lot they stand on remains in public ownership (Turner and Victorin 1996, 355–57).

Privatization did not always lead to a change of ownership of the whole building, as very poor households or households living in bad-quality flats did not buy their rental units. Local governments tended to get rid of the flats that were in the best condition, because those were the easiest to sell, whereas nonrenovated housing stock remained in the property of local governments (Poland and Hungary are examples).

In most of the countries the state-owned housing stock was managed by the state before the transition, either through companies owned by the local government or through state-controlled maintenance cooperatives. The rents and utility fees were deeply subsidized, thus arrears were rare. The management of multiunit buildings was restructured after the transition, but different countries followed different paths. At one extreme (for example, in Russia and Serbia) state management companies continued to have a monopoly on managing housing estates, which typically led to undermaintenance and huge dissatisfaction. But gradually, the new condominiums have gained the right to organize their own maintenance, although they have to compete with the public companies. At the other extreme (Romania, Hungary, etc.), the new condominiums (represented by an elected board of owners) have the right and responsibility to organize the management of the buildings, which may also lead to undermaintenance because of the lack of professional knowledge and the owners' interest in decreasing the maintenance fee. It is not rare for condominiums to be managed by individual owners who underuse the professional service providers. Both solutions have their problems, but the new homeowner associations increasingly have the freedom to choose among the private maintenance and service companies.

Newer legislation tends to handle this problem by prescribing the mandatory use of professionals, and various programs have been introduced to increase the management capacity of the new condominium managers, such as training events, licensing the administrators, and so on.

The basic problem is that there is a growing tension between poor households' ability to pay and the growing burden of housing-related costs. The latter includes both the operational cost (water, energy, etc.) and the postponed renovations. The price liberalization and service providers' monopoly have contributed to an increase in housing expenditures and, hence, to low-income owners' arrears (Bonczak-Kucharczyk 1999). This is a problem for poor owners who were able to buy their homes, but are not able to pay the operational and renewal costs.

Restitution

In Eastern European countries the majority of the urban housing stock was nationalized (confiscated) after World War II. Both the tenants of privately owned flats and owners who happened to live in their homes became tenants in the new state rental sector. Nationalization typically did not extend to single-family homes, but the threshold varied across countries. In Hungary, for example, homes with more than six rooms were nationalized, but the tenancy rights in privately owned single-family homes were transferred to the state institutions (councils).

After the collapse of the socialist system, former owners and their descendants were compensated for the confiscation of their property by restitution of their original property rights. Restitution had a technical and a political constraint. On the one hand, missing documents and the bad condition of land registries made it difficult to find evidence concerning pre-nationalization proprietors and their descendants. In Latvia, in order to avoid ambiguity concerning the date of nationalization, the property rights of the confiscated properties were returned to the persons (and to their heirs) who were owners in July 1940 regardless of citizenship. Countries typically tried to limit legal uncertainty by setting a deadline for handing in restitution claims.

On the other hand, restitution generated social conflicts between the original owners or their heirs and the tenants. As tenants' rights in the socialist housing system included the right to exchange and inherit rental units, restitution deprived the sitting tenants of these rights and, more importantly, of the right to buy their homes. The principle of restitution was accepted in every post-socialist country, but its implementation differed according to technical possibilities and the political processes. In Hungary, the original owners and their heirs only received financial compensation, because of the sitting tenants' political influence—some of whom had bought the state-owned flats (originally confiscated in the 1950s) prior to 1989. In Romania, restitution was a legal option, but it was blocked politically because of the lack of political will to transfer ownership rights to the original owners. For instance, in Transylvania there was an ethnic component to the privatization decisions: the original owners typically belonged to the ethnic Hungarian minority, whereas the sitting tenants to the Romanian majority (Dawidson 2004).

Restituted apartments became private rentals, but strong new tenant protection laws were written to guarantee security of tenure and limit rent increases by the new landlords. For example, in Croatia, tenants living in units owned by a natural person have special "protected tenants" rights. In Latvia, tenants living in restituted housing could not be evicted for the first seven years after the transition if they paid their rent and utility costs regularly (Trapenciere 2006).

In terms of quantity, restitution remained insignificant in most countries (under 1 percent of the housing stock), except in the Czech Republic and Estonia, where it affected 6–10 percent of the stock (Lux and Mikeszová 2012). However, the process had important political implications. The new landlords became politically active and formed lobby groups to have tenant protections lifted, so that they could raise the rent or evict tenants and sell the properties. The lobby groups argued that tenant protection laws deprived them of their full ownership rights, and they won their case before the European Court of Human Rights in Strasbourg (Lux 2009, 106). This decision meant that the tenants irrevocably lost the rights that they had enjoyed before the transition, which had created the quasi-market value of the apartment. The tenants living in restituted housing were not compensated for this loss.

CONCLUSION—CAN WE BLAME PRIVATIZATION FOR THE LOW LEVEL OF SOCIAL HOUSING?

Housing privatization and restitution had a long-term effect on the housing sector in post-socialist countries. Mass privatization took place in practically every country that had a substantial amount of public stock, although its speed and method varied. Privatization contributed to growing social tensions because of its regressive equity effects, even if we account for the quasi-market value of pre-privatization housing within the total privatization gain of the new homeowners.

The long-term consequence of privatization was that the share of the social housing sector shrank to a degree that made it difficult to implement social welfare policies effectively. This had two main causes. Firstly, low-income individuals became homeowners without the financial means necessary to maintain and renovate the typically obsolete stock, and without an institutional capacity for efficient cooperation. Secondly, because of constant fiscal pressure on the public budget and a lack of demographic growth and urbanization, the possibility of expanding social housing through new construction was at a minimum. Renationalization, mentioned from time to time, was not a realistic alternative. Consequently, social policy was left with two options. Firstly, housing policy needed to restructure what was left of the social housing sector (to free it from the legacy of the quasi ownership of the socialist period) and clear the path for its growth. Secondly, as the social housing sector was so small, it was necessary to create programs directed to all the low-income households in the private sector (both low-income owners and private tenants). However, neither of these options was realized.

Restitution followed a different logic, which depended on the political and technical conditions at the time of the transition. It contributed to the creation of a new private rental sector, which had its own political and economic contradictions. Privatization also contributed to the expansion of the private rental sector, but this process overlapped with the informal economy (untaxed, insecure tenancy).

Privatization (and restitution) was not a choice between the "unitary" or "dual" model (Kemeny 1995), as the unitary model was not a feasible option. To turn the socialist rental sector into a unitary model would have involved several difficult policy steps, which were not realistic under the structural constraints (fiscal pressure, new political system, privatized economy, public sector reformed, etc.) that the countries faced. My conclusion is that there was no real alternative to mass privatization (market creation strategy) because of the retrenchment of the state/public sector against the structural changes. In order to create a social housing sector from the ex-state-owned rental sector, basic changes would have been needed, including the introduction of allocation based on social need, income-related (means-tested) housing allowances, cost-based user charges, and the reduction of tenants' property rights. The political cost of enacting these changes was high, and the incentive structure was not in place to achieve them. Thus, although privatization had many deleterious consequences, it alone cannot be blamed for the state of the social housing sector in Eastern Europe today.

NOTES

1. But even in countries of the Western world it is not a simple task to separate public and private provision because of cultural and historical differences (Clapham and Kintera 1996).
2. The cooperative members could typically sell their flats independently, the cooperative being obliged to admit the buyer to cooperative membership, and these flats could also be inherited.
3. In the Czech Republic, privatization continued in the 2000s.
4. See Strategic Plan of Pardubice at http://www.mesto-pardubice.cz/en/administration2/strategic_plan2/profile2/prof_human2/prof_living2/ accessed 20 April 2009.

REFERENCES

Alexeev, M. 1988. "Market vs. Rationing: The Case of Soviet Housing." *Review of Economics and Statistics* 70 (3): 414.

Berglund, U. 2002. "Privatization, Segregation and Local Engagement: A Latvian Case Study." *Challenges and Opportunities in Housing: New Concepts, Policies and Initiatives.* Riga: CIB Working Commission 69 Housing Sociology Proceedings. http://cibworld.xs4all.nl/dl/publications/Pub281/04Chapter-2.pdf accessed January 20, 2010.

Bodnár, J. 1996. "He That Hath to Him Shall Be Given: Housing Privatisation in Budapest after State Socialism." *International Journal of Urban and Regional Research* 20:616–36.

Bonczak-Kucharczyk, E. 1999. *"Tenement Housing Sector Reform in Poland in the Recent Years—Effects of the New Solutions"* State Office for Housing and Urban Development Poland, manuscript.

Breitner, L. 1998. "Privatisation of State and Municipal Apartments: A Field Study in Latvia." Seminar paper, Sweden, Department of Economic History, Lund University.

Buckley, R. M. and Gurenko, E. N. 1997. "Housing and Income Distribution in Russia: Zhivago's Legacy." *World Bank Research Observer* 12 (1): 19–32.

Cirman, A. 2005. "Housing Finance in Slovenia: The Key Role of National Housing Fund." *Housing Finance: New and Old Models in Central Europe, Russia and Kazakhstan.* Budapest: OSI/LGI.

Clapham, D. and Kintera, K. 1996. "The Patterns of Housing Privatization in Eastern Europe." *Housing Privatization in Eastern Europe*, Westport, Connectucut, London: Greenwood.

Daniell, J. and Struyk, R. 1994. "Housing Privatization in Moscow: Who Privatizes and Why?" *International Journal of Urban and Regional Research* 18 (3): 510–25.

Dawidson, E. K. 2004. "Redistributing Nationalized Housing: Impacts on Property Patterns in Timisoara, Romania." *Eurasian Geography and Economics* 45 (2): 134–156.

Donner, C. 2006. *Housing Policies in Central Eastern Europe. Czech Republic/Hungary/Poland/Slovenia/Slovakia*. Published by C. Donner, Vienna.

Hegedüs, J. 2007. Social Housing in Transition Countries. *Social Housing in Europe*. London: London School of Economics.

Hegedüs, J., Mark, K., Sárkány, Cs., and Tosics, I. 1996. "Hungary." *Housing Privatisation in Eastern Europe*.Westport, Connecticut, London: Greenwood.

Hegedüs, J., Mark, K., Struyk, R., and Tosics, I. 1993. "Local Options for the Transformation of the Public Rental Sector: Empirical Results from Two Cities in Hungary." *Cities* 3 (2): 257–71.

Hegedüs, J. and Struyk, R. 2005. "Divergences and Convergences in Restructuring Housing Finance Transition Countries" *Housing Finance: New and Old Models in Central Europe, Russia and Kazakhstan*. Budapest: (LGI/OSI).

Hegedüs, J. and Tosics, I. 1983. "Housing Classes and Housing Policy: Some Changes in the Budapest Housing Market." *International Journal of Urban and Regional Research* 7 (4): 467–94.

———. 1996. "Disintegration of East-European Housing Model." *Housing Privatization in Eastern Europe*. Westport, Connecticut, London: Greenwood.

Hoffman, M., Haupt, B., and Struyk, R. 1992. *International Housing Markets: What We Know, What We Need to Know*. Fannie Mae Working Paper.

Housing Policy Concept, Prague, 2004. "The new housing policy concept for the capital city Prague for the year 2004 and afterward" Appendix 1 to the resolution of City Of Prague (ZHMP) number 19/12 from 24.6. 2004

Katsura, H. and Struyk, R. 1991. "Selling Eastern Europe's State Rental Stock: Proceed with Caution." *Housing Policy Debate* 4 (2): 1251–74.

Kemeny, J. 1995. *From Public Housing to the Social Market*. London: Routledge.

Lowe, S. and Tsenkova, S. 2003. *Housing Change in East and Central Europe: Integration or Fragmentation*. Aldershot U.K.: Ashgate Publishing.

Lowry, I. S. 1993. *Housing Privatization in Albania*. Washington, DC: Planning and Development Collaborative International.

Lux, M. 2003. *Housing Policy: An End or a New Beginning?* Budapest: OSI/LGI.

———. 2009. "Housing Policy and Housing Finance in the Czech Republic during Transition (An Example of the Schism between the Still-Living Past and the Need of Reform)." *Sustainable Urban Areas*. 28. Delft University Press, Delft.

Lux, M. and Mikeszová, M. 2012. "Property Restitution and Private Rental Housing in Transition: The Case of the Czech Republic." *Housing Studies* 27 (1) 77–96.

Mandic, S. 2010. "The Changing Role of Housing Assets in Post-Socialist Countries." *Journal of Housing and the Built Environment* 25:213–26.

Mandic, S. and Clapham, D. 1996. "The Meaning of Home Ownership in the Transition from Socialism: The Example of Slovenia." *Urban Studies* 33 (1): 83–97.

Mandic, S. and Stanovnik, T. 1996. "Slovenia: Fast Privatization of the Stock. Slow Reform of Housing Policy." *Economic Restructuring of the Former Soviet Bloc: The Case of Housing*. Washington, DC: Urban Institute Press.

Marcuse, P. 1996. "Privatization and Its Discontents: Property Rights in Land and Housing in the Transition in Eastern Europe." *Cities after Socialism: Urban and Regional Change and Conflict in Post-Socialist Societies*. Oxford, UK: Blackwell.

Renaud, B. 1996. *Housing Finance in Transition Economies: The Early Years in Eastern Europe and the Former Soviet Union.* World Bank Policy Research Working Paper 1565, Washington, DC.

Roberts, A. 2009. *The Quality of Democracy in Eastern Europe.* Cambridge: Cambridge University Press.

Sendi, R. 1995. "Housing Reform and Housing Conflict: The Privatization and Denationalization of Public Housing in the Republic of Slovenia in Practice." *International Journal of Urban and Regional Research* 19 (3): 435–46.

———. 2004. "The Refurbishment of Multi-Storey Housing: Social, Legal and Financial Conditions. The Case of Slovenia." Paper presented at the conference Real Estate Research in Central Eastern and South Eastern Europe, Vienna, Austria, January 15–16.

Stark, D. 1992. "Path Dependence and Privatization Strategies in East Central Europe." *East European Politics and Societies* 6:17–51.

Struyk, R. 1996. "The Long Road to the Market." *Economic Restructuring of the Former Soviet Bloc. The Case of Housing.* Washington, DC: Urban Institute Press.

Struyk, R. and Telgarsky, J. 1991. *The Puzzle of Housing Privatization in Eastern Europe.* Washington, DC: Urban Institute Press.

Székely, G. 2001. "Privatization of the Municipal Rental Stock (Az önkormányzati bérlakásszektor privatizációja)." *Statisztikai Szemle* 79 (12): 955–69.

Tadeusz, K. 1993. "Co-Operatives in Eastern and Central Europe: Poland." *ICA Studies & Reports.* Geneva: ICA.

Trapenciere, I. 2006. *European Observatory on Homelessness: Policy Update 2006 Latvia.* Riga: Feantsa.

Tsenkova, S. and Turner, B. 2004. "The Future of Social Housing in Eastern Europe: Reforms in Latvia and Ukraine." *European Journal of Housing Policy* 4 (2): 133–49.

Turner, B., Hegedüs, J., and Tosics, I. 1992. *The Reform of Housing in Eastern Europe and the Soviet Union.* London: Routledge.

Turner, B. and Victorin, A. 1996. "The Housing Policy Reforms in Eastern Europe: Case of Estonia." *Economic Restructuring of the Former Soviet Bloc: The Case of Housing.* Washington, DC: Urban Institute Press.

UNECE. 2002. *Country Profiles on the Housing Sector, Republic of Moldova.* Geneva: Economic Commission for Europe.

World Bank. 2001. *Urban Housing and Land Market Reforms in Transition Countries: Neither Marx nor Market.* Washington, DC: World Bank.

———. 2006. *Poland Housing Finance Policy Note.* Washington, DC: World Bank. http://siteresources.worldbank.org/INTHF/214578-1150377999317/20960021/RevisedHFPolicyNotePolandMarch192006-clean.pdf accessed November 20, 2010.

Yemtsov, R. 2007. *Housing Privatization and Household Wealth in Transition.* Research Paper, United Nations University. http://www.wider.unu.edu/stc/repec/pdfs/rp2007/rp2007-02.pdf accessed 15 May 2009.

3 Financing Social Housing

Wolfgang Amman, József Hegedüs, Martin Lux, and Elisabeth Springler

EMERGING NEW HOUSING FINANCE SYSTEM

Introduction—The Legacy

The definition of *social housing* in the socialist housing system is very uncertain, as public housing did not correspond to Western social housing models. State subsidized housing (both in the public and in the owner-occupied sector) was open to a wide range of different incomes and professional groups. However, a private housing market developed alongside the state housing sphere under more or less strict state control (rural self-help buildings, private condominiums, buying and selling the existing housing), which led to the emergence of a dual market. The state housing investments (public, cooperative, and owner-occupied housing) were financed through budgetary resources and through the state bank system, which operated under the control of central planning. The banks issued loans at a price and in a magnitude set by the central planning agencies. Consequently, the financing of public housing was identical to the financing of housing in general (Hegedüs and Tosics 1990).

After 1990, the socialist housing finance system collapsed. The fiscal pressure on the state budgets forced governments to cut housing subsidies drastically. Public housing investments were practically discontinued in most transition countries and subsidies to bank-financed schemes were severely cut or entirely withdrawn. Inflation increased the cost of money to the state saving banks, which augmented the pressure on the budgets—the so-called "old loan" problem (Struyk 1996).

For most transition countries, the first decade after the transition was characterized by the strongly decreasing volume of new housing construction. Between 1990 and 1997, the number of completed housing construction projects dropped by 50 percent in the five Visegrad countries, by 80 percent in the Baltic states, and by 60 percent in Russia. In the same period, the indicator of housing completions per one thousand inhabitants fell from above five (over the EU average) to 1.15 (calculation based on UN Housing Statistics).

In the early phase of the transition, the housing market was affected not only by a sharp decrease in public housing subsidies and new housing construction, but also by the mass privatization of a large part of the existing public rental housing stock, representing over 30 percent of the total housing stock in some sample countries (e.g., Slovakia, Ukraine). The ownership rate increased to over 90 percent in Hungary, 70–80 percent in Poland and the Czech Republic, and over 60 percent in Russia (see Chapter 2, this volume).

Demand for social housing has increased as a consequence of the transitional recession and growing social inequality, but the fiscal pressure on governments made large capital investments in social housing unrealistic. Consequently, the future of social housing in transitional countries depends on whether the emerging new financial institutions will prove willing and able to fund the new social landlords' housing investments; whether "social housing presents an opportunity to widen the base of their portfolios and to include a relatively low-risk stream of revenue which can be expected to rise in real terms" (Whitehead 2003, 3). The institutional stability of the emerging social landlords and whether they will be able to guarantee the necessary financial stream for the housing investments are other major questions. The goal of this chapter is to give an overview of the basic social housing finance schemes applied in selected post-socialist states and discuss options for long-term social housing finance models that may provide a solid base for the social housing sector in the region.

Distortions of the Tenure Structure: Homeownership-Based Regulations

Owner-occupied housing became the dominant tenure form across Central and Eastern Europe (CEE). Because housing subsidy systems (and tax policy) favored owner-occupation, households preferred to leave the rental sector. The uncertain future of the public rental sector (future rent levels and property rights) provided a further incentive for higher-income households to move to the owner-occupied sector. Social landlords (typically the municipalities) also tried to get rid of the social housing stock by privatization, as it placed a financial burden on the municipal budgets and led to social tension caused by the "antisocial behavior" of low-income tenants (see Chapter 5, this volume). The combination of all these factors led to the rapid shrinkage of the social rental sector.

The private rental sector remained in legal limbo in most countries: it was hardly covered by new housing legislation, and the enforcement of contracts was uncertain (Dübel, Brzeski, and Hamilton 2006; Mandic 2000; Hegedüs 2007). Housing policy focused on new condominium and mortgage regulations. The private rental sector mainly provided housing for households who did not have other alternatives: the poor, the mobile, and the young. The supply of private rental units came primarily from homeowners who acquired them during the mass public housing privatization. In countries where restitution affected a significant part of the housing stock (like the Czech Republic and Estonia), the private rental sector started to play a more significant role and eventually stabilized as an affordable alternative to owner-occupation: most of the contracts came to be concluded in written form and market rents became more affordable (Lux and Mikeszová 2012; Lux and Kährik 2012).

Legal uncertainty, financial disadvantages and a lack of institutional interest in investments made potential social housing finance very difficult. The need for social housing was channeled to the private mortgage market; the rental housing development did not represent an interesting investment opportunity for either the possible institutional landlords or the new private financial institutions.

Bank Reforms and Emerging Housing Finance

All transition countries had to undertake thorough reforms of their banking sectors. Both gradual (Hungary, Bulgaria, and Romania) and radical reform (the Czech Republic, Estonia) led to the emergence of a competitive market as well as banking crises, although with different timing. As a result, the former monopoly of state-owned savings banks was relaxed. In countries such as Serbia, Belarus, the Ukraine, Slovenia, and Lithuania, the state kept a decisive influence in the banking sector well after 2000. The new private banks, which often had foreign owners, considered the mortgage market risky, which delayed development in this area. However, as consequence of a stable macroeconomic environment and predictable legal conditions, the mortgage market developed to a profitable business by the end of the 1990s.

Because of the new mortgage finance products, the volume of outstanding loans increased dramatically in all transition countries after 2000; it went from 0 to nearly 20 percent of GDP in the Czech Republic, Croatia, Hungary, and Poland.

Housing loan funding relies on two models: the bond market accessed by mortgage banks and the commercial banks and the savings banks' deposit system.

In transition countries there were two options for mortgage bond finance. According to the option chosen by Latvia, Hungary, and Poland, legislation requires a special mortgage bank institution to issue mortgage bonds. The other option, used in the Czech Republic and Bulgaria, provides commercial banks with a license to issue bonds backed by housing (mortgage) loans. This means that universal banks can obtain a license for mortgage bond issuance as long as mortgage banking operations and assets are kept in separate legal and accounting records.

The stable increase of household income, favorable macroeconomic trends (decreasing inflation and interest rates), legal changes (foreclosure regulations), competition among banks, and the increasing surplus of financial savings in the world economy led to the rapid development of the mortgage finance system after 2000 in CEE countries. The outstanding stock of loans to households in the new EU member states nearly doubled from 12.3 percent of GDP at the end of 2004 to 22.5 percent of GDP by the end of 2007 (Walko 2008). Mortgage development was stopped by the global financial crisis. The increasing number of mortgage arrears became a new social issue especially in countries where the mortgages were issued in foreign currency and government deficits were high (e.g., Baltic states, Hungary).

Social Housing Finance Models

Governments' white papers have demonstrated since 2000 that policymakers realize the need for extending the social housing sector (Donner 2005; Hegedüs 2007). Housing policy targeted legal reform as well as quantitative goals of affordable housing provision. Sustainable solutions to the growing tension between demand for and supply of affordable housing are few and far between. However, because of privatization, low-income homeowners have become a possible target for social housing finance programs, especially energy savings and retrofit programs.

Municipal Housing and Budget Programs

In transition countries, the typical social landlord is a public management company owned by the municipality. Its financial sustainability depends on the country's rent policy, which is set either on the national level (e.g., in the Czech Republic until 2012) or the local level (e.g., in Hungary), as well as maintenance and operation schemes. The municipalities generally have little incentive to expand social/public housing, as the fiscal burden of new social rental housing competes with other municipal responsibilities, such as education, health, or infrastructure. Social/public rents are often not sufficient to even cover management and maintenance costs. The difference has to be covered by the municipalities from their general revenues. With a negative cash flow, it is hardly possible to acquire capital market financing for new construction. Moreover, the social housing sector typically generates other social and political problems.

In many transition countries, the reorganization of state authorities often shifted responsibility for housing to the municipalities without respective allocation of funds. Small municipalities feared that their social housing programs would lead to the immigration of poor people from other municipalities, which would increase rather than reduce social tensions. Small local governments thus tend to "export" problems to other places rather than effectively solve them. This "paradox of decentralization" affected households in very acute need of housing negatively, such as homeless or Roma households.

However, municipalities are generally interested in investments in their constituency, if it does not require too much public resources. Every investment generates local economic growth and typically increases the power of the local decision makers. In some cases, the financial burden of new social housing was lower than that of the existing stock, as earmarked funds from the national government were available. In transition countries such as Slovakia, the Czech Republic, Romania, and Hungary, central budget funds became the most important source for new social housing construction (see Table 3.1). To subsidize those programs, the central governments typically imposed certain conditions in terms of rent setting, allocation, and construction.

The conditions were not only different in the various countries, but also changed over time. Maximum rents (see Chapter 4, this volume) were defined either as a percentage of the "replacement value" (e.g., in Poland), as a percentage of market value (e.g., Czech Republic between 2007 and 2012), on the basis of cost-coverage (e.g., in Hungary), or were linked to disposable family income (e.g., in Romania). The actual rents are set by the local governments, and are often below the defined limit, as local governments are uncertain about the tenants' ability to pay. In Poland, for example, the average rent was around 1.5 percent of the replacement costs in 2001 (Uchman and Adamski 2003).

In the Czech Republic, most new public housing constructed after 1995 (estimated sixty thousand flats) was financed from grants allocated from the state budget. However, the original state support for municipal housing construction was in fact converted into support for co-op housing: 'tenants' paid large contributions from their own pockets; became co-op members; and, as co-op members, had relatively extensive disposal rights similar to that of homeowners. Consequently, the program led to state subsidies of

Table 3.1 Share of Public Housing in New Construction in Selected Countries in 2000, 2005, 2009

	2000	2005	2009
Czech Republic	11.5	8.4	2.0
Estonia	0.1	0.0	4.5
Hungary	1.0	1.7	0.6
Latvia	0.0	0.0	0.9
Poland	6.8	8.3	6.5
Romania	na	8.9	3.9
Slovak Republic	11.6	14.2	12.5
Slovenia	8.6	7.0	4.7

Source: EU Housing Statistics (2010), National Statistical Offices.

the construction of luxurious dwellings, dwellings for the highest-income households, secondary homes, and flats acquired purely for speculation. The program was substantially amended in 2002.

The Hungarian rental housing construction program in 2000–2004 gave a grant of up to 75 percent of the investment costs to local governments. In this period, close to thirteen thousand social dwellings were constructed, with a total grant of 240 million euros. Granting to local governments was based on a competitive selection procedure, with low construction costs as a criterion. Similarly, in Slovakia central budget grants for social housing were higher for projects with low construction costs. In Croatia the government defined maximum construction costs and land value for their social housing program (Čačić 2003). In Romania social housing construction is conducted by the National Housing Agency (ANL), which transfers the premises to local governments; they then are responsible for allocation, operation, and maintenance (IIBW 2008).

In some programs, the central governments defined allocation criteria mainly based on household income, age, household composition (e.g., young families), or professional groups. In some countries the allocation schemes are set up by the municipalities (e.g., Hungary and Romania); a more detailed comparison of models for new social/public housing construction can be found in Chapter 19.

A further important issue related to social housing construction programs was whether the new units would be eligible for privatization. In many cases, tenants became eligible to acquire their dwellings quite soon. For example, in Tallinn, a public housing program made it possible for tenants leaving restituted apartments to buy their homes after five years (Kährik et al. 2003). In Russia, privatization of newly constructed social dwellings is still practiced.

Nonprofit or Limited-Profit Housing Schemes

The cooperative sector is in crisis in most transition countries, because this tenure form is considered a version of homeownership. It has lost most of its privileges (grants, subsidized loans, free access to land, etc.) and has to compete with the private sector. However, there were several attempts, frequently supported by European donor organizations, to establish new nonprofit or limited-profit associations providing apartments for rent.

The most successful attempt in the early years of transition was Poland's TBS (housing association) program, which was based upon the French HLM model. The administration of this program was carried out by the state-held BGK Bank. The TBS could take different legal forms, such as a limited liability company, joint-stock company, or cooperative of legal persons. The majority of the TBSs were set up or initiated by local governments, in total about 450 institutions by the end of 2004. Financing required 30 percent funding from local governments, prospective tenants, or the TBS's own equity. The remaining funding was contributed by the National Housing Fund (KFM), 60 percent of which was funded by budgetary grants from the national housing budget, and the rest was mainly funded by long-term public debt contracted after 2002 from two multilateral institutions (European Investment Bank [EIB] and Council of Europe Development Bank [CEB]) in order to keep expanding the program. The interest rate subsidy in terms of net present value is in excess of 60 percent of the loan amount. The rents for TBS housing were set by the municipal councils as cost rents; but they cannot exceed 4 percent of the construction cost per year (replacement value).

The program was not exclusively aimed at lower-income groups, but rather at middle-income groups. The deposit equal to 10 percent of capital costs was provided by the tenants and therefore the selection of the tenants followed their ability to pay. The deposit was fully refundable to the tenant if the rental contract was ended and the tenant decided to move out of the flat. However, the tenants often considered themselves quasi owners. Altogether, the nonprofit housing associations have provided good standard housing with controlled rents, but the program was criticized because of insufficient targeting and excessive public costs. The total volume of the TBS program amounted up to 10 percent of total housing construction (2001) but has since expired (Zawislak 2003; World Bank 2006; Amann and Mundt 2012).

Slovakia tried to implement a limited-profit housing sector with a law on nonprofit organizations and in cooperation with the Netherlands' Matra grant program. Subsidies and tax benefits only applied to housing associations predominantly owned by municipalities with strong control mechanisms and very low building cost caps. Implementation proved to be difficult. Consequently, only two associations with quite limited activities were founded. The Matra housing organization in the city of Martin was established by the municipality to hold and maintain the public housing stock, which has not been privatized so far. Operation and maintenance of this stock must be provided by the municipality, whereas new construction and refurbishment activities were supported with loans from the Dutch financing institution DIGH (Červeňová 2005). Currently, in a similar framework with DIGH financing within the Matra grant program, a limited-profit housing association in Armenia has been established.

In the former Yugoslavia, affordable housing provision was financed from the Solidarity Funds for Housing Construction. Enterprises, institutions, and state bodies were legally required to collect a percentage of salaries to provide housing for employees. The legal base for these funds was abolished only in 2001.

In Serbia, some of these funds were transformed into municipal housing agencies, which are regarded as the basic implementing instruments of a future social housing system as defined by the Social Housing Law of 2008. In the framework of the UN-HABITAT granted Settlement and Integration of Refugees Program (SIRP), seven such agencies created low-rent dwellings for vulnerable households with highly subsidized loans on a nonprofit basis.

In Montenegro, a Fund for Solidarity Housing Development (CFSSI), following the model from socialist times, was reestablished in 1996 by the Confederation of Trade Unions. In 2008 it was transformed into a social partnership model, including the government of Montenegro, the trade unions, and the Federation of Employers on a nonprofit basis. CFSSI mainly provides affordable owner-occupied dwellings, but has also started rent and leasing schemes following an Austrian model. Financing is based on contributions from partner companies and public authorities, loans from international finance institutions (DIGH, CEB), and bank loans. Almost all Montenegrin municipalities have contractual relations with CFSSI for the provision of construction sites and infrastructure free of charge. As such, they fulfill their legal obligation to use 1 percent of their budget for social housing. CFSSI housing construction reaches up to 10 percent of total housing production in Montenegro (IIBW 2010).

There is a potential for “third sector” solutions: Private Public Partnership (short: PPP) models for housing finance and for limited-profit housing development. PPP housing legislation is one option for establishing a new business sector that targets affordable housing, particularly rental housing (UNECE 2005). Compared to public housing, PPP housing can be less costly to the state, if the necessary legal and institutional framework is in place. Thus, a well-designed PPP housing scheme may become an important tool to execute state housing policy. However, in order to establish PPP housing as a new business sector, a second strategy is necessary, that is, finance schemes that allow for affordable rents without leaving the path of market-based operations. Together, the aim is to develop social housing as a bankable product. In this respect models have recently been designed that focus on structured finance for affordable rental housing construction (Amann, Lawson, and Mundt 2009; Amann 2009).

Nonprofit or limited-profit housing associations play a major role in affordable housing provision in many Western and Northern European as well as Asian countries. It is difficult to explain why twenty years after the collapse of socialism hardly any model with similar economic sustainability has been introduced in any of the CEE countries. The introduction of such schemes in the West after World War II was characterized by strong public commitment, both institutional and in terms of financing. At that time, the markets were not able to provide sufficient quantities of housing. Today, the higher capacities of the market make it seem as though other allocation schemes were unnecessary. However, market-based housing allocation is not able to satisfy all housing needs, particularly the needs of the most vulnerable households.

Drawing on the Private Rental Sector for Social Housing Purposes

Internationally, the private rental sector plays an increasing role in social housing provision. A good example is social housing in Germany, which is heavily based on a model of regulated and subsidized private rental housing used for social purposes. The two key elements of the model, which has a more than fifty-year history, are soft rent control and housing allowances.

A solution to increase access to housing for vulnerable groups is to use social rental agencies to mediate between private landlords and households in need. The landlords' reluctance to let rental units to vulnerable groups may be managed by provision of direct or indirect guarantees. Such agencies have been established in Belgium starting in the 1970s and in the UK in the late 1980s, when discrimination of minority groups in housing allocation was identified.

For transition countries, drawing on the private rental sector for social housing issues is critical because of its highly informal functioning. Regulations concerning tenant protection, setting of rents, terms of contract, and termination of the contract are widely lacking. Due to the low share of legal written contracts, missing tenant protection, and transparency (with the exception of a more advanced private rental system in the Czech Republic), private rentals cannot fully substitute for social housing programs in post-socialist states.

There are thus only very few programs in place in CEE countries. One example is the so-called "guaranteed housing", piloted in the Czech Republic. In Hungary, a rent allowance program for rental investment was proposed (Hegedüs and Teller 2005), but it failed because the required rent guarantees were too high. In 2005, an allowance program for low-income families with children in private rental dwellings was introduced. The rent allowance paid by the central government was limited to 30 percent of the rent or 25–30 euros per month, with similar additional funding by the local governments. The program failed, partly because of the very low-income limits and partly because it required the landlord to register with the tax authority.

A basic obstacle to employing the private housing sector for social housing provision is the danger that the subsidy may be capitalized by the landlords or other private actors. But even in well-developed markets, targeted allowances or tax reliefs may lead to an increase in prices but can nevertheless provide broad affordability.

Homeownership Programs

After the large-scale privatization programs in the region diminished the social housing stock, social housing policy had to find techniques to help households to access and maintain owner-occupation. The task was to design programs targeting low-income groups that enhance access to owner-occupation or help low-income households to improve their housing conditions through renewal and reconstruction.

The advantage of these programs is that they do not need a special institutional structure and administration costs are low. The disadvantage of the programs is that they are typically poorly targeted (or not targeted at all) and thus put a fiscal burden on the economy to support a middle class that does not necessarily need state support.

Nevertheless, there are situations when homeownership programs can be considered more effective than rental programs, for example, in rural areas where there is no demand for rental housing and no skills or organizational capacities for managing and maintaining social housing. Privatized multiapartment buildings that require investment into modernization so as to avoid depreciation and marginalization are another example. In the latter case, preventing such processes through subsidy programs for homeownership can be effective and can decrease the social costs of renewing such properties in a later phase.

Most of the countries in the region had to deal with the middle- and even upper-middle income households' housing problems. Because of the collapse of the housing finance system in the 1990s, even these groups faced an affordability problem. However, the introduction of support for savings banks, interest rate subsidies and tax allowances served the higher-income groups and such created a large fiscal burden for the governments that limited their possibility to introduce targeted social housing programs. For example, in Hungary when the fiscal costs of the housing program introduced in 2000 were considered to be too high, it was the social rental program that was stopped right away, whereas homeownership programs continued (Hegedüs 2007).

Mortgage programs aim to reduce the effective interest rate paid by the borrower from a market rate. A solution applied in the region is to use a special fund to issue loans at below-market interest rates. Different sources have been used, including the revenues from privatization (Estonia, Slovenia). In Slovakia, the Housing Development Fund issues loans for eligible households at the discount rate of the National Bank in Slovakia (Zapletalova et al. 2003). Some Western countries, such as Canada, had very good experiences with mortgage insurance schemes. Similar programs in transition countries had different effects. In Estonia, after abolishing the Housing Fund, a self-managing guarantee fund, KredEx, was established in 2000 (Kahrik et al. 2003).

Another technique to reduce the effective interest rates is the introduction of tax advantages. The personal income tax may be reduced by the amount of interests paid on a loan used to finance the purchase or expansion of a dwelling occupied by the taxpayer. Among the homeownership programs, contract savings programs were particularly popular in the region.

Lump sum subsidies are a type of cash grant used to enhance housing investments by individual households. It is typically used for financing new construction, but can be given for reconstruction or even to support transaction costs. The lump sum grant is used in Hungary to support families with children for new construction and is given to condominiums in particular for thermal rehabilitation.

In Croatia, the government introduced the so-called POS program in 2001, a centralized, top-down housing construction program to help families buy their first home. The prices of such homes are considerably lower than market prices. Local authorities ensure land and infrastructure, and the state ensures favorable loans. Until 2010, almost 5,000 housing units were built in this program. The sustainability of the program could not be guaranteed, as it was tied to one political party (Tepuš 2005), and when a new government came to power in 2003, the program was no longer a political priority and consequently fewer and fewer housing units have been produced. Within the program, a partnership with local authorities for social housing construction is offered. However, only one city has used the resources for these purpose.

Housing renovation and energy saving programs become very important in current years in many countries in the region. The State Support Program in Latvia between 2007 and 2010 is a good example for such interventions.

GOVERNANCE AND THE ROLE OF INTERNATIONAL CONTRIBUTIONS FOR SOCIAL HOUSING IN TRANSITION COUNTRIES

At the national level, housing funds became an important factor. The effectiveness of housing funds depends on their size as well as their administrative capabilities. National Housing Funds have been introduced, for instance, in Poland, the Czech Republic, Slovakia, Slovenia, Romania, and Albania (Amann and Springler 2012). The Slovenian Housing Fund emerged as an important provider of finance for the social housing sector after the transition, when mortgage finance was developing slowly and housing policy was inadequate. The Polish National Housing Fund (KFM) has financed more than sixty thousand new rental units since its establishment in the mid-1990s. The administration of the fund is carried out by the state-owned Bank Gospodarstwa Krajowego (Chiquier and Lea 2009).

There has been substantial international financial support for social housing in post-socialist states. The EIB supports social housing in two major ways. Social housing may be financed directly: the EIB participates in implementing EU development aid and cooperation policies through long-term loans (UNECE 2005). It has started to actively promote social housing by redirecting funds from urban renewal projects to social housing, for example, a 200-million-euro loan for urban renewal and energy efficient social housing in Poland (Amann et al. 2006). CEB has a special focus on social housing in transition countries with a big variety of projects in Albania, Bosnia and Herzegovina, Bulgaria, Croatia, Macedonia, Montenegro, and Serbia. It promotes projects that provide assistance to the most vulnerable people while supporting a structural approach to the development of social housing schemes in the target countries (Tsenkova 2005). World Bank financial support was granted in the past to housing projects in Poland, Russia, Albania, and Latvia (Tsenkova 2005) and more recently in combination with land administration projects also to Montenegro, Serbia, and Bosnia-Herzegovina.

CONCLUSION

The social rental programs are embedded in a policy environment and thus undergo constant adjustment according to the changes of the macro-environmental conditions and social needs.

The critical question is the availability of budget resources. Support for the public rental sector was a burden on the budgets of all European countries, although the overall cost of housing programs tends to decrease as a society becomes wealthier. The transitional countries typically have a GDP per capita around 30–50 percent of the European average, whereas their real estate market prices (and rents) are around 70–90 percent of the European level. Thus, to maintain a public rental sector costs more for the transitional countries, but these expenses can be lowered in the long run. The costs of social rental programs are high, and the expenses should be thoroughly planned, based on need. An unrealistic calculation of future program costs can quickly lead to the withdrawal or termination of such programs. A specific requirement for efficient housing policy schemes is continuity over election periods, rare indeed in most transition countries.

There are several institutional forms for implementing public rental programs, and it is difficult to set priorities among the alternative solutions. We have seen that the transitional countries have attempted to make use of many various models that exist in developed countries. The key question is how to ensure that the new institutions have their own interest and capacity to survive and continue to operate, in order to guarantee the sustainability of the respective models.

Interestingly enough, many rental programs turn into ownership programs when privatization becomes an available option for the sake of a short-term (political) advantage, which causes the failure of the social rental programs. Mass-scale privatization led to the development of a general expectation or “social pressure” to privatize remaining or newly constructed units.

The financial sustainability of a program means that the new tenants will be able to maintain the apartments, that is, they can afford the rents and housing costs. Hence, it is a question of allocation (not only the poorest should have access) and putting in place an efficient housing allowance system that guarantees that housing will be maintained and managed properly and, thus, be sustainable in the long run.

The aftermath of the international financial and economic crisis showed the necessity of reinventing the downgraded social housing sectors. Although European Union and transition economies were differently affected by the international economic crisis, households suffered in all economies.

The development of social housing and its financing was of low political significance in all transition countries. Most of them followed an explicit liberal market policy model with the idea that housing provision would basically be solved by the markets. Following a strict low-tax strategy, there was no scope for social housing finance anyway. Urgent social concerns were seemingly solved with mass privatization of previously social housing stocks. Policy reform focused on preparing the conditions for commercial housing construction, mainly by introducing condominium legislation and mortgage legislation and by privatizing the banking sector. The increasing output of residential construction, resulting from the introduction of retail financing products in the early 2000s, seemed to affirm this strategy. But the economic crisis showed quite clearly that the stalled housing boom has missed demand extensively in terms of location and affordability. After twenty years of transition, hardly any of the observed countries have developed a comprehensive scheme of social housing including according financing mechanisms. International institutions, including the EU, did not help much to make a difference.

Social housing is not only a social issue. Its potential for economic or environmental development, which is highly appreciated in Western countries with integrated housing policy schemes, is hardly realized. Many transition countries have very high ownership rates despite the negative effects on household mobility and consumer choice.

Some transition countries have experienced phases of relatively high public expenditure on housing, resulting from allowance schemes and temporary initiatives in new construction. But the state expenditure rates of western or northern European countries have hardly ever been reached. Following the economic crisis, many transition countries have even reduced the previously low expenditures on social housing. The development of the private banking sector has fueled commercial housing and contributed to the house price bubble in many metropolitan areas. But it hardly influenced social housing. Unlike in the West, commercial financing has hardly been integrated into social housing finance so far. Few examples with interest subsidies for commercial mortgages had a short life span due to exhaustive public costs. The banking sector is still no partner for social housing finance. There is little progress in financing (thermal) refurbishment of the multiapartment housing stock for several reasons: lacking private funds; reluctance of the public to further subsidize such upgrades after privatization; deficient enforcement of owners' associations; and, hence, low creditworthiness for such measures.

REFERENCES

Amann, W. 2009. "New Policies to Facilitate Affordable Housing in CEE." *Housing Finance International Journal,* XXIV (2): 24–33.

Amann, W., Beijer, E., Komendantova, N., Mundt, A., , Neuwirth, G., Roy, F., Schimpel, M., and Schwimmer, W. 2006. *H!FACT—A Housing Finance Agency for Countries in Transition. Feasibility Study.* Vienna: IIBW.

Amann, W., Lawson, J., and Mundt, A. 2009. "Structured Financing Allows for Affordable Rental Housing in Austria." *Housing Finance International Journal,* XXIII (4): 14–18.

Amann, W., Mundt, A. 2012. "Institutions: Housing Developers—Developed World." *International Encyclopedia of Housing and Home.* Elsevier's Science & Technology Publishing.

Amann, W. and Springler, E. 2012. "Housing Finance Institutions: Transition Societies." International Encyclopedia of Housing and Home. Elsevier's Science & Technology publishing.

Čačić, R. 2003. "Housing in Croatia—Efforts and Results." Presentation on Ministerial Housing Conference for South Eastern Europe. Paris, 23–24 April 2003.

Červeňová, L. 2005. *The Development of the Non-Profit Housing Sector in Slovakia.* Bratislava: Faculty of Civil Engineering, Slovak University of Technology. http://www.fgw.at/publikationen/pdf/05/2005–3_4-cervenova.pdf accessed July 15, 2012.

Chiquier, L. and Lea, M. 2009. *Housing Finance Policy in Emerging Markets.* Washington, DC: World Bank.

Donner, C. 2005. *Housing Policies in Central Eastern Europe.* Vienna: C. Donner.

Dübel, H. J., Brzeski, W. J., and Hamilton, E. 2006. *Rental Choice and Housing Policy Realignment in Transition: Post-Privatization Challenges in the Europe and Central Asia Region.* World Bank Policy Research Working Paper.

Hegedüs, J. 2007. "Social Housing in Transition Countries." *Social Housing in Europe.* London: LSE.

Hegedüs, J. and Teller, N. 2005. "Development of the Housing Allowance Programmes in Hungary in the Context of CEE Transitional Countries" *European Journal of Housing Policy* Vol. 5 (2): 187–209.

Hegedüs, J. and Tosics, I. 1990. "Hungarian Housing Finance, 1983–1990: A Failure of Housing Reform." *Housing Finance International* August 2009: 34–41. http://www.housingfinance.org/uploads/Publicationsmanager/9008_Hun.pdf accessed September 15, 2011).

IIBW. 2008. *Implementation of European Standards in Romanian Housing Legislation.* Vienna: IIBW.

IIBW. 2010. Montenegrin housing legislation gap assessment. In cooperation with the Montenegrin Ministry for Spatial Planning and the Environment, financed by DIGH—Dutch International Guarantees for Housing and FWAW - Fonds Werken aan Wonen. Vienna: IIBW.

Kahrik, A., Köre, J., Hendrikon, M., and Allsaar, I. 2003. "From a State Controlled to a Laissez Fair Housing System (Local Government and Housing in Estonia)." In: Lux, M. (ed.) *Housing Policy: An End or a New Beginning?* Budapest: OSI/LGI.

Lux, M., Kährik, A. and Sunega, P. 2012. "Housing Restitution and Privatization—Aids and Obstacles to the Formation of Private Rental Tenure in Transition Countries." *International Journal of Housing Policy*, 12 (2): 137–158.

Lux, M. and Mikeszová, M. 2012. "Property Restitution and Private Rental Housing in Transition: Case of the Czech Republic." *Housing Studies* 27 (1): 77–96.

Mandič, S. 2000. "Trends in Central East European Rented Sectors." *Journal of Housing and the Built Environment* 15 (3): 217–31.

Struyk, R., ed. 1996. *Economic Restructuring of the Former Soviet Bloc*. Washington, DC: Urban Institute Press.

Tepuš, M. 2005. *Modeli stambenog financiranja (Models of Housing Finance)*. Zagreb: Albatros media.

Tsenkova, S. 2005. *Trends and Progress in Housing Reforms in South Eastern Europe*. Paris: Council of Europe Development Bank.

Uchman, R. and Adamski, J. 2003. "How to Meet Market Rules and Social Goals for Housing?" *Housing Policy: An End or a New Beginning?* Budapest: OSI/LGI.

UNECE. 2005. *Housing Finance Systems for Countries in Transition, Principles and Examples*. New York and Geneva: United Nations. http://www.unece.org/fileadmin/DAM/hlm/prgm/hmm/hsg_finance/publications/housing.finance.system.pdf accessed January 15, 2011).

Walko, Z. 2008. "Housing Loan Developments in the Central and Eastern European EU Member States." *Focus on European Economic Integration 2/08*.

Whitehead, C. 2003. "Financing Social Housing in Europe." *Housing Finance International*, June 2003: 3–8.

World Bank. 2006. *Poland Housing Finance Policy Note*. Washington, DC: World Bank.

Zapletalova, J., Antalikova, M., and Smatanova, E. 2003. "The Role of Self-Government in Housing Development in Slovakia." *Housing Policy: An End or a New Beginning?* Budapest: LGI Books, Open Society Institute.

Zawislak, Marek. 2003. "Expanding 'True Social' Sector in Poland." Presented at the UNECE Workshop on Social Housing, Prague, May 19–20.

4 Rent Regulation and Housing Allowances

Martin Lux and Alexandr Puzanov

INTRODUCTION

The state interventions during socialism created a segment of mass public (semipublic) rental housing, where rents and utility prices were by regulation kept at extremely low levels. Price regulations made it possible to suppress the wages of the economically active population and thus temporarily maintain the competitiveness of the socialist economies. Tenants who were allotted flats by the state obtained unlimited occupancy rights in the form of a so-called 'deed' to the flat—later called quasi-homeownership (Lux 2009; Hegedüs and Tosics 1998).

After 1990, the new democratic governments wanted to reintroduce private property and establish a standard market economy: there was a plan to abolish the flat ('first-generation') rent regulation regime and replace it by a new market-friendly system. Instead, massive giveaway transfer of ownership rights to sitting tenants decreased public housing within a few years to a residual and marginal share of the housing stock. Where this unprecedented banquet did not take place, the socialist type of rent regulation was preserved for another decade. New means-tested housing allowances in post-socialist states played a minor role and never became real demand-side housing policy tools. Even in countries that did not apply right-to-buy policy and restituted part of housing stock to previous owners or their descendants, the opportunity to establish a sustainable rental housing policy was wasted in the early 1990s by the slow pace of rent deregulation.[1]

The soft policy 'cushion' (preserving the status quo and protecting sitting tenants) logically could not benefit everyone and could not exist forever. State protections basically applied only to sitting public tenants or tenants in restituted housing, that is, all running tenancies. For new tenancies (new rental contracts) in the private sector the governments usually did not set any rent caps or formulate specific rules giving the new tenants effective protection. Owing to a substantial decrease in the stock of public housing, the majority of new households were forced to seek housing in the private sector. This meant that they had to find their housing under market conditions: paying a market rent and enjoying much weaker tenure protection. Especially in countries where right-to-buy policy had not been applied (Poland, Czech Republic) rental housing became divided into two segments: the 'privileged' and 'nonprivileged' (Lux 2003). Rent regulation guaranteed low rent for many high-income sitting tenants ('privileged segment'), whereas many households in need remained cut off from the possibility of getting low-rent housing and tenure security ('nonprivileged segment').

There is at least one policy implication of the inconsistent rental policy, that is, combining low rents for 'old tenancies' with high rents for 'new tenancies'. This implication is that private rental housing, a thoroughly new institution established after the change of regime, has gradually come to be regarded as a temporary and residual form of housing. Private rental housing became branded as an insecure and expensive form of tenure, where landlords make no effort to have good relations with their tenants, and it is characterized by conflicts and tensions. As a result, most citizens have sought to avoid the private rental sector. Public opinion has turned even more towards owner-occupation in all post-socialist states as rental housing as a whole was gradually becoming stigmatized.

In the countries where restitution of housing was not the approach taken all or most private landlords are former sitting tenants who benefited from giveaway privatization and found themselves at a certain stage in their family cycle with extra housing. As a result, some other features of private rental housing in post-socialist states are the 'nonprofessional' landlords, the prevalence of short-term leases, weak protection of both parties to the agreement, and the frequent use of informal leases as 'nonprofessional' landlords try to avoid taxation.

THE SCOPE AND FORMS OF RENT CONTROL IN POST-SOCIALIST STATES

Although it is very difficult to make any generalization, there are basically two forms of rent control in western countries. The first is exercised through social housing; the second regulates the private rental sector.

Even within the territory of one country we find different modes of rent setting for social housing due to the specific local conditions and changing subsidy rules in time. However, we can distinguish two basic forms of social rents: nonprofit cost rent, that is, rent covering all the capital and operational costs of social landlords after deducting public capital and/or revenue subsidies (e.g., in Austria, Netherlands, Sweden), and income-related rent, that is, rent computed as a percentage of income of eligible household (e.g., in Portugal, Ireland).

After the Second World War there were few differences between rent control for social and private rental housing. However, since the 1960s most western countries have reformed rent regulation of the private segment of rental housing. These reforms have essentially involved transforming the rigid postwar system of 'first-generation' rent regulation into the 'second-generation' system of rent regulation. What is the basic difference? Lind (2001) claims that the 'first-generation' rent regulation regime has the following three characteristics:

1. Nominal rent freezes.
2. A nominal rent trend leads to a decrease in real rent.
3. A nominal rent trend leads to a decrease in real rent or leaves nominal rent well below the level of market rent.

"Second-generation rent control is any regulation of the rental market that does not fulfil definition above. There is no nominal rent freeze, rents do not usually fall in real terms and in the long run there might be no significant difference between actual rents and market rents" (Lind 2001, 43).

In the western countries of the EU, an enormous variety of approaches of 'second-generation' rent control in private rental sector were used (Lind 2001; Haffner, Elsinga, and Hoekstra 2008; Donner 2000). The 'extreme liberal systems' of second-generation rent regulation essentially set no direct limits on the level of initial rent and subsequent rent reviews (e.g., in the UK, Ireland, *de facto* Belgium and Finland). 'Moderate systems' limit rent regulation exclusively to running leases, whereas for newly signed leases rents can be set freely (e.g., in Germany, Switzerland and Spain). In 'stricter systems' not just the rents for running leases, but also a substantial portion of newly signed leases are regulated (e.g., in the Netherlands and France). Finally, in the 'strictest systems' rents are regulated for all running and newly signed leases (e.g., in Sweden and Denmark).

Rent reviews for running leases are constrained by a maximum rent level according to the dwelling's 'quality' in the Netherlands, by a maximum rent level agreed between the municipalities and tenant representatives in Sweden, by a referential rent index in France, by the Consumer Price Index in Spain and Belgium, by a maximum 'commensurate' level of profit in Switzerland, or by the level of local reference rents in Germany. Such constraints are sometimes accompanied by the condition that shock rent hikes are not allowed (e.g, in Germany, rent cannot be increased by more than 20 percent over the course of three subsequent years).

A dual approach taken by the governments to rents in social and private sectors, observed in western European countries since the 1960s, only gradually entered the housing policy discourse in post-socialist states. Housing was supposed to offset other reform measures; it was a way to sustain political support for economic transformation. All the post-socialist governments wanted to reconfirm quasi-homeownership entitlement of sitting tenants, so the social meaning of rent regulation in post-socialist countries was more like that of the postwar era than of the 1960s onwards in western countries.

The most common hybrid introduced into the post-socialist states during the early 1990s was the complete liberalization of rents for new private contracts (new private tenancies), combined with the preservation of a very conservative type of rent regulation and socialist tenant protection for all running tenancies—including tenancies in restituted private housing if restitution had taken place in the country. This form of 'first-generation' rent control has sometimes also been extended to new tenancies in public housing (Russia, Romania).

In the early 1990s further rent reform was conditional upon the introduction of a right-to-buy policy, that is, rent deregulation was passed only if sitting tenants were also given the right to 'buy' their occupied housing and thus a chance to avoid rent increases. Surprisingly, the housing allowance was not viewed as an adequate substitute. Moreover, even if right-to-buy policies were introduced, the deregulation of rents did not necessarily mean that the rents increased to close-to-market levels. Rent deregulation in many such cases was simply a transfer of the power to regulate public housing rents from the central to the local level, but public rents remained low. Therefore, like giveaway public housing privatization, rent regulation served originally as a general tool to maintain the quasi-homeownership status of rental housing rather than being a housing policy tool to help low-income households pay affordable rent.

A COMPARISON OF RENT CONTROL REGIMES IN POST-SOCIALIST STATES

Table 4.1 shows the features of rent control in post-socialist states. First, it shows the share of rental housing out of the total housing stock and its structure in selected post-socialist states. The countries with the highest share of rental housing and, simultaneously, the highest share of public rental housing are the Czech Republic, Poland, and Russia (Bosnia and Herzegovina and Estonia have a relatively high share of rental housing but it is mainly comprised of for-profit private rental housing). Second, Table 4.1 shows the scope of rent control in each state and uses a typology of the main forms of rent control to demonstrate which form is the core approach applied in each particular country.[2]

We understand rent control as a *central (state) policy that restricts the level of rent charged by public and/or private landlords*—either by means of rent setting (tariffs), a rent ceiling, or a cap on rent increases. We also make a distinction between direct and indirect forms of rent control. Direct rent control directly sets the tariffs or caps. An indirect rent control regime sets less constraining rules on rent setting; the landlords retain considerable freedom in actual pricing. Because different contexts exist, there can be no single and universal hierarchy of forms. However, rent setting is generally regarded to be the most constraining form of direct rent control; the rent ceiling (maximum rent) is less constraining, and the capping of rent increases for running leases is even less constraining.

In four countries the rents for old tenancies in *restituted (private rental) housing* are still regulated: Czech Republic, Croatia, Slovakia, and Poland. However, new tenancies in private rental housing are exempt from any rent control regime in almost all the selected transition states, with the sole exception of Poland; the regulations do not impose any cap on later rent hikes, any limits on initial rent levels, or any regulation on the term of the contract and its renewal. In most states (Bosnia and Herzegovina, Croatia, Poland, Romania, Russia, Serbia, Ukraine) the central rent control applies to both old and new tenancies in *public housing*; in three countries (Czech Republic, Slovakia, Slovenia) rent control is limited to just old tenancies and again new tenancies in public housing are exempt. The systems that extend rent regulation to new tenancies in public housing often use public housing as social housing (e.g., in Bosnia and Herzegovina, Serbia, Romania); in the second group of countries this may not always be the case (e.g., in the Czech Republic).

It is clear from Table 4.1 that the highest share of housing stock under a rent control regime is found in Poland (18 percent), Russia (16 percent), and the Czech Republic (11 percent); at the opposite end, the lowest share of housing stock under a rent control regime is, logically, in the super-homeownership states, such as Bosnia and Herzegovina (2 percent), Romania (2 percent), Slovenia (3 percent), Serbia (3 percent), Slovakia (3 percent), and Croatia (5 percent).

In 2008–2009 there were two countries with no central rent control regime, either for old tenancies or for new contracts (and not for public or for private housing)—Estonia and Hungary. In these two countries, landlords, including public ones, are free to increase and set rents for all tenancies as they wish. In both rent control was abolished in the early 1990s in connection with mass public housing privatization. In Estonia, where compared to Hungary a substantial stock of housing has been restituted to previous owners, legislation originally only shifted power to regulate both public and private rents for running tenancies to the municipalities. However, since 2004 all rents in the private sector were deregulated by a decision of the Supreme Court. In fact, public rents in both Estonia and Hungary have remained low—in Estonia they reflect the cost principles, and in Hungary they reflect rather the various local political interests.

In Russia, rent in public housing (whether running or new tenancies) is set by normative acts issued by local governments, which must be in accordance with the indirect central regulation of municipal rent setting. Central regulations deal with the binding components of rent (two components: *pure rent* and payment for repair and maintenance); the cost principle of public rent setting (*pure rent* should cover the reconstruction costs of a house/flat, and the second component, payment for repair and maintenance, should cover the costs of housing-related services); and the specific status of low-income households (they do not pay the *pure rent* component). Another specific indirect form of rent control comes from the fact that the utility service fees (affecting 70–80 percent of monthly housing related payments) and annual caps on tariff increases are set by the regional authorities. Although both of these practices rank among the less constraining forms of rent control, and although they are limited only to public housing, their combined use makes Russia a country with one of the most conservative ('first-generation') rent control regimes in the region. The situation in Ukraine is very similar to that in Russia. However, there public tenants pay only repair and maintenance costs and there is no 'pure rent' component of rent payments. Consequently, the level of public rents remains very low in both countries.

At the opposite end of the pole, since 2005 the rent control regime in Poland has acquired the character of a 'second-generation' rent control regime. Since 2005, the only central restrictions on municipalities and private landlords relate to rent increases, and caps are not set as central tariffs but instead as the 'justifiable' growth level (e.g., the increase in rent can be justified by the refurbishment of the flat, low capital profit of the landlord, higher costs to repay a mortgage loan for the landlord due to inflation, etc.). In the case of a dispute justifiability is decided by the court. Recently, rents increased to a level closer to market value and the system of rent regulation is now much like the regime in Switzerland. Despite the fact that it applies to all tenancies, Polish rent control is 'market-friendly'.

Until 2005, the Polish regime was one of the most conservative rent control systems in the region—rents for all running tenancies (both public and private) were capped at 3 percent of the dwelling replacement value (reconstruction costs). However, in the well-known case of *Hutten-Czapska versus Poland*, the Grand Chamber of the European Court of Human Rights in Strasbourg ruled strongly in favor of private landlords in Poland: "the decision disapproves strong rent control, proposes government restitutionary compensation for landlords and requires an effective eviction law, leaving the responsibility for the tenants affected by this to the state" (Ball 2010, 1). Poland was thus forced to make a substantial change to the rent control regime by a decision of the European Court for Human Rights.

Next to Poland and Russia, the last country with a relatively large rent-controlled housing stock is the Czech Republic (11 percent of the housing stock, including old tenancies in the private rental sector). Deregulation of controlled rents started in 1992 and the maximum regulated rent was stipulated in relevant government decrees: since 1999, when regulated rents were still several times lower than market rents, the maximum regulated rent stopped rising in real terms and since 2002 also in nominal terms. The process of rent deregulation did not restart until 2007, when a special act on rent deregulation came into force. Like in Poland, until 2007 and despite several decisions of the Czech Constitutional Court deeming rent regulation unconstitutional, the system in the Czech Republic was one of the most conservative regimes in the region—rents for running tenancies remained practically frozen from 1999.

The main motive for restarting the deregulation of rents in 2007 was a decision of the Strasbourg court in the *Hutten-Czapska versus Poland* case. The Czech government became concerned about losing a case with private landlords like that in Poland, which could lead to the government having to pay large financial compensation to landlords. At that time thousands of Czech private landlords were already preparing a joint action against the Czech state and had submitted it to the Strasbourg court. Rapid rent deregulation started in 2007. The act established an intermediary period during which the maximum rents for running tenancies were set to increase to 5 percent of the market value of the property (the average market value is set per m^2 for each municipality based on transfer tax data collected by tax offices). The intermediary period should have ended in 2010, but it was extended to 2012 in large urban centers in response to the economic crisis. Rents should therefore soon be deregulated (the state will withdraw from this field), and a 'second-generation' rent control regime will be established. This regime will set only a cap on rent increases to the level of 'locally relevant rent' (i.e., basically the free market rent typically paid for the same kind of dwelling in the same location); any disputes over the locally relevant rent is settled in court. The system will therefore be similar to the German system of rent control.

In other selected post-socialist states rent control is limited to public housing, which is, firstly, marginal in scale and, secondly, often defined as social housing. The most conservative form—flat-rate tariffs differentiated somewhat by specific coefficients—is used in Serbia (3 percent of the housing stock under rent control regime), Slovakia (3 percent of the housing stock), and Romania (2 percent of the housing stock). In Romania, rents are set according to a government decree, in which basic cost tariffs are differentiated by specific coefficients that reflect the category of flat and its location. The tariffs are amended each year at the end of January and adjusted in relation to the inflation rate in the previous year. However, tenants eligible for social housing may in fact pay an even lower rent than tariffs: the maximum rent payable by tenants in social housing is 10 percent of the gross monthly income of a household. The difference between that amount and the tariff rent is subsidized by the municipality. In Slovakia the tariffs are announced in government decrees and based on the Price Act.

In the remaining post-socialist states the rents in public housing are capped by maximum rent levels. These maximum rents are calculated as a percentage of estimated (assessed) dwelling value—2.5 percent of the dwelling value in Bosnia and Herzegovina (2 percent of the housing stock under a rent control regime) or 4.68 percent of the dwelling value in Slovenia (3 percent of the housing stock)—or they are computed as a percentage of the replacement costs—0.54 percent of replacement (construction) costs in Croatia (5 percent of the housing stock).

Table 4.1 Main Parameters of Rent Control in Selected Post-Socialist States, 2010

	BA	CZ	HR	EE	HU	PL	RO	RU	SK	SI	RS	UA
Rental housing as % of housing stock (2008/2009)												
- public housing	2.0	11.0	2.5	4.0	3.7	8.5	2.0	15.5	2.8	1.8	3.4	4.7
- private nonprofit housing*	0.1	-	-	-	-	2.0	-	3.0	-	2.0	0.0	-
- private for-profit housing	20.0	14.0	8.4	13.0	4.0	9.0	6.7	8.0	1.5	1.2	7.3	n.a.
Total	**22.0**	**24.0**	**10.9**	**17.0**	**7.7**	**19.5**	**8.7**	**23.7**	**4.3**	**5.0**	**10.7**	**n.a.**
Form of rent control												
Direct 1: Central rent setting							■		■	■	■	
Direct 2: Central caps on rents (maximum rents)	■	■	■				■			■		
Direct 3: Central regulation of rent increase						■		■				■
Indirect: Central rules on public rent setting								■				■
No rent control				■	■							
New contracts in existing public housing under rent control	YES	NO	YES	NO	NO	YES	YES	YES	NO	NO	YES	YES
Est. % of rental housing under rent control out of total in given segment												
- % public housing	100	70	100	-	-	100	100	100	100	80	100	100
- % private nonprofit housing	100	-	-	-	-	100	-	0	-	80	-	-
- % private for-profit housing	0	25	20	-	-	80	0	0	7	0	0	0
% of total housing stock	2	**11**	5	-	-	**18**	2	**16**	3	3	3	5

*Does not include hybrid forms, such as co-op housing, only pure rental housing provided by private nonprofit organizations (housing associations, nonprofit enterprises).

Notes: BA: Bosnia and Herzegovina; CZ: Czech Republic; HR – Croatia; EE – Estonia; HU – Hungary; PL – Poland; RO – Romania; RU – Russia; SK – Slovakia; SI – Slovenia; RS – Serbia; UA – Ukraine.

The amount of new public or nonprofit housing built after 1990 is marginal. New public or nonprofit housing often had the character of social housing and was intended for a specific target population; consequently, here rents are again controlled by the state. However, rent control in new public or nonprofit housing reflects the level of state subsidies and/or the specific conditions of subsidy programs and it is set as a cost rent. The cost of new construction, however, may be high, so rents in any newly built public or nonprofit housing are often higher than in existing public housing (with the exception of Romania or Russia, where the same rent regulation principles apply to both existing and newly built public housing).

An example of more extensive new social housing construction in the region is the TBS nonprofit housing scheme in Poland, where the maximum rent is centrally regulated (the relevant legislation on this was passed in 1995) at 4 percent of the dwelling's replacement value (i.e., the average construction costs annually declared by regional councils). The same applies, for example, to Slovakia: the maximum rent in new public housing built after 2001 is 5 percent of the acquisition cost. Other examples of specific *ad hoc* rent regulation schemes applied to new public or nonprofit housing include flats built in the Czech Republic under ministry programs directed at 'supporting housing' and 'social housing', flats built in Hungary under the Szécheny government program, or public flats built in Serbia for refugees from the ex-Yugoslav republics.

As mentioned in the preceding, the pace of 'legal' rent deregulation is not necessarily connected with the pace of 'price' deregulation. The central regulation of rents was quickly dissolved only in those countries that applied a generous right-to-buy policy (Estonia, Russia, Ukraine, Hungary), whereas it remained strong for a long time in countries where this policy was rejected (Czech Republic, Poland). There are several exceptions to this rule—Romania, Slovakia, and all post-Yugoslav republics—where rents for public housing continued to be regulated by the central government. However, real price deregulation (rent increase) and thus the real shift to a 'second-generation' rent control regime for running tenancies first appeared, paradoxically, in the countries that avoided right-to-buy policies: the Czech Republic and Poland. However, the main reason is not the absence of a right-to-buy policy but rather the restitution of the housing stock. In the Czech Republic, Poland, and also in Estonia, the restituents were powerful enough to lobby for a change in the rent control regime and they succeeded by taking legal action against the state.

HOUSING ALLOWANCES IN SELECTED POST-SOCIALIST STATES

A means-tested housing allowance is one of the most important instruments of housing and welfare policy in developed European states, especially in the field of rental housing. It complements social housing and is part of the social security system of each country. With respect to housing policy, this is a demand-oriented instrument. Indirectly, it may also affect the supply. Increasing the disposable income of the population by providing an allowance stimulates housing demand; the reaction to an increase in demand should be a corresponding increase in the supply. The introduction of housing allowances therefore "reflected housing policy rather than social security concerns" (Kemp 1997, 16).

Housing allowances were introduced in the western countries from the middle of the 1960s (Germany 1965) onwards, but especially during the 1970s (Great Britain 1972, France 1977) and 1980s. The basic principle of housing allowances is to provide eligible households from the rental or owner-occupied housing sectors with a benefit equal to the difference between the actual and the normatively set level of household housing-cost burden, defined as the share of housing expenditures out of total household income. When calculating the housing allowance, three factors in particular are usually taken into account: household income, housing expenditures, and household size (an international comparison of different models in western countries is found, for example, in Kemp 2007).

Table 4.2 presents an international comparison of several aspects of housing allowances in sample post-socialist states. There is no housing allowance in Serbia or Bosnia and Herzegovina. In Romania, only a 'heating allowance' exists, which provides compensation for unpredicted increases in the price of fuels used for central heating systems and is paid directly to the local thermal energy providers. In several other post-socialist states the estimated share of households receiving a housing allowance is very low: less than 1 percent in Slovenia; 2 percent in Estonia, the Czech Republic, and Croatia; 3 percent in Poland; and 5 percent in Slovakia and Ukraine. The housing allowance is more widely received only in Russia (11 percent of households) and Hungary (8.5 percent of households). The situation in Hungary is relatively new, and the housing allowance has played this more significant role since 2004.

In many countries the first housing allowance scheme was established relatively soon after the regime change, but generally it underwent various amendments in later years, especially after 2000. Usually the eligible households are also the recipients of the housing allowance; only in Slovenia and Poland are the allowances paid directly to landlords (initially this was also the case in Russia). In all countries, except Slovenia, the allowances are paid both to tenants and homeowners; they are therefore tenure neutral (in Croatia since 2001).

The source of allowance financing varies: in approximately one-half of sample countries the allowances are paid entirely or mainly out of the state budget (Czech Republic, Estonia, Ukraine, Slovakia, Hungary), in one country they are paid mainly out of the regional budgets (Russia), and in the remaining countries they are financed exclusively or mainly out of the municipal budgets (Poland, Slovenia, Croatia). In two of the countries in which most expenditures relating to housing allowances are paid by the municipalities some form of cofinancing from other sources exists: in Slovenia the allowances for private market tenants are cofinanced by the state budget and in Croatia (for the gas allowance) by the regional budgets. Allowances are also cofinanced in Hungary—about 10 percent of the total amount comes from the municipal budgets; in Russia part of the total housing allowance due in less-developed regions is cofinanced out of the federal state budget.

This situation is not constant in time. As Table 4.2 shows, with the exception of Poland, most post-socialist states have seen a strengthening of centralization (bottom-up change) in the financing and regulation of housing allowances. In some countries at least part of the total housing allowance due has over time been overtaken from the municipalities by the regions (Russia, Croatia) or the state (Slovenia, Hungary). In Hungary there was a radical change in financing and competence in 2004, when the state almost fully took over the role that had been played by the municipalities to that time. And in Russia, also in 2004, the financing responsibility was fully transferred from the municipalities to the regional level. The opposite trend has been observed only in Poland, where in the 1990s the municipalities received about half of the total allowance due from the state budget, but now they bear all the costs themselves; after the 2004 tax income distribution reform they began receiving a higher share of collected tax income, but became fully responsible for paying the housing allowance.

If there is one feature common to the housing allowances schemes in all the selected post-socialist countries it is their marginal significance. Their role is limited to income maintenance for the lowest-income families; they are not an effective demand-side housing policy instrument. The restrictive conditions attached to the housing allowance, such as the explicit income ceilings (Estonia, Poland, Slovenia, Croatia, Hungary) that limit household eligibility, demonstrate this. The housing allowance is often governed by social security legislation (Estonia, Croatia, Hungary, Ukraine, Czech Republic, Slovakia) rather than specific housing legislation (Russia, Slovenia, Poland); in Estonia it is part of the subsistence benefit and in Slovakia part of assistance to people in material need.

Consequently, the housing allowance is more of an auxiliary tool that helps low-income families cover the costs of increasing utility prices (such as prices for energy, gas, heating, water supply) than it is a substitute for rent regulation or public housing privatization (Hegedüs and Teller 2005, 189). This fact explains why housing allowances are usually (with the sole exception of Slovenia) tenure neutral, that is, why they are allocated not only to tenants but also to 'poor' homeowners. This situation has changed little since 2000.

Another shared feature is the paradoxical fact that almost all housing allowance models in sample countries are geared towards already protected tenants or homeowners (except in Croatia): 'privileged' tenants, 'social' tenants paying regulated rent, or homeowners who got their housing cheaply through giveaway privatization. Although official rules introduced more recently usually do not distinguish between different types of tenants or homeowners (for example, the explicit exclusion of 'unprivileged' tenants was ruled out in Russia in 2002 and in Slovenia in 2008), restrictive conditions, such as income and housing cost ceilings, are clear signs that the allowance targets mainly 'old' and protected tenants and homeowners.

In the private sector, tenants that pay market rents (and, respectively, owners that are repaying mortgage loans) are still, although recently more implicitly, excluded from receiving effective assistance in the form of the housing allowance in the overwhelming majority of sample countries. Their incomes are generally higher than income ceilings (otherwise they could not pay the housing market price) and market rents are often well above the cost ceilings or tariffs applied in the housing allowance formulae. Even though the rent-to-income ratio of 'unprivileged' tenants is often substantially higher than the normative rate of burden set in the allowance formulae, they receive no allowance or they receive only a type of specific allowance (Slovenia).

Moreover, most existing housing allowance models do not take into account real housing costs but instead use notional cost tariffs (Hungary, Slovenia, Ukraine, Russia). In Slovakia, the amount of the housing allowance is a simple one-figure tariff, and notional costs are set at a low level, reflecting the situation in the 'privileged' sector; here the exclusion of households that pay market housing prices is the most apparent.[1] In addition, these simple tariffs barely reflect regional differences in market rents and prices, and this again confirms the role of the housing allowance as a social benefit that covers a part of maintenance fees and utility costs (utility costs do not vary regionally too much).[2] In Estonia, however, real housing costs are taken into account to determine the amount of the housing allowance, but they are limited by ceilings (maximum values); the ceilings are set by the municipalities. In Poland real housing costs are included in the calculation of an allowance, with only indirectly set ceilings (comparable costs in municipal housing). The Czech Republic now has the least constraining allowance formula: since 2007 real housing costs are included and, thanks to rent deregulation, the ceilings are set at levels close to rents/costs in the private market rental sector.

The normative rate of burden of a housing allowance is defined as the share of household income that a household is expected to spend on housing. In other words, it determines the minimum financial contributions of a household to its housing expenditures not directly (in absolute values) but indirectly, in the form of a percentage of the total household income. The standard normative rate of burden varies among post-socialist countries, ranging from 15 percent (Ukraine) and 18–22 percent (Russia), to 30 percent (Hungary and Estonia) and 30–35 percent (Czech Republic). It can

Table 4.2 A Comparison of Selected CEE Housing Allowance Models, 2010

	Housing allowance is a special benefit designed to cover housing costs	Housing allowance is governed by housing legislation (HL) or social security legislation (SSL)	All tenures are eligible for the housing allowance	Explicit or implicit income ceilings for housing allowance eligibility	Who provides funds for housing allowance payments?	Trend in housing allowance financing after its establishment	The share of households receiving housing allowance out of total number of households (2008 or 2009, in %)	The main recipient of housing allowance
CZ	Yes	SSL	Yes	Implicit	State	No change	2.5	Household
HR	Yes	SSL	Yes	Explicit	Municipalities, special heating allowance from regions	Moderate centralization	2.4	Household
EE	No (part of subsistence benefit)	SSL	Yes	Explicit	State	No change	2	Household
HU	Yes	SSL	Yes	Explicit	State and small part (about 10%) municipalities	Strong centralization	8.5	Household
PL	Yes	HL	Yes	Explicit	Recently exclusively municipalities	Strong centralization	3	Landlord
RU	Yes	HL	Yes	Implicit	Regions with differentiated state subsidies to weak regions	Strong centralization	10.6	Household
SK	No (part of social assistance in material need)	SSL	Yes	Implicit	State	No change	4.9	Citizen in material need (eligibility is jointly assessed with other family members
SI	Yes	HL	No, only tenants	Explicit	Municipalities with small state subsidies for special allowances to private market tenants	Moderate centralization	0.8	Landlord
UA	Yes	HL	Yes	Implicit	State	No change	5	Household

Note: CZ: Czech Republic; HR – Croatia; EE – Estonia; HU – Hungary; PL – Poland; RU – Russia; SK – Slovakia; SI – Slovenia; UA – Ukraine.

vary according to the composition and size of the household (e.g., Czech Republic, Estonia) or household income (e.g., Poland).

The 'taper' shows the amount by which housing allowance decreases when the income of a household increases by one currency unit. In most of the sample countries, the taper was relatively gentle, but the models in Estonia, Hungary, Slovakia, and Russia were the exceptions. Their allowance models have a high taper, or there are specific thresholds after which the allowance is sharply reduced. This kind of situation can lead to a poverty or unemployment trap.

CONCLUSIONS

There are only a few countries in our sample of post-socialist states where the rent in some private housing units is regulated by the state. This pertains mainly to rent in restituted housing stock. Basically, new tenancies in the private rental sector are concluded freely on the market—often black market, because many landlords do not want to declare income from rent on their tax return. Conversely, public rents are usually subject to a specific regime of central rent control—either direct rent setting, rent capping, or rent increases. In countries where regulation is applied to both sitting and new public tenants, public housing tends generally to be viewed as social housing. In countries where new public tenancies are exempted from rent control this may not always be the case. There are three countries in our sample where rent control is imposed on more than 10 percent of the housing stock (Poland, Russia, Czech Republic); and there are two countries in our sample where central rent control has disappeared entirely (Estonia and Hungary).

In our analysis we discovered that the pace of 'legal' rent deregulation in the 1990s was closely connected with (or even dependent on) the introduction of a right-to-buy policy. The central regulation of rents was quickly eliminated or decentralized only in those countries that applied a generous right to buy policy (Estonia, Russia, Ukraine, Hungary), but it remained strong in those countries where this policy was rejected (Czech Republic, Poland). However, the real deregulation of prices (rent reform) and thus the real shift to a 'second-generation' rent control regime for running tenancies first occurred, paradoxically, in the countries that avoided right-to-buy policies: the Czech Republic and Poland. The main reason for this was the restitution of the housing stock and the fact that private restituents in these two countries successfully challenged the state regulation of rent in international court.

There are specific rent regulation schemes that are applied to rental housing built after 1990 and subsidized out of the public budget but generally this housing accounts for just a small part of the total housing stock, except in Poland, Slovakia, and the Czech Republic. In Poland this relates to dwellings built under nonprofit TBS schemes, and in the Czech Republic and Slovakia it involves municipal dwellings built under various government programs.

The decentralized housing allowance system of the early 1990s was later, except in Poland, transformed into a more central model of financing. Increased centralization of the financing and regulation of housing allowances has been typical across most post-socialist states in our sample (especially for Hungary and Russia in 2004).

The marginal significance of the housing allowance is a shared feature of the selected post-socialist countries. Although it is impossible to fully evaluate a housing allowance scheme without detailed knowledge of the given country's social security system (such as how it calculates the living minimum or subsistence benefits), the role of the housing allowance in selected post-socialist states is clearly limited to income support for the lowest-income families, rather than being an effective demand-side housing policy instrument. Its main purpose is not to enable rent (housing) reforms but rather to compensate lower-income households for increases in utility prices.

Another shared feature is that almost all housing allowance schemes are oriented towards tenants who already enjoy tenure protection and towards homeowners: 'privileged' tenants, 'social' tenants, and homeowners who got their own housing through giveaway privatization. Tenants that pay market rents in the private sector are still, explicitly or implicitly, excluded from obtaining effective help in the form of the housing allowance (except under the recent system introduced in the Czech Republic).

New tenancies in the private sector are not protected by rent control or by effective tenure security legislation. The market rents in the private rental housing are often several times higher than rents in public (nonprofit) housing, even in countries where rents in public housing are no longer centrally regulated (Hungary, Estonia). Young families often have little chance of obtaining public or social housing because the tenancy turner in such housing is low and there is relatively little public housing left since the giveaway housing privatization. Despite this fact, the housing allowance generally provides them with no effective help with their high housing costs.

There are at least two clear policy implications from rental housing segmentation. One is that such a policy will logically result in all citizens preferring (and even being forced) to become homeowners, because homeownership is then the only secure and accessible form of housing tenure. The second implication is that rental housing is becoming stigmatized as a residual and temporary form of housing: residual for people on low or unstable income and temporary for students and young singles. This situation will only strengthen the housing system's orientation towards owner-occupied housing in the future.

NOTES

1. Politicians deliberately chose housing as a policy 'cushion', which was intended to soften the blows of the more painful effects of economic transformation.
2. As stated earlier, rent regulation applies especially to old tenancies because new tenancies in private rental housing are exempt from any rent control

in all post-socialist states; in some states, however, new tenancies in public housing are subjected to rent control.

3. Notional housing expenditures are rarely applied in EU housing allowance models. Instead, the ceiling (maximum costs) is often used, whereas actual costs are taken into account in the calculation of the benefit. Above the level of the ceiling, a household must pay for all other expenditures with its own resources.
4. In Russia the standard notional costs set by the regions are differentiated by the municipalities themselves, but this differentiation does not take into account differences in free market rents, but rather differences in utility costs.

REFERENCES

Ball, J. 2010. "'Where Will European Property Law Go Next?' Tenancies and Property after *Hutten-Czapska* v *Poland* and *FEANTSA v Slovenia.*" Paper presented at COBRA Conference, Paris, July 2–3.

Donner, C. 2000. *Housing Policies in the European Union.* Vienna: Christian Donner.

Haffner, M., Elsinga, M., and Hoekstra J. 2008. "Rent Regulation: The Balance between Private Landlords and Tenants in Six European Countries." *European Journal of Housing Policy* 8:217–33.

Hegedüs, J. and Teller, N. 2005. "Development of the Housing Allowance Programmes in Hungary in the Context of CEE Transitional Countries." *European Journal of Housing Policy* 5:187–209.

Hegedüs, J. and Tosics, I. 1998. "Rent Reform—Issues for Countries of Eastern Europe and the Newly Independent States." *Housing Studies* 13:657–58.

Kemp, P. 1997. *A Comparative Study of Housing Allowances.* London: Department of Social Security.

———, ed. 2007. *Housing Allowances in Comparative Perspective.* Bristol: Policy Press.

Lind, H. 2001. "Rent Regulation: A Conceptual and Comparative Analysis." *European Journal of Housing Policy* 1:41–57.

Lux, M., ed. 2003. *Housing Policy—An End or a New Beginning.* Budapest: LGI/OSI.

———. 2009. *Housing Policy and Housing Finance in the Czech Republic during Transition. An Example of Schism between the Still-Living Past and the Need of Reform.* Amsterdam: Delft University Press.

5 Social Landlords and Social Housing Management

József Hegedüs and Nóra Teller

INTRODUCTION: TRENDS IN SOCIAL HOUSING MANAGEMENT

A broad concept of housing management encompasses the entire set of institutions that implement programs to help needy households meet their housing needs. In this chapter, we will use a narrower interpretation of this concept, limited to social housing agencies and their regulating institutions. This approach thus does not include targeted income support programs that mitigate low-income households' affordability problems. That topic is covered by Chapter 4 in this volume. Social housing management in this more narrow approach includes activities such as housing allocation, maintenance, renewal, rent setting, rent collection, arrears management, asset management, business administration, and so on (see Priemus, Dieleman, and Clapham 1999; Gruis and Nieboer 2004; Gibb and Trebeck 2009).

The social housing sector in the developed world went through major changes in the last three decades, characterized not only by a shift in the tenure structure (Harloe 1995, among others), but also by changes in housing management (Ruys, Bruil, and Dix 2007). Social housing systems differ from each other in terms of the sector's size and its organizational forms. According to the mainstream approach (Gibb 2001; Boelhouwer, van der Heijden, and van de Ven 1997; Czischke 2009), the main types of organizations are state-owned housing, municipality-owned housing, and different forms of cooperatives and nonprofit organizations. The "content" of the services provided by social housing agencies (allocation, tenant rights, affordability, rent allowances, etc.) has changed according to the behavior of the management companies, the strategies of the potential beneficiaries (households), and the policy environment (legal framework, subsidy programs, etc.).

Social housing management in the more developed part of Europe faces a paradox, as the sector has to increase its efficiency while guaranteeing its social mandate (Burke 2004). The sector must become more open to market processes both in terms of investment and operation because the subsidies to the social housing sector have gradually been reduced. Management companies and social landlords have to change their strategy accordingly:

they either have to privatize part of the stock to decrease the financial burden or offer services for better-off households who can afford the increased housing costs.

Such a policy shift took place, for example, in Holland and Sweden. Direct subsidies to housing cooperatives (Holland) and municipal housing enterprises (Sweden) have been eliminated, and means-testing played less and less of a role in the allocation of housing, because the rent allowance system achieves, via social targeting, the goal of decreasing inequality among the tenants. Interestingly enough, redirecting the support from the social landlords directly to the beneficiaries leads to a real "unitary system" (Kemeny 1995), which means that social landlords have to compete with the private landlords for the tenants who enjoy an income benefit in the form of a means-tested rent assistance or housing allowance. This policy shift tends to result in the shrinkage of the social rental sector, because rent increases will strengthen the households' preference for homeownership, especially if the subsidy system is biased towards ownership, thus leading to a "residual social housing system".

Another important trend was the emergence of a "very social housing" sector as in France, where social landlords serving very poor households took over social tasks (crime prevention, youth programs, arrears management, etc.) that were formerly the responsibility of other specialized institutions (Levy-Vroelant and Tutin 2007).

Analyses of the social housing sector should not neglect the role of institutions and programs that are not directly connected to the traditional social landlords. Social rental agencies in Belgium and Holland, which function as intermediaries between needy households and the owners of the private units, are a good example for this specific form of housing management (De Decker 2002, 2009). Furthermore, rent allowance schemes for tenants in the private rental sector in Germany give an example for a social housing subsector that is not dependent on social landlords, but has an important effect on the housing system.

This chapter will focus on the development of new forms of social housing management; the role of the new social landlords; and on the sources of tension in the changing social housing sector (allocation, rent arrears, renovation). In order to understand these issues in context, we will discuss the degree to which the sector managed to leave the legacy of the socialist housing system behind (Tsenkova and Turner 2004) in the transition process.

SOCIAL HOUSING MANAGEMENT IN THE TRANSITION PERIOD

Although the size of the social rental sector varied between socialist countries (Turner, Hegedüs, and Tosics 1992), they all implemented some form of the Eastern European Housing Model (EEHM), which relied on large state or cooperative management companies to administer the owner-occupied housing estates as well as the public rental stock.[1] The subsidized housing costs (rent and utilities), which were independent of actual economic costs, formed part of the shortage economy (Kornai 1980). This resulted in permanent excess demand, which limited the tenants' "voice option". Long waiting lists were typical of the socialist housing system, and allocation was based both on "positional" advantages and need factors (Hegedüs and Tosics 1996). The revenues (rent and utility fees) did not cover maintenance and operation costs, and as housing was not an economic priority, the sector was consequently underfinanced, which led to a degradation of the stock. The management companies paid very little attention to the tenants' complaints regarding the physical condition of the stock, which led to high levels of dissatisfaction with public rental housing in the region.

However, there were important differences between countries under the EEHM due to the differing political and organizational structure of the socialist states. There were two basic approaches. The first model was characterized by a "sectorial" structure, where the ministries organized the social services of the employers (and their families) through large state-owned enterprises. The second model was based on a territorial structure, where the deconcentrated units of the socialist state had specialized institutions for providing social services, typically through the council system. Housing cooperatives were managed either within the council system (for example, in Hungary) or through the ministries (for example, in Russia).

The sector was restructured after the transition, but the process differed from country to country depending on privatization and decentralization (see Chapter 2, this volume).

The basic question was how the social landlords and the changing legal environment would change the nature of the public rental sector. Would means-tested rent allowances replace the rent-subsidy system based on unitary low rent? Would the extended property rights of the tenants disappear? Would need be a major factor in the allocation process? These questions have not been fully settled yet, as the public rental sector is still going through the gradual process of transition. Many elements of the socialist housing system survived the early phase of the transition because of the vested interest of the sitting tenants. However, the social landlords did come to have more freedom in setting their own strategy, constrained mainly by the political costs of rent increases, evictions, and so on.

Following privatization, the new owners of the housing stock had the right (as in Hungary, the Czech Republic, and Slovakia) to select among different forms of building management. The management of the privatized buildings was under the control of the elected representatives of the housing association or condominium, who could personally manage the building or hire a specialized management company. Consequently, the state-owned management companies lost their monopoly to operate and maintain the stock. In fact, this even meant that the public management companies could lose the right to manage state-owned housing units, if these units were in condominiums where the majority of the apartments were privately owned. (We will discuss the problems associated with such "mixed ownership" later in this chapter.) Privatization also meant that the number of housing units owned by local governments decreased drastically, and it thus made economic sense for small municipalities to merge the social housing management companies with other local service providers (real estate managers of the markets, cemeteries, district heating, etc.). However, in some countries, privatization did not lead to the collapse of the old state management companies, as the new owners did not have the right to change the management (for example, in Russia, Armenia, or Ukraine).

> In the Czech and Slovak Republics, the old state management agencies were monopolistic, inefficient, and paid little attention to tenant complaints. Reforming them has been a popular theme among the region's local officials. One district in Prague terminated all of the functions of the state management agency and publicly requested proposals from private firms to fill the breach, fully aware at the time that no such firms existed. Firms were literally created overnight and ultimately 25 new firms answered the government request (Kingsley and Mikelsons 1996, 199–200).
>
> In Hungary, prior to 1990, 36 large management companies operated 83 percent of the public housing stock. In 1990 the central state subsidy for management companies was eliminated and the corporate law required local governments to restructure their enterprises as joint-stock companies. An examination of these companies in 1991 showed that most companies had made streamlining changes to these organizations, including breaking them into several companies (Hegedüs, Mark, and Tosics 1996, 123–24).
>
> In Slovenia, there was a rapid privatization of management services. Prior to housing privatization, only a small number of local monopoly firms had been vested various powers by the owners of housing stock, be they firms, municipalities, or private individuals. These firms collected the rent and managed the housing stock. After 1991 the municipal maintenance firms were privatized and a large number of new firms emerged to compete for contracts with the older firms (Mandic and Stanovnik 1996, 165).

SOCIAL HOUSING MANAGEMENT FORMS

As a consequence of the general trend towards decentralization, the management of the remaining public housing stock was transferred to the municipal governments (Dabla-Norris 2006). We will now describe the two major types of housing management, carried out by local governments and nonprofit organizations.

In a decentralized system, the municipality (a council committee or a department in the town hall) has the right to make all decisions concerning property rights. It thus decides about privatization, investments, allocation of vacant units, rent levels, and rent allowances (although the last two functions can also belong to the central government—see Chapter 4, this volume). Although it is formally the municipality's task to set the local social housing strategy, management companies can informally acquire decision-making powers through administrative functions and participate in preparing proposals on rent structure and rent allowances, or even proposals for national grant allocation tenders. The reasons for this are technical rather than political. The municipalities simply do not have the capacity to carry out all the administrative and management tasks delegated to the local level.

The management companies are under pressure from local governments to improve the financial performance of the public sector, although the companies' formal responsibility is only the management of the stock. Thus, management companies have a strong incentive to improve rent collection levels, decrease rent arrears, and thus get rid of the "problematic tenants". The nonpaying tenants, typically the poorest households who accumulate unmanageable debts, have very few alternatives to consolidate their financial situation. They can only scale down housing, which means moving to worse housing conditions, in low-served areas, to poor settlements. The process can lead to large-scale evictions and rent increases, which affect pockets of poverty in some countries and more mainstream social housing in others (FRA 2009). However, there are political constraints on the "rationalization" of public housing: for instance, local governments try to avoid evictions, because they are politically very unpopular. To solve this problem, some local governments pass the conflict on to private companies: housing units can be sold (with sitting tenants) to a private developer, who can evict the tenants without political problems—and any responsibility to find new housing for the tenants.

As mentioned earlier, some municipalities merged housing management companies with other local service providers, such as district heating or trash collection companies. The resulting companies typically cross-subsidize the public rental sector with the revenues from nonresidential units and other profitable activities, because the social rental sector is financially not self-sufficient.

The second major form of housing management is the nonprofit model. This model is widespread in Western Europe, where it had a long history of government support. Today, international donor agencies try to implement the models that worked in their home countries in Eastern Europe, with varying success. The main focus of these projects is newly built housing.

The Polish TBSs ("social building associations"), established in 1996, are based on the French HLM model. A TBS is a private entity that works closely with local governments to provide nonprofit subsidized social rental housing (World Bank 2006). Interestingly, in small cities, TBSs sometimes manage the communal stock as well their own stock to help diminish housing management costs for the local government. However, according to a critical study by the World Bank (2006, 20; emphasis ours), the TBS model represents a quasi-homeownership intervention rather than a long-term social rental development scheme:

> The rental associations or cooperatives are required to provide 30 percent equity, the Fund financing up to 70 percent of the project. This down-payment may derive from the tenants, *who as a result consider themselves as quasi owners and are selected through this qualification.* The funding of the KFM [the state bank, J.H.-N.T] depends excessively on budgetary grants from the national housing budget.

This conclusion is supported by a recent change in the legal framework that raised the possibility for the owner to privatize the TBS units. The TBS model was very dependent on support from the central budget, which was a major constraint on its development. Moreover, the central government does not enforce its regulation of the sector, which leads to distortions in the system due to the interests of the tenants and the municipalities. For more on Poland, please see the Polish case study in this volume.

In Slovakia, a Dutch grant program, Matra, helped create a nonprofit housing organization in the city of Martin in 2005 (Kandlbauerova 2004; Cervenova 2005). The project failed after three years because the municipally owned cooperative that originally managed 678 municipal dwellings was privatized—the local government wanted to save the cost of operating the program. This case demonstrates the extent to which social landlords in transition countries depend on the local government finance structure. The pressure to reconcile social and market functions appears at the local government level, which is under constant fiscal pressure from the central government, as funding is reduced and mandates are underfunded. Thus, local governments have to sacrifice some social programs, like housing, which are not based on central funding, in order to maintain their financial stability.

In Serbia, the Settlement and Integration of Refugees (SIRP) program was developed and implemented by UN-HABITAT from 2003 to 2008 (see the Serbian case study in this volume).

> Beneficiaries pay a grant-in-aid as rent, depending on the degree of their social vulnerability, and are not entitled to purchase the flat. [. . .] These flats may become the base of the Social Housing Residential Fund. The physical environment and the social environment are equally important; together, they endow the supportive environment. [. . .] So far, this project has been launched in 19 municipalities in Serbia, with 271

> apartments built for some 650 vulnerable persons. The experience made with this approach to social housing shows that people accommodated in this manner are socially integrated; they are not dependent on institutionalised relief, less of a burden for the state, need fewer health services and, most importantly, enjoy a higher quality of life. The project promotes solidarity and builds a sense of belonging between the inhabitants and the community (Zarkovic 2004, 1–2).

The preceding quote provides a clear description of the aims of such social housing projects. However, in the process of implementation, programs come under the pressure of local interest groups: the local governments want to limit spending on the projects (as in the case of the Matra project), and the tenants expect to have the apartments privatized (as in the case of the SIRP project, see Chapter 15, this volume, for details).

In Slovenia, a new nonprofit form of housing provision was created in 2003, which is subsidized through the Housing Fund. The Slovenian local housing funds are strongly controlled by the municipalities, and cannot be considered quasi-independent institutions (see Chapter 17, this volume).

Although these new, "quasi" independent nonprofit solutions have always had a high priority in international experts' and donor agencies' evaluation of Eastern European housing policy programs, the factors that could guarantee the autonomy and sustainability of this form of housing management are missing. These nonprofit organizations have not succeeded in establishing themselves as independent social landlords, capable of promoting their own political and financial interests. Thus, the municipalities remain the dominant social landlords in the region.

SOCIAL CONFLICTS IN PUBLIC HOUSING MANAGEMENT

Although the social housing sector shrank, the demand for social rental housing increased significantly because of growing affordability problems in the post-transitional societies (Baharoglu 2003). The new social landlords faced tension arising from the gap between the growing demand for social housing and the population's diminished opportunity to access social rentals.

The basic question for the social landlords is how to allocate the scarce vacant units so as to satisfy social needs, market mechanisms, and fiscal constraints. Social landlords generally use two kinds of allocation procedure. The municipality (or the management company, if it has been delegated the task) either maintains a waiting list and allocates the new or vacated units according to a point system or it invites applications for potential tenants according to specific eligibility criteria. The use of waiting lists is decreasing, because the number of people on the waiting lists is so large that it makes the allocation process very complicated. However, the selection of the beneficiaries on a tender basis makes the *ad hoc* selection process unpredictable and open to corruption as well as undue political influence. There can also be irregularities in the allocation process if households with "positional advantages" have easy access to better-quality accommodation. A typical example of allocation bias towards specific better-off groups is that local governments often give high priority to key workers in the allocation procedures.

There is a paradox of allocation in the subsidized social sector: needy households cannot afford the cost of an apartment with district heating, bathroom, and so on, because of the ineffectiveness of the housing allowance systems. Furthermore, the municipalities' hands are tied: national regulations prohibit them from allocating "substandard" apartments to the beneficiaries. This means that a household selected according to needs criteria measured by household size, income, housing conditions, and so on, is often unable to pay the costs of a better-quality apartment and thus rapidly accumulates debt. Consequently, the municipalities prefer to have solvent tenants from the lower-middle class who do not create an additional financial burden. Sometimes, tender procedures are designed so that tenants compete based on who can offer to cover higher rent levels or can contribute to the renovation of the typically run-down housing unit more than the competitors.

The allocation policy of the local governments is strongly influenced by decentralization, that is, incentives built into the intergovernmental fiscal relation system. Typically, municipalities are responsible for social programs for the poorest, such as income supplement schemes and social housing, which are never fully compensated by transfers from the central government. This creates an adverse incentive for local governments dominated by the middle class to underserve or even to "export" the poorest population to other entities. For example, in Hungary, attempts to "export the poor" have included special grants offered to poor or vulnerable households to move away, or rich Budapest districts acquiring housing for their poor in other parts of the city. Urban reconstruction and rehabilitation programs based on various levels of gentrification inevitably shift the composition of the population towards the middle class.

High housing costs and increased energy prices lead to growing affordability problems for the poor. The arrears issue represents a conflict within the social housing sector in most transition countries. Based on EU-SILC data, the share of households facing difficulties in paying the rent may reach 50 percent of the tenants in certain countries (Hungary, Poland, etc.). This means that low-income households are not able to pay their housing costs, even if they rent at a low price.

Although the behavior of the municipalities follows economic rationality, this does not in itself explain the entire phenomenon, because municipalities are political institutions as well as economic entities that, in principle, have a social mission to fulfill. For example, some municipalities initiate social housing programs by decreasing funding for other projects (see country reports in this volume). Changing tenancy rights offer the municipalities another tool to bring together their social mandate and real estate management tasks: fixed-term contracts are starting to replace the open-ended contracts that were typical of the socialist system in most countries. However, this is a gradual process, and "old tenures" still represent a majority of the stock (e.g., in Slovakia, approximately half of the public housing stock rented out with open-ended contracts, whereas estimates in Hungary are at 95 percent).

As a consequence of privatization, municipalities were left with low-quality housing stock, which stood in need of major rehabilitation. Investment levels and new construction in the social housing stock remained low in the last two decades (see Chapter 3, this volume) because governments could not take on the fiscal burden and because of a lack of political support for social housing policy. The shrinkage of the social housing sector has led to a special residual rental model, where the worst housing is inhabited by low-income people. However, even this small sector (5–10 percent of the stock) is mixed in terms of its position in the housing system depending on the spatial arrangement of the stock and the type and quality of public housing investment in the socialist era.

The urban social housing stock throughout the region consists of three types of neighborhoods. Firstly, tenement houses in larger urban areas built in the beginning of the 1900s, which are typically in the worst condition, because the housing units in better condition were purchased by the sitting tenants or returned to their former owners in the privatization and restitution process. Housing units in urban settlements originally built as social housing (small floor area, without basic amenities) belong to this type. The units in the housing estates built from the 1950s until the end of the 1980s belong to the second type of social housing. These are characterized by a higher level of housing consumption (good location, sufficient layout, with central heating and bathroom), but also relatively high maintenance costs. Individual apartments in better locations, which for one reason or the other have not been privatized, make up the third type of social tenancies (less significant in terms of numbers). Each of the three types represents a different challenge for the efficient management of the stock.

The possible dangers of "mixed ownership" were a topic of debate during the privatization process. Mixed ownership poses a major problem for housing policy because it significantly reduces the effectiveness of social housing management and limits renovation options. Local governments thus preferred to privatize entire buildings, although this was limited by privatization laws. However, mixed ownership keeps social segregation within bounds, whereas buildings in full public ownership that house only marginalized households easily develop unmanageable social problems. Thus, although the mixed ownership model is more expensive, it has also proved to be more effective.

Table 5.1 Management Characteristics of the Public Rental Sector in Selected Countries in 2009–2010

	Eligibility	Priority	Management and Allocation	Rent Levels	Arrears
Bosnia and Herzegovina	"Social housing" is undefined, and supported housing provision is reserved for refugees to date.	Returnees and refugees, war victims and their families.	In theory, local-level municipalities manage the stock (or their partner NGOs/organizations that run the programs), but there are no to few housing units to allocate.	Set by law, min. 1.5% max 2.5% of the "estimated housing value", but there are discounts for war veterans and victims, applied after 2007.	No data.
Croatia	Local decrees set eligibility criteria, and eligible households are included in waiting lists.	Vulnerable families, e.g., with disabled members.	Municipalities and management companies run the stock; allocation is the responsibility of the municipalities.	The government decides upon the general level, and there is a formula that has to applied for each dwelling.	It is a substantial problem, app. 30% of the tenants are in arrears, despite very low rents, enforcement is very weak.
Czech Republic	Specific allocation criteria are applied according to substock, e.g., financed from various schemes, but basically low-income people are preferred (based on means-testing); no central regulation is applied	No central regulation, it is low-income people who are prioritized.	Only public authorities allocate housing (crisis housing is to a large extent run by NGOs with own allocation rules).	By the end of 2011 the rent control on old tenancies will be abolished, rents for new rental contracts are set by the municipalities.	Significant, especially for the Roma, but also for others; app. 30% of the rent is due. Eviction can take years, arrears management is with municipalities.

Estonia	People with low income and no means to solve their housing needs (there are waiting lists).	The neediest households, such as elderly people or tenants of "restituted" homes, disabled persons.	Only public authorities allocate housing.	Fixed with the landlord case-by-case based on the maintenance fee and utility fees, dwelling related tax, owner equity.	App. a third of all debts is due for over three months, one-twelfth of all rents are outstanding.
Hungary	No central regulation, but income limits and no own housing property are mostly applied criteria, but detailed conditions are defined at local level with huge variations within the country.	No central regulations, but normally priority is given to families with children.	Only public authorities allocate housing.	Municipalities decide upon the rent levels, in the newest stock developed with state grants, rent levels are set through the contract design.	No exact data, but generally, 30–60 % of the tenants are indebted in the public sector.
Poland	There is no single rule, but most municipalities apply income brackets as eligibility criteria, low- to middle-income households would fit in one of the subgroups of social housing (central rules apply to a part of the substock, to others it is only local regulations), in others more low-income people.	Homeless, low-income families and families who were evicted	There are various players, depending on substock; allocation varies according to substock.	Rent levels differ according to the substock of the social housing sector, e.g., rent in so-called "social apartments" is very low, typically 50% of council rents.	44.5% of council rental tenants are in arrears (app. 440,000 households).

Continued

Table 5.1 Continued

	Eligibility	Priority	Management and Allocation	Rent Levels	Arrears
Romania	Low-income families, but allocation criteria are set locally within the frames of the housing law.	Disadvantaged people, young people leaving social care establishments (after eighteen years of age), disabled persons, young married couples up to thirty-five years old, people with average income, evicted tenants from restituted housing, persons from houses affected by natural disasters.	Only public authorities allocate housing. Municipalities are responsible for the management, day-to-day tasks are subcontracted in larger municipalities.	Rent level in social rental apartments is determined by a complicated formula, but should in no case exceed 10% of the disposable household income.	One-third of all dwellings in larger cities to one-quarter in smaller cities.
Russia	The state and public authorities set the rules, but the actual owners of the stock can set exact income limits, housing space per person to be put on the waiting list. If there are no special requirements for categories set by federal or regional laws or presidential decrees, the rules are established by the municipality. The practice is to include not only poor in the waiting list.	Orphans graduating from state institutions, people who lost their previous social rental housing units, etc.	Municipalities allocate dwellings based on waiting lists.	Set directly in nominal price by municipal legal acts, differentiated by types of buildings. Average maintenance costs are cost-based.	Rent collection is about 95%, there is eviction procedure for debts for over six months, but it is seldom enforced.

Serbia	There is no official definition, whom social housing should target, and the current legislation is too broad.	It basically encompasses the average income (middle-class) population with affordability problems.	Municipalities allocate housing, but there is a legal option for nonprofits to run social housing stock, for which there are no examples.	Rents are administratively set, intransparent, some housing by international donors apply cost-based formula.	No data.
Slovenia	Slovenian citizens having certain income levels (low income but still able to afford rents) and poor housing conditions.	Families with more children, families with fewer employed members, to youth and young families, to handicapped persons and their families, to citizens with longer periods of being employed and without proper housing or in subtenancy, and to claimants whose profession or activity is considered as important for specific local community.	Only public authorities allocate housing.	Defined as % of the value of the home, which also has a methodology, covers upkeep and maintenance, management costs, depreciation, capital costs—each of them to a certain ratio. the value of the home excludes the cost of land and infrastructure.	No data, the eviction procedure is via court.
Slovakia	The actual selection of tenants and concrete procedure of selection is upon discretion of the municipalities, and they may apply a diversity of ways to allocate new rental dwellings, i.e., waiting lists, lottery, etc.	Individuals who are not able to ensure housing with their own effort under market conditions.	Only public authorities allocate housing.	New regulation in force since 2011 allows for gradual increase of the rent and termination of the rent contracts by the owners for "old rentals", and for new rentals (app. half of the stock), the Ministry of Finance	No data.

Continued

Table 5.1 Continued

Slovakia				regulates the rent, which cannot exceed 5 percent of procurement costs of the flat per year; the owner can set a lower rent, but must ensure management, maintenance and repairs of the building.	
Ukraine	There are several subgroups of the population eligible for registering for waiting lists for social housing schemes.	Invalids of war, victims of the nuclear disaster of Chernobyl, orphans and children leaving foster care, disabled children without parents and in specialized foster care arrangements, families with five or more children.	Municipalities allocate housing as they conduct the registration in the waiting lists.	Rent levels are set based on the tenants' income and assets, the composition of the household, and the physical characteristics of the dwelling. In theory, the fee paid should cover the rent as well as maintenance costs of the building, and the fees for communal services. There is a maximum limit the tenant should pay (20% of the monthly income).	No data.

Source: for Bosnia and Herzegovina, Croatia, Russia, and Ukraine: country case studies. For the remaining countries: country case studies in this volume and table from EC 2011.

For example, in the former East Germany, the majority of the public housing sector remained under the control of housing cooperatives. Generous state subsidies enabled the full renovation of the stock. An important lesson is that the decision-makers (governments, social landlords) did not take a potential decrease in social housing demand into consideration, which resulted in a million renovated housing units standing empty in former East Germany.

CONCLUSION

The transition process in Eastern Europe led to the development of new forms of public housing management. The principal question was whether the municipalities would be able to transfer their housing stock from public housing characterized by an across-the-board rent subsidy, extended property rights of the tenants, flexible allocation process, low-level services, and so on, into a social rental sector where the allocation process is clearly regulated and transparent, where the rents provide basic cost recovery, and a targeted (means-tested) rent allowance guarantees affordability for low-income households.

The new social landlords—the municipalities and, to a lesser extent, nonprofit organizations—have not been able to create such a system on their own. A "perverse" consequence of decentralized social policy without adequate financial incentives (e.g., a grant structure that can compensate horizontal inequities) is that the municipalities with the highest poverty levels have the highest need for social housing, but the lowest financial means (and incentives) to implement it.

The new social landlords have to combine two conflicting functions: property management and a social mission. This is not an unmanageable conflict, but a system of efficient intergovernmental fiscal relations is needed where the cost of the social functions is allocated among the different level of government so as to control the perverse behavior of the social landlords (for example, the privatization of low-quality rental units). The greatest challenge throughout the region is thus to reconcile rent levels that do not even cover the cost of substandard maintenance with property management principles. The social housing sector is a "loss-making" activity, which is not or only partly compensated for with central government grants. The problems of underfinancing, arrears, and social issues pose major risks for the sustainability of the sector.

The lack of responsible and regulated social landlords is a key cause of inefficiency in many Eastern European social housing systems. In the coming years, European Union funding may help create a more responsible social housing sector in the region by imposing new regulations and goals.

NOTES

1. We will primarily concentrate on the public rental sector, although many of our claims also hold true for the owner-occupied housing estates of the socialist period.

REFERENCES

Baharoglu, D. 2003. "Public Housing in an Era of Privatization, a Solution, or a Process of Slumification in Transition Economies?" Paper presented at the World Congress, Cities & Markets, Vienna, October.

Boelhouwer, P., van der Heijden, H., and van de Ven, B. 1997. "Management of Social Rented Housing in Western Europe." *Housing Studies* 12 (4): 509–29.

Burke, T. 2004. "Governance and Social Housing: Can Good Governance Be Bad Practice?" Paper presented to the International Housing Conference 'Housing in the 21st century: Challenges and Commitments', Hong Kong, China, 02–04 February 2004

Červeňová, L. 2005. *The Development of the Non-Profit Housing Sector in Slovakia.* Bratislava: Faculty of Civil Engineering, Slovak University of Technology. http://www.fgw.at/publikationen/pdf/05/2005–3_4-cervenova.pdf accessed March 20, 2009.

Czischke, D. 2009. "Managing Social Rental Housing in the EU: A Comparative Study." *European Journal of Housing Policy* 9 (2): 121–51.

Dabla-Norris, E. 2006. "The Challenge of Fiscal Decentralisation in Transition Countries." *Comparative Economic Studies* 48 (1): 100–31.

De Decker, P. 2002. "On the Genesis of Social Rental Agencies in Belgium." *Urban Studies* 39 (2): 297–326.

———. 2009. "Social Rental Agencies: Still a Splendid Idea?" *European Journal of Homelessness* 3:215–30.

EC 2011. Study on Social and Health Services of General Interest in the European Union Prepared for DG Employment, Social Affairs and Equal Opportunities DG EMPL/E/4

FRA. 2009. *Housing Conditions of Roma and Housing and Travellers in the European Union. Comparative Report.* Luxembourg: Office for Official Publications of the European Communities.

Gibb, K. 2001. *Trends and Change in Social Housing Finance and Provision within the European Union.* Glasgow: Department of Urban Studies, University of Glasgow.

Gibb, K. and Trebeck, K. 2009. "Different Roads? Evidence about the Changing Provision of English Social Housing." *International Journal of Housing Markets and Analysis* 2 (4): 373–91.

Gruis, V. and Nieboer, N. 2004. *Asset Management in the Social Rented Sector: Policy and Practice in Europe and Australia.* Dordrecht: Springer / Kluwer Academic Publishers

Harloe, M. 1995. *The People's Home?: Social Rented Housing in Europe & America.* Oxford: Blackwell

Hegedüs, J., Mark, K., and Tosics, I. 1996. "Hungarian Housing in Transition." *Economic Restructuring in the Former Soviet Bloc: The Case of Housing.* Washington, DC: Urban Institute Press.

Hegedüs, J. and Tosics, I. 1996. "Disintegration of East-European Housing Modell." *Housing Privatization in Eastern Europe.* Greenwood, London.

Kandlbauerova, A. 2004. "Responsibilities for Housing Development on Different Institutional levels in Slovak Republic." Presented at the UNECE Conference on Social Housing Vienna, November 28–30.

Kemeny, J. 1995. *From Public Housing to the Social Market: Rental Policy Strategies in Comparative Perspective.* London: Routledge.

Kingsley, T. and Mikelsons M. 1996. "The Czech and Slovak Republics: Housing as a 'Second Stage' Reform." *Economic Restructuring of the Former Soviet Bloc: The Case Study of Housing.* Washington, DC: Urban Institute Press.

Kornai, J. 1980. *Economics of Shortage.* Amsterdam: North Holland Press.

Levy-Vroelant, C. and Tutin, C. 2007. "Social Housing in France." Social Housing in Europe. London: London School of Economics.

Mandic, S. and Stanovnik, S. 1996. "Slovenia: Fast Privatization of the Stock, Slow Reform of Housing Policy." *Economic Restructuring of the Former Soviet Bloc: The Case Study of Housing.* Washington, DC: Urban Institute Press.

Priemus, H., Dieleman, F., and Clapham, D. 1999. "Current Developments in Social Housing Management." *Netherlands Journal of Housing and the Built Environment* 14 (3): 211–23.

Ruys, P.H.M., Bruil, J., and Dix, H. 2007. "Modes of Governance in the Dutch Social Housing Sector." *Annals of Public and Cooperative Economics* 78 (3): 381–413.

Tsenkova, S. and Turner, B. 2004. "The Future of Social Housing in Eastern Europe: Reforms in Latvia and Ukraine." *European Journal of Housing Policy* 4 (2): 133–49.

Turner, B., Hegedüs, J., and Tosics, I., eds. 1992. *The Reform of Housing in Eastern Europe and the Soviet Union.* London: Routledge.

World Bank. 2006. *Poland Housing Finance Policy Note. March 19, 2006.* Washington, D.D.: World Bank.

Zarkovic, B. 2004. "Living solidarity—an obligation to tradition and to future" UNECE Symposium on social housing, Vienna, 28–30 November, 2004 http://www.europaforum.or.at/site/HomepageUNECE/Paper_Session1_Zarkovic.pdf accessed February 23, 2011

6 Housing Exclusion of the Roma
Living on the Edge

Catalin Berescu, Mina Petrović, and Nóra Teller

INTRODUCTION

In this chapter, we aim to explore the mechanisms of direct or indirect housing exclusion policies, and link them to the general exclusion of Roma (Kemeny 2001). We claim that the post-transition period significantly accelerated the downward mobility of many Roma households, who were among the first victims of the social and economic changes in the whole region. We conclude that housing exclusion is a result of broader social exclusion processes, and that current social housing policies—even if integrated with other measures—are often hampered, on the one hand, by institutional disinterest and, on the other hand, by the lack of political will and financial support by national governments. Thus, current social housing policies further exacerbate exclusion. Even when implemented, the measures can barely handle the complex marginalized social, economic, and cultural situation of the Roma in the region.

In the first section of the chapter we examine the discourse of housing exclusion of the Roma. Then we show the housing situation of the Roma in Serbia, Romania, and Hungary and explore how it has been changing throughout the past two decades. The consecutive section elaborates on the policy responses and their challenges. In the conclusion we highlight some of the factors that hamper effective interventions targeted at the housing inclusion of the Roma, with a focus on these three countries.

ANALYTICAL FRAMEWORK: THE HOUSING EXCLUSION DISCOURSE

The housing exclusion discourse is fed by the human rights approach, on the one hand, and a research strand focusing on the causes of housing deprivation, on the other hand.

In the human rights–based discourse, *housing exclusion* refers to a form of, a route to, or a threat of individual housing exclusion (normally as a complementary term to access to adequate and affordable housing[1]), which can be further exacerbated by housing discrimination through spatial segregation, forced evictions, and exposure to hazards (Busch-Geertsema, O'Sullivan, and Pleace 2010). The causes for housing exclusion are multiple: deregulation of the housing market and the withdrawal of states from social housing provision are seen as central elements (Edgar, Doherty, and Mina-Coull 2000). Equally substantial are welfare policies, labor market policies, and housing policies, which are in continuous interaction, simultaneously and variably influencing the choices and strategies of households. Thus, they all have a concurrent affect on housing vulnerability (Stephens et al. 2010).

The research strand of the discourse is set by the social exclusion literature, including the redistributionist discourse, the moral underclass discourse, and the social integrationist discourse; all emphasizing different grounds of exclusion, power relations, and goals of interventions (Watt 2000, 15, relying on Levitas's classification from 1998).

Relying on the social integrationist discourse, and acknowledging that discourses can change in time and among public policy areas as well (Marton 2004), we largely ascribe the exclusion of the affected communities to structural factors, with an additional qualification. We claim that the limits of the concept of *individual* housing exclusion hinder the understanding of Roma housing exclusion, which is well documented as a group-level phenomenon throughout several European countries (FRA 2009b; Council of Europe 2009; EC 2010). Thus, many features of exclusion affect Roma communities rather than individuals. In that sense housing exclusion of these groups is connected to both concepts of poor people and poor areas (Powell 2000).

HOUSING EXCLUSION OF THE ROMA IN CENTRAL AND EASTERN EUROPE

Many Roma face housing exclusion in Central and Eastern Europe (CEE) (FRA 2009b; Council of Europe 2009; EC 2010). This statement, however, is as weak as the parts of its constituent phrases: in empirical research, there is no single definition for *Roma* (Ladányi and Szelényi 2001; Bárány 2002). In addition, and more importantly, in the European context, there is barely "a" Roma group. It is a heterogeneous, stratified, geographically, linguistically diversified ethnic minority in many countries, which is claimed to be the most considerable in size in Romania and Bulgaria in the European area (World Bank 2005; Rughinis and Fleck 2008).

Taking into account all of the preceding, in this chapter, we refer to the Roma in Romania, Hungary, and Serbia as a minority comprising several subgroups that are linguistically, culturally, and socially heterogeneous. Still, in all three countries, many Roma live in marginalized situation, face unemployment, and rely on social welfare provision, as well as experience

Table 6.1 Current Living Conditions of the Roma in Hungary, Romania, and Serbia

	Hungary	Romania	Serbia
Size of total population	10.2 million	19 million	7.3 million
Size of Roma population (unofficial)	550,000–600,000	1.5–2.0 million	250,000–450,000
App. ratio of Roma population*	5–6%	7–9%	3.5–6%
Basic demographic characteristics**	Larger family size, considerably lower life expectancy than that of non-Roma mainly due to unhealthy living conditions, decreasing fertility, but still higher than that of non-Roma in all countries (estimates vary between one and a half times to two times higher).		
Urban/rural proportion of Roma population	Rural: 60% Urban: 40% Highest concentration in northeastern and southwestern Hungary.	Rural: 60% Urban: 40% But even in rural areas, many Roma live on the outskirts or separate settlements.	Rural: 47% Urban: 53% But half of them in urban–rural fringes, highest concentration in Belgrade and big cities primarily in south Serbia.
Issues of education	Many segregated schools, very low participation in secondary and basically no representation in higher education.	Segregated schools, high dropout rate of Roma.	63% without completed primary education, enrollment in primary schooling 66% but dropout rate 73%, enrollment in secondary schooling is only 10% with 38% dropout rate, practice of moving Roma from regular schools to ones for children with learning disabilities (80% of pupils are Roma).
Issues of labor market participation	High unemployment rate.	App. 23% of the respective age-group is active in the labor market.	High unemployment rate—four times higher than in overall population, (app. 20% of Roma aged thirty-five to forty-four were employed full-time, compared to 60% of general population).

Continued

Table 6.1 Continued

Housing conditions	Poor housing conditions, app. 6% of Roma live in spatially completely segregated settlements, app. 1,600 segregated neighborhoods housing app. 300,000 people of which: 14% isolated 66% peripheral plus one hundred ghettoized villages and two hundred villages are in process of ghettoization.	App. 2,000 settlements comprising one million people, very poor infrastructure and housing condition, level of spatial segregation of ghettoes: 37% isolated, 52% peripheral, 57% monoethnic, 16% delimited by natural or artificial barriers.	App. six hundred Roma settlements (70% of Roma population), mainly small in size but highly segregated neighborhoods, 35% are illegal, 35% partially legalized, 43.5% are slums.

*Mean unofficial size of Roma population compared to size of total population; http://www.policy.hu/olmazu/StatisticnumberRoma.pdf, Roma in detail.
**Country data are of indicative nature, compiled from different databases even within countries, thus not comparable.
Source: Hungary: Domokos (2010); Romania: National Census, EUROMA cross-country report on housing issues, NSRF reports; Serbia: Jaksic and Basic (2005) and FRA (2010) and OSF (2010).

discrimination in the labor market and in education (FRA 2009b; Council of Europe 2009; EC 2010). Many Roma live in segregated, underserved neighborhoods and in overcrowded and poor housing, and have health problems and lower quality of life (Pallai 2009). Poverty is reproduced among the Roma to a large extent, and socialization into deep/extreme poverty has been going on for at least the second generation after the transition.

Table 6.1 depicts the current living conditions of the Roma in the selected countries.

Although the origins of housing conditions of the Roma are diverse, policies under state socialism and the transition period have had a decisive impact on today's conditions.

In Hungary, before the transition, the housing shortage in cities and regulated moves to cities caused a "postponed urbanization", whereas poor labor force could only move to surrounding villages, which trapped poor Roma and non-Roma. After the transition, many poor people left their urban dwellings due to increased housing costs, and the poor and Roma flowed into urban transition zones with poor housing (MTA 2004). At the same time, those employed in industries and commuting on a monthly basis to large cities moved back to their villages after the industrial plants had been closed down.

After the transition, social housing got privatized to the tenants. At the same time the remaining 3–4 percent of dwellings, composed of the lowest-quality stock housing, represented social rentals for the most vulnerable ones (Székely 2001), among them Roma families especially in urban areas. In some cities urban rehabilitation programs led to a series of population-change investment projects and finally to gentrification, pushing them out from urban neighborhoods to the outskirts or remote villages. Devaluation of housing in Roma neighborhoods sped up the process. Based on the most recent Roma survey from 2011, a fifth of all Roma live in segregated neighborhoods, which indicates that segregation has increased (Ladányi and Szelényi 1999; Teller 2011). Roma settlements are concentrated in eastern and northeastern Hungary (in 1993: 50 percent of them). Rural housing conditions are especially poor, being more overcrowded and less equipped with infrastructure than the average (Kemény 2000).

In Romania, after slavery from the thirteenth to the nineteenth century and having been forcefully settled after World War II, Roma were settled in villages and in urban areas in the historic centers or public housing estates without having benefited from any land reform. They often dispersed into blocks of flats. Roma were temporarily located in historical centers that should have been later displaced by socialist city centers. Or, as it happened in Transylvania, they were housed in former Saxon houses as the owners left for Germany and were forced by law to give up the houses.

After the revolution, the Roma were heavily affected by the restitution process and they either had to leave the homes or remained as unprotected dwellers, facing rent increases, indebtedness, and eviction. Many of them live as squatters; only 60 percent have clear legal forms for the dwelling they live in. There are high levels of residential segregation, which affects school segregation and exclusion from the labor market (Sandu 2006; Berescu and Celac 2006). The housing conditions of the most excluded ones range from overcrowded rundown prefab housing on the outskirts of towns, dilapidated houses in historical centers, and villages cut off from public services to improvised housing placed on wasteland and exposed to heavy pollution. The latter ghettoes are the result of forced evictions due to rent arrears or unclear legal titles (FRA 2009a; Sandu 2006; Berescu and Celac 2006; Dan 2004).

In Serbia, during socialism, only a small fragment of employed Roma were granted housing, as socially provided housing was targeted at higher social groups (see Chapter 15, this volume). In addition, they were settled in the lowest-quality housing and scattered across the cities in "non-Roma" areas, facing latent assimilation. The majority relied on self-built and often illegal housing construction, which resulted in the creation of settlements with poor housing and infrastructure facilities. In 2002, there were 593 settlements, of which 72 percent were partially legalized or not legal at all, and 43.5 percent were slums. Around 60 percent of Roma live in unhealthy and unsafe environments, around 30 percent have no access to public water supply, and 70 percent have no access to sewage (Macura 2006; Jaksic and Basic 2005).

Today, only 5 percent of the Roma live in public tenure (compared to 3 percent of the population in general), and most of these housing arrangements are emergency lodgings, like abandoned barracks used to house workers during large construction undertakings. The Centers for Social Care utilizes these for housing the most destitute Roma families (officially as a temporary solution) (Republican Statistical Office 2007; UNDP 2006).

The Roma tend to move towards the big cities and concentrate in existing settlements on peripheral sites or form new shantytowns in search for better opportunities. The migration of Roma displaced from Kosovo since 1999 exacerbated this process. Therefore, unclear legal status (insecure housing situation with high risks of forced evictions) and the unhealthy living conditions are the most stringent problems. Those in rural areas are more disadvantaged; however, the spatial proximity to urban infrastructure does not have a positive effect on their living conditions either. Poor housing and unemployment are strongly correlated to low education achievements and poor health status, referring to the complexity of the Roma housing exclusion phenomenon (Miladinovic 2008, Djordjevic 2004).

To sum up, despite some differences in the nature of the housing issues of the Roma in Serbia, Romania, and Hungary, there are common patterns of the genesis of housing exclusion, as follows: forced settling of Roma communities (in Romania the nomadic groups) during and after World War II, continuous segregation, and a strong impact of the economic changes of the transition. Considerably worse living conditions compared to the average, dilapidating housing and insecurity of tenure, and unclear legal arrangements are common to all countries, similarly to the regional variations within the countries. Large number of Roma settlements in Serbia, recently speeding up segregation developments in Hungary in the northeast, the rapid growth in heavily underserved areas in Serbia and Romania, and the rise of urban ghettos characterize housing exclusion of the Roma.

PROCESSES OF EXCLUSION

In most post-transitional countries, the status of the Roma has always been disadvantageous if compared to the population of similar education and labor history. Extensive socialist industrial development relied on low-skilled labor force, promoting or forcing moves to urban industrial areas also for many Roma people.

The industrial branches that absorbed masses of low-educated Roma were typically in heavy industry and mining, with comparably low payments for generally unskilled work. Even in the years of massive expansion, access to housing was problematic and largely state controlled even in the private housing sector (Mandic and Clapham 1996). New (public) urban housing supply was ensured via prefab housing estates, with limited access for the Roma in Hungary (Szelényi and Konrád 1969) but with better access in Czechoslovakia (Temelova et al. 2011) and Romania. The Roma in Yugoslavia relied more on informal, self-built housing.

Economic transition reshuffled this structure. Employment possibilities for unskilled labor force were cut from one day to the other, and the inflow of poor households began into lower segments of the housing market and to cheaper areas. The downward perpetuation of these areas sped up with a considerable spatial concentration of poverty due to better-off households moving away (Skifter Anderson 2003).

At the same time, decentralization of housing policy, housing privatization, and the privatization of housing services (water, heating, and management) took place in most of the countries (Hegedüs and Teller 2007). This caused immediate increase in housing maintenance and utility costs. The gains from privatization were not accessible for all social strata. Many families did not have valid rental agreements at the time of privatization, for example, due to squatting or rent arrears. Rental agreements could also be missing because their homes were built illegally and could not be legalized accordingly due to the lack of, or as is the case in Bulgaria, according to, newer legislation. In some places, the registration of tenants was also not up-to-date due to large numbers of people lacking identification documents. All these challenges are characteristic for Roma families in all three countries. Moreover, generally there has been strong disinterest in keeping the high-cost groups or granting them access to local service delivery where there is a risk of nonpayment or antisocial behavior (Teller 2009).

Rather, housing policies tend to aim to keep the better-educated and younger population in place to avoid the aging and moving away of the better-off households. Therefore, pushing off "high-cost", "high-risk" tenants is reportedly on the agenda in many municipalities in many of the post-transitional countries, exacerbating housing exclusion of vulnerable groups, among them poor Roma (Hegedüs 2007).

Typically in the 2000s, besides heavily supporting middle-class homeownership via a diversity of housing finance tools, there were some national housing policy interventions targeted at the lower strata of society. These aimed at a small-scale, still ever so important, extension of the social housing stock, and increased targeted or means-tested support for lower-income homeowners, as well as refurbishment programs of housing estates in numerous post-socialist countries, but not Romania and Serbia. Still, the Roma could benefit only indirectly from such tools. Although in some cases they were directly targeted by national funding, it depended on local implementation solutions whether they got included or not.

POLICY RESPONSES TO ROMA HOUSING EXCLUSION IN HUNGARY, ROMANIA, AND SERBIA

In various countries, local- and national-level programs have been aiming to solve the housing issues of segregated and disadvantaged Roma communities, and they have tried to tackle at least some aspects of housing exclusion. The interventions range from clearing legal titles; through infrastructure investment; to coordinated actions of income generation, education, community development, and housing development. The success, relevance, scope, and sustainability issues of each of the interventions are different, similar to the variety of regional differences and housing situations they address.

The evolution of housing interventions started with the NGO sector, prominently supported by international organizations, such as World Bank, UNDP, Soros Foundation, OSCE, and international charities. Some of these punctual programs were focusing on inhuman and unhealthy living conditions and forced evictions, but they could not tackle general housing exclusion patterns or mass reproduction of extreme poverty among excluded Roma groups.

In Hungary, in 2005 the national government launched a Roma Settlement Integration Program focusing on small to medium-size villages throughout the country. During its five years of operation, the program was extended and improved, finally reaching approximately forty communities with a funding of about 14.6 million U.S. dollars. The program design was based on combining interventions from various fields (training, social work, infrastructure investments), it was assisted by external mentoring, and in very few cases it implemented desegregation measures (Petrovacz et al. 2010).

Despite several challenges, the interventions have had tangible integration effects in most settlements. Where it did not, for example, in Szentgál, a small village close to Lake Balaton, it was more about the local consensus among the political elite and the Roma self-government. This consensus could not be changed, and it resulted in a fostered spatial isolation of the Roma. Generally there was a strong local resistance to spatially integrate the Roma and let them purchase or rent housing in the central parts of the villages. Also, the lack of creation of employment opportunities to sustain improved living conditions has been a major shortcoming of the program. In some other villages, where the local government was more supportive to (or at least not challenging) the targets of the program, the state-funded program could serve as a first step to include the Roma in village life. This was achieved by helping them move to the integrated parts and getting access to paid jobs, as it happened in Sirok, a touristic village in northeastern Hungary. Here, the municipality facilitated the process by making public employment options available for Roma, for example, delivering hot meals to the elderly in the village. It also forbore to claim rent for the use of the community house's building for the purposes of the project and the follow-up activities. A local NGO (with strong methodological support by a regional NGO) took the lead. Beneficiaries in Sirok were rehoused in refurbished secondhand homes throughout the village, and most of them were involved in the renovation works.

What remains a problem, however, is the lack of (state-funded) follow-up activities in many of the villages, and the lack of jobs to get people to sustain their increased housing costs. The state-level housing policy has not been supportive of embedding similar interventions in its framework. The directions of most recent policy developments targeting Roma housing issues are not clear, either. The atmosphere of discrimination and latent or violent actions against the Roma, however, has been becoming stronger especially since 2009–2010, without having received effective policy responses.

In Romania, to date there is little undertaken at the state level to tackle issues deriving from unsettled housing conditions and extreme housing poverty. As a comparison, local and international NGOs have been more active. For example, in Balţeşti, a village with approximately 10 percent Roma population, a small-scale program was organized by the Soros Foundation, Habitat for Humanity, and the local municipality. The village had to address a typical after-transition challenge: most of the industrial plants were closed; hence, many people lost their jobs and earnings. Roma craftsmen cannot sell their products, and they cannot use their carts due to recent legislation that limits the access of carts on public roads. Local agriculture is not developed; still, many people get day-paid jobs during the summer. To tackle the most severe housing conditions, the municipality assigned plots for housing investments and provided assistance with the building permits. The selection of beneficiaries was carried out by the actors together, and they participated in (re)constructing their and their neighbors' homes. Professional assistance and supervision is provided, and currently there are negotiations about establishing a grassroots enterprise for garbage collection. There are few options for channeling adults into vocational training programs, as many lack elementary education. The uniqueness of this program lies in the fact that program planning is based on the participation of beneficiaries. So is the implementation phase, which includes their workforce in the construction work to keep the program costs low. Still, whereas living conditions will substantially improve, there will be little spatial desegregation. Rather, the expected outcome is an increased participation of Roma children at school, presuming that improved living conditions will lead to less stigmatization, healthier life, and acceptance by the majority population.

On the contrary, the Pata Rat settlement's case, close to the garbage pit of Cluj, shows how the local administration's decisions can have a deteriorating impact on families' lives. The settlement has two parts. One houses approximately six hundred people ("Dallas"), and is an informal settlement of improvised shacks. Here, people make a living from recycling and garbage collection. The other part is located on Cantonului Street, which is the result of a mass eviction by the city hall. There, people live on a narrow piece of land between a railway track and a truck road (Berescu and Celac 2006; Rughinis 2004). During 2010 part of "Dallas" was demolished and fifty Roma families from there and other integrated parts of the city were forced to move to near the garbage pit, 6 kilometers away from the city, lodged in "houses" with seven to eight people in a room with common toilets for every four "apartments". This case provides an illustration of the process that has recently more and more characterized housing interventions relating to the Roma. New constructions in the last ten years resulted in substandard social houses in improvised, improper locations like former farms (Piatra Neamt, Roman) and other forms of segregated neighborhoods (Dorohoi, Mangalia, Cluj). These are widespread solutions of municipalities to "resolve" housing exclusion of the Roma by further spatially excluding them from city life.

In Serbia, Roma housing strategies have been based on self-built activities, also in the post-transition context of rising unemployment and affordability problems. From 2000, a number of pro-Roma national strategies and laws were initiated, but their implementation and enforcement has failed.[2]

A number of pilot programs were run by foreign donors and the NGO sector, primarily focused on improving Roma housing conditions, but with limited long-term effect on overcoming housing exclusion as a multidimensional phenomenon. "Best practice" examples are founded on the readiness of public authorities to support the programs, the inclusion of community members in processes that affect their living conditions, and the location of settlements. Housing interventions were primarily based on family work contribution, with professional assistance and provision of construction materials from the donors. Roma neighborhoods located in peripheral urban areas were more successfully upgraded than those close to city centers.

One of the most successful (although partly) regenerated Roma settlements is Orlovsko Naselje (Eagle's Nest) in Belgrade. Its regeneration started in the early 1990s. Here, the focus of the interventions was, on the one hand, to provide basic housing in the framework of a settlement renewal process (starting from needed political decisions and planning activities to complete infrastructure development and housing adaptations). On the other hand, interventions aimed to integrate the settlement into the self-government system by establishing a neighborhood administration and accomplishing increased tolerance of the surrounding population. Other social and economic aspects of the program were neglected due to lacking financial resources; thus, no work was initiated on children's education program and training of adults, legalization of individual houses, or developing social infrastructure (kindergarten, etc.) (Macura et al 1997). However, the new recycling plant was opened in the settlement in 2010 to ensure regular earnings for at least a part of the local population

In Serbia, the 1990s and 2000s witnessed the enlargement of Roma shantytowns in close proximity to well-served urban neighborhoods. The informal settlement under the Gazela Bridge in New Belgrade received no attention by the municipality before European Investment Bank (EIB) and European Bank for Reconstruction and Development (EBRD) financed infrastructure investment urging the city administration to act and resettle the neighborhood.[3] After the first failed resettlement attempt in 2005, the city administration sought solutions for assimilation and socialization of the Roma. Four more years passed when the city hall came up with a new settlement's plan to house four hundred families from this neighborhood, but no acceptable site for the new settlement could be found in any of the proposed neighborhoods because of strong local resistance. Then a new "action plan" was announced to place families in flats scattered throughout the city, with an argument that it would prevent the creation of an isolated ghetto. The Roma NGOs opposed this plan by arguing that this would limit Roma's access to recycling activities as well as accessibility to training programs and other social services. The plan of buying social housing for families provoked strong public debates that used arguments related to housing affordability and the perception of the Roma as undeserving poor.

In the end, without any clear explanation, the city gave up the plan, and in August 2009 employed a short-term Resettlement Action Plan based on container housing when the works on Gazela Bridge reconstruction became urgent. The inhabitants were resettled to peripheral locations in container housing, without any previous consultation, employment options, or education facilities for children. The donors did not intervene; they "only" expressed awareness that Serbian authorities have difficulties justifying the more favorable treatment of the Roma in comparison to other vulnerable groups, and they accepted the solution applied by the municipality.[4]

To sum up, the resettlement program was thwarted by widespread prejudice against the Roma and authoritarian political actors who underpin stigmatization, but also by hesitating international and local actors and low social capital of the Roma. Despite several positive examples in other cities in Serbia, which are limited in scale and scope, wider issues of housing exclusion have not been tackled in a complex way, primarily due to missing adequate systemic approach to social inclusion in general.[5] Thus, it could be said that real effect for the settlements has been moving from slums of despair to poor settlements of hope, which confirms that structural factors reinforce the reproduction of poverty.

CONCLUSIONS: LESSONS OF THE ROMA HOUSING POLICY RESPONSES IN HUNGARY, ROMANIA, AND SERBIA

Roma are discriminated in the sphere of housing at individual, community, and institutional levels. There are two dimensions of this discrimination: it is both historically determined as well as driven by the economic transition problems and the significant rise of racism in our societies (FRA 2010, 36).

In Hungary, more recently, Roma housing integration has been addressed through a complex approach. Nevertheless, the outreach of the programs was far too little compared to the mass of people living in segregated neighborhoods and low-quality stock. Currently ongoing debates on how to progress with Roma housing integration programs show that public housing solutions can be considered as viable options in a nonrural context, where municipalities have the capacity to run a housing stock. Thus, a large portion of the issue will be resolved only in the long run.

In Romania, new constructions in the last ten years resulted in substandard social houses in improvised, improper locations, which cannot serve as spatial arrangements facilitating integration. Municipalities have not developed any interest in searching for other options. Furthermore, keeping the Roma issue more or less invisible, also in spatial terms, is a broadly accepted policy at the local level. National-level plans were developed; however, their implementation was almost symbolic and mainly oriented towards infrastructure investments that brought little benefit to the communities.

In Serbia, nominally, Roma housing exclusion has been considered a multidimensional phenomenon with impacts on employment, education, and health. Nevertheless, in practice the programs were primarily focused on improving housing and environmental conditions in Roma settlements. Most of the programs have been financed by foreign donations, which limited the sustainability of results. Effects of restricted public resources are exacerbated by the marginalized social position of Roma and discrimination at the individual level. Social housing programs apply inadequate targeting and do not reach the poorest; thus, the number of Roma beneficiaries has been underrepresented. At the same time, social rental housing as such has been stigmatized due to the role it has played in Roma (re)settlement.

Civil and institutional resistance to programs improving Roma living conditions shows the local political risk of getting engaged in pro-Roma housing programs. Increased social distance and widespread poverty among the majority population made the Roma stigmatized and perceived as undeserving poor—for whom social expenses are deemed to be a waste of resources, or projects are perceived as a privilege at the expense of the majority.

Institutional discrimination becomes evident in prolonging, postponing, or rejecting programs and activities that could improve Roma lives and in the weakness of the national strategies not accompanied by plans and budgets. Even if poor Roma living conditions get improved, this is regularly through new ghettoes, without an option for social mix. Moreover, marginalization is (co)produced by municipalities that tolerate illegal construction on public land but are reluctant to deal with it officially, that is, to legalize settlements and integrate them within the broader city framework.

The sustainability of program results is challenged in all countries, because better housing conditions mean increased housing costs, which only can be covered by earnings. Thus, although Roma housing interventions try to break the circle of poverty, no foundations for long-term sustainability are offered. The current welfare settings are incapable of supplementing the effects of the programs and counteracting the effects of labor market discrimination (Kertesi 2005; Cerami 2010).

Despite attempts to combine several policy interventions, desegregation is seldom set as a goal in the programs. This is related to the fact that the housing inclusion of the Roma has to deconstruct physical, mental, and political barriers put up by the local communities and neglected, if not fostered, by the national policymakers. Thus, reproduction of severe housing exclusion remains unhindered, and social integration loses a very important pillar. As long as housing projects are not accompanied by efforts to increase inclusion in education, health protection, and employment, the exclusion of the Roma will be reproduced irrespective of partial environmental and housing improvements.

NOTES

1. The right to adequate housing (Art.11 [1]) 1991.12.13. CESCR General comment 4. (General Comments), http://www.unhchr.ch/tbs/doc.nsf/0/469f4d91a9378221c12563ed0053547e?Opendocument accessed May 15, 2012.
2. The Law on Protecting Rights and Freedom of National Minorities from 2000 recognized the Roma as a national minority; the Poverty Reduction Strategy (2003) envisaged removing of any kind of discrimination towards the Roma in employment, education, health, and housing policies; Law on Planning and Development (2003, 2009) introduced efforts to ease upgrading of Roma settlements, and so on. Finally in 2010 the Strategy for Improving the Status of the Roma in Serbia was adopted. The Housing Action Plan was developed and adopted by the Republican government within the context of Roma Decade Project. Several quantitative aims were defined for 2005–2015: developing of planning documents and property regulation for 240 Roma settlement; resolving the urgent situations and/or resettling slums in thirty settlements; sustainable rehabilitation and improvements of living conditions in 120 settlements (see www.mrc.org.rs/publikacije/pub_s_06.pdf, accessed May 26, 2012). The Law of Housing, for example, is completely outdated, and there is no National Housing Strategy, which completely undermines the fact that Law on Social Housing was adopted recently, which in itself pays no adequate attention to housing vulnerability of specific social groups, like the Roma (see Chapter 15, this volume).
3. Both EIB and EBRD have clear preconditions that local authorities should follow when resettlement is needed. These conditions include: consultations about the available options, provision of legal support to families, and adequate and sustainable alternative options. Metal containers are not considered as a sustainable and permanent option, but as a short-term solution that has to provide adequate sanitary conditions as well as access to schools and health and social care. This solution must be of limited duration and employment opportunities should be integral part of the resettlement process (see www.eib.org/project/news/gazela-bridge-rehabilitation-project.htm accessed May 26, 2012).

4. Therefore, authorities took containers as a form of social housing and stated that Roma families can use them only until they are in a socially deprived category, afterwards they would have to leave them and the units would be given to those in social need. Such statements provoked fear that after five years of the announced program the city will seize to subsidize rents and families will be forced to relocate to illegal settlements again.
5. For example, in Serbia, quite a number of the Roma are not registered in vital statistics and do not have any administrative evidence necessary for obtaining civil status and claiming basic human/social rights. This issue has become increasingly important in acquiring the right to social housing, which has been abused by local governments in order to diminish the pressure of the Roma population for scarce resources.

REFERENCES

Bárány, D. Z. 2002. *The East European Gypsies: Regime Change, Marginality, and Ethnopolitics*. Cambridge: Cambridge University Press.

Berescu, C., Celac, M., Ciobanu, O., Manolache, C. 2006. *Housing and Extreme Poverty*. The Roma Communities Case. Bucharest: Ion Mincu University Press.

Busch-Geertsema, V., Edgar, B., O'Sullivan, E., and Pleace N. 2010. "Homeless Policies in Europe: Lessons from Research." FEANTSA.

http://www.feantsa.org/files/freshstart/Consensus_Conference/Research/FEA%20020-10_EN_final.pdf accessed May 18, 2012.

Cerami, A. 2010. "The Politics of Social Security Reforms in Czech Republic, Hungary, Poland and Slovakia." *A Long-Good Bye to Bismarck? The Politics of Reforms in Continental Europe*. Amsterdam: Amsterdam University Press.

Council of Europe. 2009. *Ensuring Access to Rights for Roma and Travelers, the Role of the European Court of Human Rights*. Strasbourg: COE.

Dan, A. 2004. *Accesul la locuire în România astăzi*. (The Acces to Housing in Romania today) in Calitatea vieții nr. 3–4/2003, http://www.iccv.ro/oldiccv/romana/revista/rcalvit/pdf/cv2003.3-4.a07.pdf accessed August 20, 2011.

Djordjevic, B. 2004. *Romi od zaboravljene do manjine u usponu*. Nis: OGI.

Domokos, V. 2010. *Szegény- és cigánytelepek, városi szegregátumok területi elhelyezkedésének és infrastrukturális állapotának elemzése különböző (közoktatási, egészségügyi, településfejlesztési) adatforrások egybevetésével (Analysis of the Location and Infrastructure Supply of Poor Neighborhoods and Roma Settlements Based on the Comparison of Data Sets of Education, Healthcare and Regional Development Analysis)*. Report commissioned by the National Development Agency. Hungary.

EC. 2010. *Roma in Europe: The Implementation of European Union Instruments and Policies for Roma Inclusion—Progress Report 2008–2010. Commission Staff Working Document*. Brussels: EC.

Edgar, B., Doherty, J., and Mina-Coull, A. 2000. *Support and Housing in Europe: Tackling Social Exclusion in the European Union*. Bristol: Policy Press, the JCSHR and FEANTSA.

European Roma Information Office. *Survey on Ethnic Data Collection—Risk or Opportunity?* http://erionet.org/site/upload/surveys/Data%20Collection%20Survey.pdf accessed January 15, 2010.

FRA. 2009a. *EU-MIDIS Report*. Vienna: Fundamental Rights Agency of the EU.

———. 2009b. *Romania RAXEN National Focal Point Thematic Study Housing Conditions of Roma and Travellers*. Vienna: Center for Legal Resources.

———. 2010. *European Union Agency for Fundamental Rights*. Annual Report 2010. Conference Edition. http://fra.europa.eu/fraWebsite/attachments/AR_2010-conf-edition_en.pdf accessed May 18, 2012.

Hegedüs, J. 2007. "Housing in Hungary." In: Schanclon, K. and Whitehead, C. (eds.) *Housing in Europe*. London: London School of Economics.

Hegedüs, J. and Teller, N. 2007. "The Privatization of the Housing Stock in Eastern Europe—The Case of Hungary." *Home Ownership: Limits to Growth*. Amsterdam: IOS Press.

Jaksic, B, and Basic, G. 2005. *Umetnost prezivljavanja: Gde I kako zive Romi u Srbiji (The Art of Surviving: Where and How Roma Live in Serbia)*. Belgrade: Institut za filizofiju i društvenu teoriju.

Kemény, I. 2000. "A magyarországi romák (The Roma in Hungary)." *Változó Világ 31*. Budapest: Press Publica.

Kemeny, J. 2001. "Comparative Housing and Welfare: Theorizing the Relationship." *Journal of Housing and the Built Environment* 16 (1): 53–70.

Kertesi, G. 2005. *A társadalom peremén: Romák a munkaerőpiacon és az iskolában (At the Margins of Society: Roma in the Labor Market and Education)*. Budapest: Osiris Kiadó.

Ladányi, J. and Szelényi, I. 1999. "Szuburbanizáció és gettósodás (Suburbanization and Ghettoization)." *A cigányok Magyarországon*. Budapest: MTA.

———. 2001. "The Social Construction of Roma Ethnicity in Bulgaria, Romania and Hungary during Market Transition." *Review of Sociology* 7 (2): 79–89.

Levitas, R. 1998. *The Inclusive Society: Social Exclusion and New Labor*. Basingstoke: Macmillan.

Macura, V. 2006. "Inclusion of Roma Population through Housing and Settlements Improvement." *Four Strategic Themes for the Housing Policy in Serbia*. Belgrade: SIRP.

Macura, V., Cvejić, J., Ferenčak, M., Petovar, K.l. 1997. *Eagle's Nest—Roma Enclave: Concept of Sustainable Renewal and the Results*. Belgrade: Publikum.

Mandic, S. and Clapham, D. 1996. "The Meaning of Home Ownership in Transition from Socialism: The Example of Slovenia." *Urban Studies* 33 (1): 83–97.

Marton, G. 2004. "Constructing the Meaning of Social Exclusion as a Policy Metaphor." *Social Constructionism in Housing Research*. Aldershot: Ashgate Publishing Limited.

Miladinovic, S. 2008. "Etnicka i socijalna distanca prema Romima." *Socioloski pregled* 43 (3): 417–37.

MTA. 2004. "Települési és lakásviszonyok, költözések (Settlements and Housing Conditions, Mobility)." *The Roma in Hungary 1971–2003*. Budapest: MTA.

Open Society Foundations. 2010. *No Data—No Progress: Country Findings, Data Collection in Countries Participating in the Decade of Roma Inclusion 2005–2015*. Washington, DC: OSI.

Pallai, K., ed. 2009. *Who Decides? Development, Planning, Services, and Vulnerable Groups*. Budapest: OSI/LGI.

Petrovacz, R., Somogyi, E., and Teller, N. 2010. *Telepeken és telepszerű lakókörnyezetben élők integrációs programjának értékelése (Evaluation of the Integration Program Targeting at Segregated Neighborhoods and Settlements)*. Budapest: Metropolitan Research Institute.

Powell, M. 2000. "Towards a Geography of People Poverty and Place Poverty." *Policy and Politics* 29 (3): 243–58.

Republican Statistical Office. 2007. *Living Standard Measurement Survey in Serbia*. Belgrade: RSO.

Rughinis, C. 2004. *Social Housing and Roma Residents in Romania*. Budapest: Open Society Institute and Center for Policy Studies. http://pdc.ceu.hu/archive/00001919/01/rughinis.pdf accessed May 18, 2012.

Rughinis, C. and Fleck, G., eds. 2008. *Come Closer: Exclusion and Inclusion of Roma in Present-Day Romania*. Bucharest: Human Dynamics.

Sandu, D. 2006. *Roma Social Mapping. Targeting by a Community Poverty Survey*. Bucharest: World Bank.

Skifter Andersen, H. 2003. *Urban Sores: On the Interaction between Segregation, Urban Decay and Deprived Neighbourhoods*. Aldershot: Ashgate Publishing Limited.

Stephens, M., Fitzpatrick, S., Elsinga, M., van Steen, G., and Chzhen, Y. 2010. *Study on Housing and Exclusion: Welfare Policies, Housing Provision and Labor Markets*. Brussels: European Commission, Directorate-General for Employment, Social Affairs and Equal Opportunities.

Székely Gáborné, J. 2001. "Az önkormányzati bérlakások privatizációja (The Privatization of Public Housing)." *Lakásviszonyok III. Társadalomstatisztikai Füzetek* 31:32–51.

Szelényi, I. and Konrád, Gy. 1969. *Az új lakótelepek szociológiai problémái (Sociological Problems of the New Housing Estates)*. Budapest: Akadémiai Kiadó.

Teller, N. 2009. "Vulnerable Groups and the Effects of Selected Local Government Service Delivery Policies in Three Hungarian Cities." *Who Decides? Development, Planning, Services, and Vulnerable Groups*. Budapest: OSI/LGI.

———. 2011. *Adaptációs csapdák. Hipotézisek a romák lakásmobilitásáról az NCSSZI 2011–es romaadat-felvételének lakásváltoztatási kérdéseire adott válaszok és a korábbi cigányfelvételek lakásmobilitási adatai alapján.* (*Pitfalls of adaptation. Hypotheses about housing mobility patterns of Roma based on the 2011 NCSSZI survey questions and previous Roma data collections*). Budapest: NCSSZI.

Temelová, J., Novák, J., Ourednícek, M., and Puldová, P. 2011. "Housing Estates in the Czech Republic after Socialism: Various Trajectories and Inner Differentiation." *Urban Studies* 48 (9): 1811–34.

UNDP. 2006. *Social and Economic Position of Roma and IDPs in Serbia*. Belgrade: UNDP.

Watt, P. 2000. "Discourses of Social Exclusion: An Analysis of Bringing Britain Together: A National Strategy for Neighbourhood Renewal." *Housing Theory and Society* 17 (1): 14–26.

Word Bank. 2005. *Poverty, Social Exclusion and Ethnicity in Serbia and Montenegro: The Case of Roma*. http://web.worldbank.org/WBSITE/EXTERNAL/COUNTRIES/ECAEXT/EXTROMA/0,,contentMDK:20888098~menuPK:616000~pagePK:64168445~piPK:64168309~theSitePK:615987,00.html accessed May 18, 2012.

Part III

Country Case Studies

7 Bosnia and Herzegovina
Limits of the Human Rights Approach to Social Housing

József Hegedüs, Gorana Stjepanović, and Nóra Teller

INTRODUCTION

In Bosnia and Herzegovina, the transition process was postponed by the five-year Balkan War, which necessarily shifted the policy focus away from addressing the conditions and consequences of the transition towards managing the postwar 'return' process.[1] At the very least, transition-related policy challenges were considerably exacerbated by the postwar reconciliation and adjustment processes. The attempt to return to the prewar situation as set out in the 1995 Dayton Agreement was the most important strategic direction; all other policies had to play a subordinate role to this.[2]

As a consequence, there has been a delay of more than a decade in getting the transition development processes back on track. More importantly for our focus, there are only a few options for the creation of social housing policy in Bosnia and Herzegovina that are not heavily based on the human rights approach.

Although there is a wealth of information on the postwar return process and reconstruction in Bosnia and Herzegovina, data on the housing situation in the country are scarce and this necessarily limits the robustness of the findings presented here. More so, as the documents and data available for the two (plus one) entities—the Federation of Bosnia and Herzegovina, Republika Srpska and the Brcko District—vary in depth and scope, and last census data available date from before the war.

The framework for the analysis is the human rights approach to housing. It derives from the Universal Declaration of Human Rights (Article 25.1), which sets out that:

> Everyone has the right to a standard of living adequate for the health and well-being of himself and of his family, including food, clothing, housing and medical care and necessary social services, and the right to security in the event of unemployment, sickness, disability, widowhood, old age or other lack of livelihood in circumstances beyond his control.

This document is supplemented by various further international agreements, such as the Council of Europe's European Social Charter of 1961 (Article 16), its Protocol of 1988 (Article 4), the Revised European Social Charter of 1996 (Article 31), and the International Covenant of Economic, Social and Cultural Rights (Article 11). Most of these documents are not binding, but state policies must nonetheless be formulated in conformity with the responsibilities assumed by all signatories to the document (Freeman 2011). This means that in countries that opt for a human rights–based approach to housing, the formulation of social housing policy is subject to economic and social rights objectives rather than representing a tool to enhance social cohesion or housing mobility among those who cannot satisfy their housing needs in the open housing market.

First, this chapter discusses the major postwar challenges and development trends in Bosnia and Herzegovina. Then, it focuses on the limits of activities undertaken by donor and international organizations as the main actors behind housing programs since the war, and highlights what housing needs these programs can answer and what challenges remain beyond their scope. In the third section we elaborate the essential barriers to robust social housing policy development in Bosnia and Herzegovina, which, on the one hand, largely derive from the prevailing human rights–based approach applied in housing and social housing policy, as defined by the post-Dayton institutional circumstances, and, on the other hand, to some extent are inherited from the prewar situation. We conclude by highlighting some challenges that social housing policy in Bosnia and Herzegovina should address in the near future.

MAJOR POSTWAR CHALLENGES AND DEVELOPMENT TRENDS[3]

The population of Bosnia and Herzegovina has decreased from the prewar 4.5 million to an estimated 3.8 million in 2006. The 1990–1995 war resulted in hundreds of thousands of war victims and missing persons, and approximately half a million people fled the territory of Bosnia and Herzegovina to other parts of former Yugoslavia and to several West European countries like Austria and Germany. The emigration process continued even after the Dayton Agreement. The Office of the High Representative, the institution representing the effective leadership in postwar Bosnia and Herzegovina, set up by the allied forces under the Dayton Agreement, estimated that 1.3 million citizens of Bosnia and Herzegovina are living and working outside the country (UNDP 2007). This mass of people represents a great source of income for family members who have remained behind, helping to increase consumption and invest in housing (Mansoor and Quillin 2006).

Out-migration and domestic migration of inhabitants have caused significant demographic changes. These changes can be summed up as changes to the ethnic structure of the population (that is, the share of Croats, Bosniaks, and Serbs), geographic distribution, age, and the population growth rate (Ibreljić et al. 2006). Domestic migration flows are estimated to have affected nearly a quarter of the population. Around one million refugees have been forced to migrate within or out of the country. Half of them (at least on paper) returned to areas where they were in the minority before the war (Ministry for Human Rights and Refugees [MHRR] 2006).

The return process largely involved the in-kind 'restitution' of housing. The housing demand of people who were still registered as returnees (forty-five thousand in 2008) represented an unresolved housing issue for the state administration, which obliged itself to offer housing to, or, more concretely, to restore the property rights and the housing of returning families in compliance with the terms set out in the Dayton Agreement. These terms are based on the human rights approach to housing.

In Bosnia and Herzegovina, approximately one-third of all housing units were damaged in the war (425,000 units out of 1.3 million), and according to data collected by the MHRR in the postwar years, 80 percent of all housing affected had been completely demolished. Wartime damage impacted different areas in Bosnia and Herzegovina to a varying extent, depending on where the front line was and for how long. In the Federation as a whole, 33 percent of the housing stock was damaged and 6 percent destroyed; whereas in Republika Srpska, in the west and north of the country, 29 percent of the stock was damaged and 5 percent was destroyed. Only three-fifths of the damaged stock had been restored and renewed by the end of 2006, which presented the state, obliged to fulfill the Dayton return requirements, with a serious challenge (MHRR 2006).

Besides large losses to housing stock, there were two other significant processes that left municipal governments without public housing resources that could be used to provide affordable housing to the public. One was the return process itself, wherein internally displaced persons and refugees were offered in-kind housing compensation, and the second one was give-away housing privatization.

The large-scale privatization of publicly owned housing began in 2000 in Bosnia and Herzegovina, with the introduction of the Act on Privatization of Publicly Owned Housing.[4] Privatization essentially involved transferring housing assets to sitting tenants or to those who held the tenancy right before the war either for free or for up to approximately 10–15 percent of the dwelling's market value, depending on the entity (the part of the country). In the Federation, privatization was free of charge, in Republika Srpska tenants could buy their housing for 10–15 percent of its market price, and in Brcko District tenants had to pay around 10 percent of the market price. All in all, approximately 26 percent of the total stock that was previously in public ownership was converted from 'social' to private property.[5]

In theory, revenue from the privatization process should have been used for the development of social housing or housing policy in general, but, owing to the lack of a regulatory framework (there is no mention of 'social' housing in the legislation) and the limited amount of revenue accumulated from such low-price privatizations, the opportunity to use revenue from the socialist 'patrimony' to pay for future housing development was lost. The privatization of publicly owned housing was a political tool to assuage the impoverished Bosnian society, or what Struyk (1996) referred to as a shock absorber.

To conclude, both the needs of returnees and the general destruction caused by the war explain why housing reconstruction remained the strategic goal of various policies designed to answer the housing needs of returnees. However, besides the demand generated by the general return process, there were other sources of pressure on the housing market. The economic recovery—even though accompanied by large-scale unemployment and the formation of a busy informal market (ETF 2006)—began in urban areas and caused a housing shortage in those cities damaged most by the war. These pressures, however, did not result in unsolvable challenges. The out-migration of large population groups and the aforementioned demographic trends—even if they caused huge population growth in some areas—did not put so much demographic pressure on the housing market as to result in unaffordable rent levels and general overcrowding.

Based on data collected in their 2008 assessment, Hegedüs and Teller (2008) concluded that housing costs—especially for those who live in the private rental sector—represent a considerable burden, amounting to over a third of a family's average monthly income (including informal activities in the labor market). Nevertheless, they found that housing affordability issues had more to do with the problems in the social welfare system in general. Moreover, besides the general income benefits, local benefit schemes were marginal both in scope and scale (Ninković and Papić 2007). The welfare system was under constant change in the second half of the 2000s, and reforms had to address, among other things, the weak targeting of welfare resources. More concretely, welfare services had to move away from programs and policies where 75 percent of beneficiaries were estimated not to be poor, which contributed to the fact that only 4 percent of the poor population received some form of targeted social assistance (World Bank 2003, 103–9). Around ten years after the war, in 2004, 17.8 percent of the population or approximately 680,000 people were considered to be poor (Šabanović et al. 2006).

ACTIVITIES OF DONOR AND INTERNATIONAL ORGANIZATIONS—THE POST-DAYTON PLAYERS

The return process was basically dependent on the support of donor and international organizations, because these were the channels that drove substantial funding into the housing sector and took the lead in embedding the return process in state operations. The Organization for Security and Co-operation in Europe [OSCE] played a prominent role is this development and was the first to raise the issue of developing a strategic framework for social housing in the postwar context (OSCE 2007).

Because the return process involved extensive in-kind housing compensation, it generated enormous investment into housing in the country. Aid revenue equaled an estimated 20 percent of GDP in the postwar years, falling to around 5 percent of GDP at the end of the 2000s (Nedić 2006; Lierl 2007). Interestingly, however, and in line with the principles of the human rights approach of overcoming the damage caused by the war at any 'price', 80 percent of the investments were directed towards heavily damaged rural areas (Hegedüs and Teller 2008).

The generally lower demand for rural housing was coupled with an increase in the number of housing market transactions. This can be seen as an immediate effect of the inflow of aid into housing. As the return process was tied to reestablishing the 'original' ethnic mix from before the war, many returnees decided to sell their houses after they obtained funds or aid for (starting or finishing) the reconstruction and move elsewhere, to ethnically more homogenous parts of Bosnia and Herzegovina or simply closer to their relatives or jobs. Reportedly, many people kept their reconstructed housing as holiday homes.

Donor agencies had a prominent role both in the reconstruction process and in designing and offering alternative housing programs for specific target groups. However, a common weakness of these programs was that they dealt with immediate crisis solutions and did not take into account long-term management and targeting perspective or issues of sustainability.

'Generating' building stock that could be used as social rental housing was the most challenging task, and different projects and institutions tried tackling it with various solutions. In some projects, for example, NGOs or municipalities made temporary use of unclaimed dwellings that had not been reallocated in the compensation process. In most cases, newly constructed dwellings owned by the given NGOs or other organizations were offered as social housing, usually for no rent (often households did not even have to pay the utility fees).

In Ilijaš, a city of fifteen thousand, located in the Federation not far from the border with Republika Srpska, Hilfswerk Austria, for example, launched a project in cooperation with the office of the UN High Commissioner for Refugees to help several female victims of the war.[6] The project was co-funded by the relevant territorial government and housed the women and their children in an integrated part of the community in a multifamily building with social assistance services. In Mostar, the fifth largest city in Bosnia and Herzegovina, and one with a unique ethnic and religious mix both before and since the war, the city government supported converting the 'collective center' for refugees into zero-rent social housing with floating support services. In Zenica, once a major industrial city, the Swiss

Humanitarian Agency and German Pax Christi organization ran homes for the elderly together with the Canton government and the Canton's financial support, which offered not just housing and social and health services, but also supplementary housing allowance schemes for the elderly (Hegedüs and Teller 2008).

Another important and recent project was called 'Social Housing in B&H', organized by the Catholic Relief Services (CRS) and jointly financed by the Netherlands, the Bosnia and Herzegovina state-level government and CRS. The project was designed to provide social housing in sustainable communities for at least 130 vulnerable households (approximately 370 individuals). This project was to be implemented in at least three municipalities and would be accompanied by floating services. These services would cover support for income generation and the reintegration of beneficiaries of the project, creating links between beneficiaries and local communities and building capacity for participation in the development and implementation of social housing and coordination of the long-term participation of local authorities and other stakeholders in the management of buildings. Beneficiaries of the constructed buildings were users of collective centers and unsettled accommodation from any parts of Bosnia and Herzegovina, returnees and professionals prioritized as essential to the new return communities. This pilot program was to offer four models of social/nonprofit housing for lease, each specific to the type of ownership structure, local capacity and conditions, and the target groups. To date, sixty-three housing units have been built and allocated in two municipalities, and forty-eight more in Drvar and Jablanica are awaiting a service permit. This project is an example of how including the dimension of social mixing in the project hopes to enhance the sustainability of the project.

In Republika Srpska, and more specifically in its capital, Banja Luka, some small steps have been taken to provide housing for persons disabled by the war and their families. The Ministry of Labor and War Veterans was the engine for the development of a program established in 2008: the Program of Housing Disabled War Veterans and Families of Victims,[7] in which the government promised to provide funding to obtain housing 5,606 households in the mentioned groups for war victims, pledging a sum of 34 million U.S. dollars over the period 2008–2010. The Republika Srpska government also pledged 17 million U.S. dollars for infrastructure on construction sites in order to help municipalities to take part in the program, as the municipalities have to provide location, technical documentation, and building and service permits for these housing investments, the total cost of which is estimated to equal 30 percent of the total investment costs in housing in Bosnia and Herzegovina.

Another significant development in Republika Srpska was the introduction of mortgage loans for housing. With a decrease in financial risk resulting from the entity's engagement in the program, banks were given an incentive to lower the interest on loans and this helped to increase housing affordability. In the framework of a supported loan program, these mortgage loans were provided through the Investment Development Bank (*Investiciona Razvojna Banka*), which granted low-interest credits. The basic interest rate was a little more than half of the average interest rate on mortgage loans (5.6 versus 9 percent), subsidized by 3.6–4.8 percent, with a 20 percent down-payment rate and a maximum twenty-year annuity. Monthly installments amounted to 350–550 U.S. dollars. As this sum is close to the average wage earned by the middle class in Bosnia, these loans were only affordable to mid- and high-income groups. Nevertheless, this scheme actually affected the housing market on a secondary basis: new buyers (mostly by selling their old flats) increased the supply in the housing market. Among the criteria for obtaining a subsidized loan are again 'merits' connected with the civil war: families of victims of the war, people disabled in the war, and civilian victims of war are given priority, as are families with four or more children and inhabitants from undeveloped municipalities (3.6 percent). In addition to this social targeting, support can also be given to 'key workers': young, highly educated married couples and families with three children (4.3 percent); young couples with one highly educated adult; and families with two children (4.8 percent) also, to some extent, benefit from this program. Subsidized mortgage loans are granted for the structural extension of existing housing if the total living area per person does not exceed 20 square meters. The number of households that benefited from these loans was small, but compared to the previous access of the aforementioned groups to mortgage products, it is still significant. The total number of households that received a loan was 755 in 2009 and 1,022 in 2008, which is approximately 0.25 percent of all households.

Homeownership programs were widely applied also through other policy tools. In Canton of Sarajevo, for example, in 2009 a project was launched based on granting access to permanent housing with a subsidized purchase price. The government of the Sarajevo Canton pinpointed two locations for housing construction and 185 flats were built. Eligibility criteria for this project were defined in a Canton-level decree and considered the applicant's age, education level, size of the household, participation in the civil war, and so on. Based on these criteria, the Canton government creates a ranked list (actually a sort of waiting list) of applicants and then according to rank on the list invites candidates in to confirm their commitment to buy one of the flats. After signing this agreement to buy, the government leaves the candidates at least thirty days to get the necessary down payment, which is approximately 1,120 U.S. dollars per square meter (the market value of an average flat is 2,000 U.S. dollars per square meter). Presuming that the most attractive are the ones 50 m2 in size, this gives us a housing price of approximately 56,600 U.S. dollars. Considering the level of the average wage in Bosnia and Herzegovina, we can assume that this scheme offers 'affordable homes' to mid- and high-income groups rather than to vulnerable households.

Nevertheless, besides targeting relatively higher-income households via ownership programs, there have been various attempts and efforts towards answering the housing needs of vulnerable households and finding the niches for potential interventions in a highly unaccommodating legal environment that has primarily been focusing on fulfilling the Dayton criteria and completing the return process.

Some of the projects should be seen as direct answers to the severe social and economic conditions that hit many households during and after the war and as part of the reforms that have been under way since the year 2000. But as we may surmise from the preceding, most of the efforts have been steered towards meeting the needs of those who were involved in the civil war, irrespective of their income level. Many other vulnerable groups, such as disabled, the elderly, single parents, and so on, are largely left out of these programs.

ESSENTIAL BARRIERS TO SOCIAL HOUSING POLICY DEVELOPMENT

The return process has been the most decisive challenge ruling any housing policy developments in Bosnia and Herzegovina in the after-war context. In conformity with this, the property law regime was biased towards return. In practice this meant that the right of the returnee was set above any rights that might have accrued to the occupant of the property.

The Dayton Agreement set out that all returnees have a right to their assets. Thus, the local authorities did not have the right to keep the property right of the not privatized, socially owned apartments of those tenants who were not returning in practice. Also at the local level, compensation in kind overruled any other options.

What is even more important, as Džepar-Ganibegović (2003, 35–36) points out, is that there are no constitutional competencies for either housing or social issues at the state level: "There are ministries of physical planning and construction, as well as ministries for social affairs in both Entities, but these have neither competencies nor capacity to deal comprehensively with the housing and social sectors and develop intersectoral policy programs."

Moreover, setting up the states within the state (that is, the 'Entities') with their own real estate cadastres, registration procedures, and so on, delayed the process of addressing other challenges. Like in other Balkan countries (see Chapter 15, this volume), illegal construction has put limits on the scope of urban and regional planning and the area available for the development of housing and social housing. Other constraints include the slow pace of legalization of informal housing, the low quality of self-help construction, and the considerable amount of unfinished housing construction.

To sum up, in the current legal and economic environment the future direction of development of the social housing system and social housing policy is still unclear, but there is a great need to shift away from the human rights–based approach adopted as part of the return and compensation processes towards securing housing tenure and mobility for those in need. Today in Bosnia and Herzegovina, an impoverished country where economic development has not been yet fueled by market liberalization, public consumption has declined and there are strict budget limits and severe constraints to any such development.

CHALLENGES FOR THE NEAR FUTURE

In the transition process, after the postwar reconstruction, the housing problems of many groups (the Roma, homeless, young families without supporting families, first-generation urban migrants, etc.) have become critical. These issues have created a need to introduce special housing programs especially for such groups and move away from exclusively targeting war victims and their relatives. This could be brought about more efficiently if various types of housing programs, such as those already piloted by several NGOs or internationally run housing projects, could be combined. Low-cost homeownership and rental and housing allowance schemes can be useful for selected groups to a varying extent (Hegedüs and Teller 2008).

However, this should be accompanied by at least two parallel governance changes. The first relates to the state administration, the second to illegal construction. Firstly, Bosnia and Herzegovina has a very complicated and very rigid administrative-political structure. Achieving efficient social housing policy for vulnerable groups presupposes adequate changes on the level of general housing policy and the development of a legal framework specifically for social housing policy. In both Entities the focus should be on making the necessary institutional changes in order to enhance the state's capacity for designing specific programs for socially vulnerable groups and securing the financial resources for such programs. Secondly, the funds for social housing should be established. Resources could come—at least in part—from direct and indirect taxation and be directed into more targeting housing subsidies. Nevertheless, unless the cadastre and registration system is complete and illegal construction is curtailed, the creation of a social housing policy is unlikely and there will be no basis for the long-term planning of public services and for addressing the spatial and quality aspects of housing.

Taking into account the large informal economy, the financial strategy of social housing policy needs to follow a step-by-step approach, starting with close-ended programs and moving to entitlement-based programs that address the needs of vulnerable households, then to ensuring the success and survival of the results of the programs. Last but not least, the return process will soon reach a conclusion, which will allow for a shift in the focus of social housing policies towards the sustainability issues of housing in Bosnia and Herzegovina, as there are almost no funds available for urban regeneration, refurbishment, or housing allowance schemes in general. The new focus will also provide an opportunity to create a transparent and affordable rental housing sector, which, at the same time, will bring the social housing challenges faced by Bosnia and Herzegovina closer to those faced by other transition countries around 2010.

NOTES

1. The return process covers the interventions to facilitate reestablishing the ethnic and demographic situation that characterized Bosnia and Herzegovina before the war.
2. Available from http://www.ohr.int/dpa/default.asp?content_id=379 accessed May 18, 2012.
3. The main source of information is field research conducted in the spring and summer of 2008 by József Hegedüs and Nóra Teller, presented in Hegedüs and Teller (2008), conducted with the assistance of Dina Karahasonovic and Nermina Dzepar-Ganibegovic, to whom we are especially grateful. The original report is available at http://www.mhrr.gov.ba/PDF/Izbjeglice/2.%20Needs%20of%20%20Social%20Housing%20in%20Bosnia%20and%20Herzegovinapdf.pdf accessed May 18, 2012.
4. For example, for the Republic Srpska Entity, such legislation was introduced by the National Assembly of Republika Srpska with the Act on the Privatization of Publicly Owned Housing in 2007 (Zakon o privatizaciji državnih stanova 2007), *Službeni glasnik RS*, No. 72/07.
5. Formerly, social ownership was closer to private ownership in its practice—much like in other former Soviet countries (Philpott 2006).
6. For more information see http://www.hilfswerk.at/hwa/projekte/osteuropa-und-balkan/bosnien-und-herzegowina/soziales-wohnen accessed May 18, 2012.
7. In Serbian: Program stambenog zbrinjavanja porodica poginulih boraca i ratnih vojnih invalida I-IV kategorije u Republici Srpskoj.

REFERENCES

Džepar-Ganibegović, N. 2003. "An Outline of Pilot Project for Social Housing in Canton Sarajevo". *Workshop on Social Housing.* Prague: United Nations Economic Commission for Europe.

ETF. 2006. *Bosnia And Herzegovina.* ETF Country Analysis for Ipa Programming in the Field of Human Resources Development.

Freeman, M. A. 2011. *Human Rights: An Interdisciplinary Approach.* Cambridge: Polity Press.

Hegedüs, J. and Teller, N. 2008. "Need of Social Housing in Bosnia-Herzegovina." *A Report Prepared in the Framework of the Follow Up on the Functional Review of the Return Sector in Bosnia and Herzegovina. Project.* http://www.mhrr.gov.ba/PDF/Izbjeglice/2.%20Needs%20of%20%20Social%20Housing% 20in%20Bosnia%20and%20Herzegovinapdf.pdf accessed May 18, 2012.

Ibreljić, I., Kulenović, S., Kadušić, A., and Smajić, S. 2006. "Migration Flows in Bosnia and Herzegovina after 1992." Presented at the 46th Congress of the

European Regional Science Association (ERSA), Volos, Greece, August 30–September 3.

Lierl, M. 2007. *Transfer Payments, Individual Income Composition and Inequality in Bosnia and Herzegovina*. Syracuse: International Relations and Economics, the Maxwell School of Syracuse University.

Mansoor, A. and Quillin, B., eds. 2006. *Migration and Remittances. Eastern Europe and the Former Soviet Union*. Washington, DC. World Bank. http://siteresources.worldbank.org/INTECA/Resources/257896-1167856389505/Migration_FullReport.pdf accessed May 18, 2012.

Ministry for Human Rights and Refugees. 2006. *Housing and Urban Profile of Bosnia and Herzegovina. An Outline of Devastations, Recovery and Development Perspectives*. Sarajevo: Ministry for Human Rights and Refugees, Department for Housing Policy and Analytical Planning.

Nedić, G. 2006. *Financial and Technical Assistance in the Reconstruction and Development of Post-Conflict Bosnia and Herzegovina*. Working Papers 073, September, Global Development Network Southeast Europe (GDN-SEE), the wiiw Balkan Observatory.

Ninković, R. and Papić, Z. 2007. *Reforming the Systems and Structures of Central and Local Social Policy Regimes in Bosnia and Herzegovina*. Sarajevo: Independent Bureau for Humanitarian Issues in Bosnia and Herzegovina.

Organization for Security and Co-operation in Europe. 2007. *Report on Roma Informal Settlements in Bosnia and Herzegovina*. Sarajevo.

Philpott, Ch. B. 2006. "From the Right to Return to the Return of Rights: Completing Post-War Property Restitution in Bosnia Herzegovina." *International Journal of Refugee Law* 18 (1): 30–80.

Šabanovic, E., Memić, F., and Đipa, D. 2006. "Efficiency of Targeting of Social Transfers in Bosnia and Herzegovina." PowerPoint presentation. http://siteresources.worldbank.org/PGLP/Resources/EdinSabanovicetal.pdf accessed May 18, 2012.

Struyk, R., ed. 1996. *Economic Restructuring of the Former Soviet Bloc*. Washington, DC: Urban Institute Press.

UNDP. 2007. *The Silent Majority Speaks (Snapshots of Today and Visions of the Future of Bosnia and Herzegovina)*. http://europeandcis.undp.org/cpr/show/161BE7CD-F203-1EE9-BD4C1FDAE001EFBC accessed May 18, 2012.

World Bank. 2003. *Bosnia and Herzegovina: Poverty Assessment*, vol. 1, *Main Report*. Washington, DC: World Bank.

8 Croatia

The Social Housing Search Delayed by Postwar Reconstruction

Gojko Bežovan

INTRODUCTION

This chapter provides insight into housing policy development in Croatia and describes the emergence and implementation of social housing programs after 1990. In this chapter, *social housing* will be defined as rental housing with rents at below-market value. This part of the housing stock targets low-income households and households that, for various reasons, are receiving social assistance.

From the start of the 1990s new democratically elected governments declared that housing is not the responsibility of the state and that the market is the most efficient approach to housing provision. This liberal approach had two important consequences: the privatization of public housing stock and the decentralization of housing policy. Sitting tenants were given the right to buy their flats and housing management companies were privatized. Concerning decentralization, housing became the responsibility of the local authorities, but no concept precisely defining how they should proceed to meet the housing needs of the local population was ever formulated.

Croatia, as a former Yugoslav republic, performed economically well during communism (Družić 2004). However, the war in 1991–1995 had a disastrous impact on the country's subsequent socioeconomic development and caused numerous housing problems, such as the need to provide housing for displaced persons and refugees and deal with the damage caused to the housing stock and infrastructure. During the war 25 percent of the country was occupied by foreign military forces and more than 50 percent of the territory was affected by war operations. This chapter seeks to describe the unique course of development of social housing in a country that pursued a liberal housing policy after 1990, while simultaneously having to deal with the painful effects of the long post-communist Balkan wars.

In the first section the chapter presents historical development and provides a short overview of the main macroeconomic and social facts. A comparison of the main trends and changes in housing policy after 1990 with current housing policy problems provides the framework for understanding the achievement of Croatia's social housing programs. The chapter then describes and evaluates the social housing programs applied during the transition. Evaluations of the effectiveness and efficiency of the country's social housing programs are based on empirical evidence. The conclusion summarizes the main findings and recommends areas for future research.

THE HISTORICAL, MACROECONOMIC AND SOCIAL CONTEXTS

National enthusiasm about the prosperity of Croatia, after the first free multiparty elections in the spring 1990, sank in 1991 when the war for the independence of Croatia broke out. The war had a substantial impact on the country's macroeconomic and social development. For example, in 1993 GDP fell to 41.5 percent of its level in 1989.

From 1991 to 1995 Croatia bore the effects of war and saw a drastic decline in economic activity and an increase in social problems (Puljiz 2008). The government, with the support of international aid organizations, had to provide shelter for several hundred thousand displaced persons and refugees.[1] Around 8 percent of the housing stock was damaged or destroyed during the war. Croatia's war economy was struck with high unemployment and rising inflation and the quality of life deteriorated rapidly.

The social policy that the government introduced in 1993 to tackle the most acute problems, in partnership with local authorities and civil society organizations, established safety nets at the local level. The Governmental Stability Program, announced and introduced in the same year, stopped inflation and laid the foundations for stabilizing the macroeconomic situation. In the late 1990s the most important reforms, primarily of the pension and health systems, were made with the conditional support of the World Bank and the International Monetary Fund.

The war also influenced demographic trends: a part of the population moved to neighboring or to developed countries. Between 1991 and 2001, the population size decreased by 7.25 percent, and other demographic indicators, such as birthrates and fertility rates, worsened (Puljiz 2008).[2] Political discontents left unresolved by the war led to the rise of a nondemocratic government that survived until the late 1990s, and this fact isolated Croatia from the EU integration process and the economic assistance of the European Union.

Real economic recovery came in 2000, and since then GDP growth has equaled 4–5 percent annually. In 2008 a slowdown was recorded resulting from the impact of the global economic crisis: annual GDP growth was only 2.4 percent in 2008 and in 2009 GDP declined by 5.8 percent (in 2010 by 2 percent). This economic downturn had an impact on the labor market: the registered unemployment rate was 13.2 percent in 2008 and rose to 19.6 percent in January 2011.

In recent years, income inequalities and the poverty rate have stagnated or grown slightly. The at-risk-of-poverty rate in 2008 was identical to the rate in 2007 (17.4 percent), but the relative at-risk-of-poverty gap increased from 21.9 percent in 2007 to 24.9 percent in 2008. World Bank (2010) simulations show a rise in the absolute poverty rate in 2009 as it grew to 13.5 percent from approximately 10 percent in 2008.

THE HOUSING POLICY LEGACY FROM THE SOCIALIST PERIOD

Housing became a political issue in the 1920s, when there is evidence of the first social housing programs in Zagreb, the capital city. The city built a number of social housing facilities called 'city houses' with small flats of one or two rooms, mostly for socially excluded families (Radovčić-Mahečić 2002).[3] Several foundations and civic associations were also involved in building social housing in that time. As a measure of social protection, Zagreb applied a certain form of rent control, and the city also had a program for the middle class that built small detached houses on public plots (provided free of charge).

After 1945 housing policy was a part of the centrally planned economy. Some private housing was nationalized, but some homeownership was preserved, so that families were allowed to own a maximum of two larger or three smaller dwellings. In the private rental sector the state set up strong tenure security for tenants and rent control similar to what is applied in public housing. A radical shift in housing policy occurred in the 1960s: housing policy was decentralized to the level of the local authorities and later, under the ideology of workers' self-management, to the level of state companies.

From the 1960s, housing provision was planned and implemented at the municipal level (the local authorities) by 'self-management interest communities for housing and infrastructure'.[4] Employees paid a monthly housing contribution to the state companies' 'collective consumption fund'. Profitable companies also contributed to this fund from their profits at the end of each year. There were regulations as to how companies and working organizations then allocated money from this fund. Housing commission, as a workers' council, was responsible for maintaining a waiting list of employees, who applied for: (a) the allocation of a rental flat; (b) loans to buy a flat; (c) loans to build a detached house; or (d) loans to improve the condition of an existing housing unit.[5]

Most of the money from the collective consumption fund was channeled to the local 'self-management interest communities for housing and infrastructure' to construct new rental flats. These flats were then the property of state companies or the working organizations at the companies where tenants were employed. Tenants were given a rental contract that often included the obligation to work for the given company for ten years. By the 1980s, however, practices governing the allocation of dwellings had become very dubious (Bežovan 2008).

According to the law, an additional obligation was that collective consumption funds operated by companies or working organizations had to contribute to housing allowances and to the specific municipality fund that would be used for the construction of social housing, which was referred to as 'flats of solidarity'. The waiting lists for the allocation of social dwellings were maintained by the municipalities, and socially excluded families in particular qualified for access to social housing under the program. In late socialism this was the only social rental housing program targeting low-income people, and it offered a very limited number of newly built housing units.

Alongside the housing provisions described in the preceding, there was also a co-op housing program supported by several by several special provisions.[6] Finally, the construction of flats for sale on the free market never stopped in former Yugoslavia, and in the 1980s a free market in newly constructed flats contributed to pluralism in housing provision. By the end of the 1980s the following housing policy programs existed in Croatia:[7]

- State company housing construction was planned at the local level and financed from the collective consumption funds.
- Marginal social housing construction for people with lower income in the form of 'flats of solidarity', which were planned at the local level and financed from municipal funds.
- The housing allowance was planned and implemented at the local level.
- Housing loans were provided under favorable conditions from the collective consumption funds.
- Housing loans were provided by banks under favorable conditions.
- There were subsidies in the form of VAT exemptions on the purchase of building materials and favorable land and loan access for the construction of co-op housing.
- There were subsidies for the purchase of building sites.

During socialism there was no properly defined and politically recognized concept of social housing targeting lower-income households; the 'flats of solidarity' program that did exist was small in scale and was operated only as a part of local housing policy, especially in larger cites. This fact highly influenced the involvement of the state in the provision of social rental housing in the new market environment after 1990. The long-term decentralized housing policy and existence of a private housing market during late socialism can be seen as two other distinct institutional aspects that may help explain the government strategies adopted after 1990. Path dependence in housing policies has also been recognized in other transitional countries (Hegedüs 2007a).

THE MAIN TRENDS IN CROATIAN HOUSING POLICY AFTER 1990

The first government established after the political changes in 1990 announced the implementation of comprehensive housing reform. Employee housing contributions were canceled, as was the role of companies in the provision and management of housing for their employees. The withdrawal of the state from the sphere of housing provision, the quick privatization of existing public housing to the ownership of sitting tenants, and the strengthening of free market conditions were the main reform goals at the beginning of the 1990s (Bežovan 2008). However, the transfer of housing policy competence away from former state companies into the hands of the municipalities was hindered by the lack of financial resources of the municipalities (the abolition of the old system was not accompanied by the introduction of other subsidy rules). Consequently, local housing policy could not *de facto* be effectively realized (Lux 2003, 408). Such circumstances can be seen as a 'political deficit' in the process of setting up local housing policies.

The most important part of the housing reform implemented during the 1990s in Croatia, like in other transition countries (Hegedüs et al. 1996), was the sale of public housing to sitting tenants: the giveaway privatization of public housing. Public housing represented 25 percent of the total housing stock, most of it located in larger in larger towns (in Zagreb it formed 45 percent of the housing stock).[8] Privatization started in 1992 and over the next two years a major part of the housing stock was sold to sitting tenants at a substantially discounted price.[9] By the end of 2004, 317,831 flats had been sold; 38 percent were purchased in a single payment and 62 percent in installments.[10]

Table 8.1 Housing Tenure Structure in Croatia and in Zagreb, 2001

	Croatia		Zagreb	
Housing tenure	Households 1,477,377	100.0%	Households 275,464	100.0%
Homeownership	1,225,235	82.9	222,697	80.8
Private renting	49,259	3.3	11,742	4.3
Social housing	42,195	2.9	9,630	3.5
Renting part of the flats	12,570	0.9	2,630	1.0
Housing with relatives	110,008	7.4	23,375	8.5
Others	38,110	2.6	5,731	2.1

Several social groups became the victims of right-to-buy, whereas the political elites benefited considerably from it, as they obtained high-value housing units for small amounts of money (Bežovan 2008). The new political elite allocated themselves attractively located and spacious public housing units and, later, bought them at a discount.[11] Part of the income from privatization was supposed to be spent on social housing construction and for the social groups that were negatively impacted by the denationalization (restitution) process.[12] However, this legal obligation was fulfilled only by a small number of local authorities (Bežovan 2004). The sale of public housing stock substantially changed the housing tenure structure in Croatia (Table 8.1).

As mentioned, the war in Croatia caused numerous housing problems. The scale of new housing construction during the war and during the first years after the war seriously decreased. The priorities of housing policy were housing renovation and the provision of accommodation for the victims of war (Radić 2004).[13] A subsidy program for war veterans and victims led to the construction of approximately 6,364 housing units between 1997 and 2010. These flats were built in partnership with local authorities (which provided land and infrastructure) and central government (which covered construction costs). Families who had a member killed in the war and war veterans with 100 percent disability got flats for free.

War veterans with a lower level of disability were eligible to purchase full ownership of these flats, and depending on the level of their disability they obtained a subsidized housing loan for this purpose. The value of the land and infrastructure was not calculated into the property's selling price, and the price was reduced by the percentage of the veteran's disability.[14] This program was a partial 'substitute' for a real social rental housing program.

The housing allowance was recently made part of Croatia's social care system and it is the responsibility of the local authorities.[15] Until 1996 there was also no VAT on housing construction. The introduction of VAT on building materials and services in 1996 (initially 22 percent, now 23 percent) increased the price of newly built housing units. Additionally, a housing savings program was introduced in 1998, with a state savings premium of 25 percent on annual deposits (1,250 HRK [221 U.S. dollars] per depositor saving 5,000 HRK [884 U.S. dollars] per year). In a period of austerity (2005) the state savings premium was reduced, and it now amounts to 15 percent of annual deposits, that is, 750 HRK (132 U.S. dollars).[16] Approximately 10 percent of the country's citizens participate in the housing savings program. According to Tepuš (2006), this program is not very competitive in the housing market. As the beneficiaries of this program mainly come from well-off households living in good-quality housing, there is now a public debate about the usefulness of the scheme.[17]

In 2001, the government introduced a state-subsidized housing construction program as a centralized program of help for first-time buyers, the so-called POS program. It was promoted by one political party (Tepuš 2005).

The prices of housing units built under the POS program are considerably lower than market prices and the program represents a kind of middle-stratum support for access to owner-occupied housing. Local authorities willing to take part in the program must make a public call and establish priority criteria for dwelling allocation. Local authorities provide land and infrastructure, the cost of which should be no more than 40 percent of the total construction costs of a flat. Eligible buyers need to have sufficient purchasing capacity: debt service should not exceed 30 percent of their net household income, and they must be able to secure a down-payment of 15 percent of the dwelling price. The maximum loan maturity is thirty years. The interest rate is around 5 percent per annum. By the end of January 2011, 5,054 flats had been built under this program.[18]

This program also facilitated social housing construction for low-income households and vulnerable social groups.[19] The government offers low-interest loans and the local authorities are again responsible for securing land and infrastructure. In this case, the loan is repaid by the local authority. However, so far only one city used these resources for social housing.

The main problem of the POS program lies in its direct top-down political control. This program has been largely implemented without any planning or deep assessment of housing needs. Often, too-large flats have been built when there was no demand for them from eligible households. Moreover, the quality of the construction work and the building materials used under the POS program has been poor. And there have been abuses: members of well-off families living in their parents' property have bought flats built under the program and then leased them or resold them for a profit.[20] The POS program is not well targeted to those in need, and it is very inefficient and has been 'abused' for market speculations.

Since 2003, the transfer tax for persons who are buying their first housing (first-time buyers) has been waived. The first-time buyer does not have to pay 5 percent of the value of the housing unit as a transfer tax at the time of dwelling purchase. However, the main tax incentive for first-time buyers is that all investments related to the purchase of a housing unit, including interest rates on housing (mortgage) loans used for the purchase, are accepted as income tax–deductible expenditures. Rent paid on the free market (documented with a written rental contract) is also deductible from income tax.[21] Total annual tax exemptions are capped at 12,000 HRK (2120 U.S. dollars) per year and per person. Recent research gives the evidence that tax incentives are becoming increasingly important for first-time buyers (Bežovan 2008). However, as part of antirecession measures, the law was changed, and since 2010 tax incentives for housing and rent deduction do not qualify as tax deductions.

Housing construction boomed until 2009, both in the capital and in the country as a whole (Table 8.2). The boom was driven by demand from well-off families who considered housing a safe investment for generating a stable income in the future. The decline in the housing market in 2009 was

Table 8.2 Number of Newly Built Permanently Inhabited Flats in Croatia and Zagreb, 1991–2009

	Croatia		Zagreb	
Year	Number of flats	Index	Number of flats	Index
1991	12,623	100	4,740	100
1992	7,767	62	2,813	59
1993	8,343	66	2,162	46
1994	9,710	77	2,417	51
1995	7,359	58	1,906	40
1996	12,624	100	1,784	38
1997	12,516	99	2,118	45
1998	12,557	99	2,245	47
1999	12,175	96	2,482	52
2000	15,988	127	2,530	53
2001	12,580	100	2,580	54
2002	18,047	143	3,341	70
2003	17,877	142	4,627	98
2004	18,763	149	4,015	85
2005	19,995	158	4,771	101
2006	22,121	175	6,139	130
2007	25,609	203	8,895	188
2008	25,368	200	8,744	184
2009	18,740	148	4,923	103
2010	14,942	118	3,938	83

influenced by economic recession and a rise in interest rates. The limited availability of mortgage finance and general credit crunch brought housing prices down.[22] Under pressure from the banks that provide project finance to housing developers, the government introduced a special incentive in the summer of 2010: favorable loans for the first-time buyers if they buy unsold newly built housing stock. The very limited reaction to this incentive shows how deep and structural the crisis in the housing market was.[23]

THE POLICY CONTEXT OF SOCIAL HOUSING PROVISION

After privatization and restitution, very few housing units remained in the hands of the local authorities and state-owned companies. These flats were smaller in size (55 square meters in average), poorly maintained, and old. In total this stock of housing amounted to about fifty thousand units: 2.5

percent of the total housing stock. Like in other transition countries, this part of the housing stock is mainly occupied by "socially and economically marginalized people" (Tsenkova 2003, 203). As Hegedüs has written (2007b, 174), "[it] is the most dilapidated part of the housing stock and where the poorest households are concentrated".

The Act on Housing Rent from 1996 gave public housing that had not been sold in the giveaway privatization the status of housing with protected rent.[24] In fact, this measure turned residual public housing into real social housing. The local authorities own the housing units, and the central government sets the level of rent. The rent in social housing is low, just 2.61 HRK per square meter (0.46 U.S. dollars), an amount not sufficient even to cover basic dwelling maintenance. Some tenants are not willing to pay even this low rent, and public landlords have no means of effectively dealing with the rent arrears.

The private rental sector, which involves about 120,000 flats (8.4 percent of total housing stock), has traditionally been part of the gray economy. Although there are regulations on landlord–tenant contracts, in 2005 only seventeen thousand such contracts were registered.

The introduction of the Act on Social Care in 1998 established Croatia's current housing allowance system. Local authorities—municipalities and towns—are responsible for allocating funds for social care in their programs. A single tenant or family whose monthly income in the past three months did not exceed 500 HRK (88 U.S. dollars) per capita may qualify for the housing allowance.[25] The housing allowance is subject to space (dwelling size) limits. These limits are very restrictive and give the allowance a residual meaning: only a small number of households are eligible for the housing allowance.

Additionally, a household (person) is not entitled to a housing allowance if it owns or co-owns a house, flat, or weekend cottage. The monthly housing allowance maximum is 250 HRK (44 U.S. dollars);[26] exceptionally, the allowance can be higher, up to the limit of 500 HRK (88 U.S. dollars): this is just in case the local social (services) department recommends it as the only way to avoid separating children from their family. Since 2001, homeowners are only entitled to a special allowance for heating costs.

According to amendments to the law from 2001, the local governments are responsible for funding the housing allowance and the regional governments are responsible for paying the heating allowance that are *de facto* financed from the state budget.[27] The maximum heating allowance is 880 HRK (155.5 U.S. dollars) per year and per household. In 2009, only 1.8 percent of households received a housing allowance; 2.4 percent of households are eligible for both allowances. Compared to other central European transition countries, only Slovenia has a smaller share of households that receive a housing allowance (Hegedüs and Teller 2005).

From 2001 to 2009, a relatively constant number of housing allowances per year was recorded. The average monthly housing allowance was equal to 165 HRK (29 U.S. dollars) in 2005. The average monthly heating allowance was 72 HRK (12.6 U.S. dollars). Together, the average total allowance was 237 HRK (41.8 U.S. dollars). In fact, it is comparable to the average size of the housing allowance in Poland, Slovakia, and the Czech Republic (Hegedüs and Teller 2005, 190).

Management companies, which in larger towns are often owned by the municipality, are responsible for the management of the housing stock in cooperation with residents. All homeowners pay monthly contributions to a 'reserve fund' and implement a plan of maintenance and investments. Tenants in the social renting sector generally pay a rent that is lower than the contribution to the reserve fund. This means that the municipalities, as the landlords of social dwellings, have to pay extra money to the reserve fund from their own budgets.

THE RESULTS OF EMPIRICAL STUDY OF SOCIAL HOUSING

As part of a study of social housing practices in Croatian cities conducted in early 2008 in cities with more than twenty thousand residents a mail survey was sent to thirty-one cities and responses were received from twenty-six of them.[28] The study's research methodology involved a questionnaire survey designed to collect relevant information on social housing practices (existing public housing stock after privatization and newly built social flats) in cities and also information about plans and attitudes towards social housing. In addition, four case studies on social rental housing were carried out in four cities (Zagreb, Velika Gorica, Varaždin, and Karlovac).[29] Interviews with the mayors of each city and the officials responsible for housing provided data for assessing housing as a political priority and governance issue. The following are some of the results of the study.

Most social housing units are located in larger cities: Zagreb—7,657 units; Rijeka—476; Varaždin—390; Osijek—369; Velika Gorica—284; and Split—249. Over the past ten years, the number of social housing units has increased very slowly in five of the surveyed cities, remained stable in eight cities, and decreased in nine. Given that the number of social housing units increased in only five cities, it is clear that a limited social housing program (under the POS program) cannot meet the increasing demand for social housing.

The study checked on whether the sitting tenants in social housing were given again the option of buying the housing units they live in.[30] Nine cities decided to sell these housing units. A look at the practices of such sales shows that speculative interests are often behind the transactions: these housing units, after renovation, are often resold for a higher price. By contrast, Karlovac has recently started to sell old and poorly maintained flats to the sitting tenants. The city has no resources to improve the quality of these flats, and this was mentioned as the main reason for the decision to sell them.

Some cities complain that as a result of rent control rents are insufficient to cover maintenance costs and they have to bear the costs of managing and maintaining these housing units. Recently, the city of Zagreb formulated a proposal to sell these housing units due to the financial losses from maintaining them. The decision contains provisions to prevent speculations: in the case of resale, the city has the preemption right. Here it is evident that the ability to overcome the deficit in governance (Tsenkova 2003, 203) is crucial for the housing sector overall.

It was expected that cities would invest in new social housing construction. The funds from the sale of public housing owned by cities should have been spent on social housing construction. However, only twelve cities have invested into social housing construction during the past ten years.[31] Relative to the size of the cities, the most social housing was built in Varaždin (140), Zadar (126), and Osijek (105). The cities usually buy housing units on the market, and thus pay a higher price for them than what they would have spent to build them.[32]

A relatively large number of social housing units (approximately nine hundred) and public rental units (approximately five hundred) have recently been built in Zagreb.[33] Support for the construction of public rental housing should be distinguished from the program for social housing. Young families with more children, whose income above the locally set ceiling makes them ineligible for social housing, are eligible for new public dwellings. The rents in this housing are higher than in social housing, but they are lower than in the private rental market. This public rental program in Zagreb has the capacity to become a model for similar programs in other larger cities. The mayors and officials of three other cities from the case studies see public rental housing as more important than social rental housing. In their view, public housing is an investment in a competent labor force and represents an opportunity to attract young professionals to work in public services (schools, health and social services, police, local administration). Public rental housing is understood as an investment in real development, whereas social renting housing is seen more as a 'necessary evil'.

From the study it is obvious that without any incentive from the national level of housing policy it is not to be expected that the cities themselves will invest more in the development of social housing. In general, the role of the central government is crucial for social housing development and sustainability (Hegedüs 2008). The existing POS program does not provide any real incentive for social housing construction.[34]

Priority lists exist in nineteen cities,[35] based on means-testing, so the households that should get social housing in the next several years have already been selected. As mentioned earlier, the low level of rent makes social housing projects unsustainable. In the survey, city representatives were asked to express their view on several statements (Table 8.3). Social rents are low and cannot be compared to the market rent. For example, market rent on an average attractive location in Zagreb is approximately

Table 8.3 Level of Agreement with Statement on Social Housing Project Sustainability

	Yes	No	No answer
Protected rent should be increased	12	7	7
A considerable number of protected tenants are not poor households	10	8	8
Level of rent should be determined by the cities, owner of housing	18	2	6

50 HRK per square meter (9 U.S. dollars). Consequently, the market rent for an apartment of 40 square meters amounts to 2,000 HRK (353 U.S. dollars), and social rent for the same apartment in the same location is 104 HRK (18 U.S. dollars).

Researchers have often heard local authority employees make the claim that social tenants are not always poor households. The representatives of ten cities support this opinion. Evidence shows that allocation of housing units with social rent to scientific, cultural, and public workers is practiced in nine cities. The city of Zagreb has allocated 142 such housing units during the past ten years; Split allocated forty-one and Zadar forty-six housing units.

Does this mean that the criteria for the allocation of social housing should be more targeted or possibly even prescribed by the national law (Lux 2003, 416)? In general, the development and administration of targeted programs is a serious issue (Hegedüs 2007a): some cities highlight problems related to rent arrears. From the debate in professional circles and from the information in the media, it is evident that, as a part of social care programs, cities should have a certain number of flats as shelters for homeless families. The survey results show, however, that twenty-three cities are without any such services, and three cities did not provide an answer to this survey question. One city stated that they have so-called emergency housing and described it as a room with a bathroom for families in urgent housing need.

The homeless, an increasingly vulnerable group in Croatia, can count on a social care program in seven cities (Zagreb, Rijeka, Split, Osijek, Zadar, Karlovac, and Varaždin). In three cases, the cities organize and pay for the costs of shelters, and in three cases they do it in cooperation with civil society organizations. Homelessness is a new social risk caused by a number of factors (Bakula-Anđelić and Šostar 2006; Šikić-Mićanović 2010). Civil society organizations, providing advocacy and mobilizing additional resources, are more efficient than cities in providing social services for this socially excluded population.

Roma households, an ethnically excluded population, have a good chance of obtaining social housing. However, what local authorities are mostly doing is improving the infrastructure and housing conditions in their settlements. Housing officials from the cities feel that this strategy is more appropriate for the lifestyle of the Roma than giving them social flats. The demand for social rental housing in the four case study cities is estimated at between 3 percent and 5 percent of the local housing stock. Mayors and local government officials indicate that the main obstacle to solving housing problems is sufficient housing stock for the elderly.[36]

In the survey, city representatives were asked to write their thoughts on the issue of social housing. Smaller cities do not envision including social rental housing among their responsibilities. The cities of Zagreb and Varaždin have assumed these responsibilities whereas two other cities, Karlovac and Velika Gorica, have not. One representative of a city with more than forty thousand inhabitants concluded by saying: "There is no social housing or planned social housing, nor is there a housing policy in our city. Housing in the city depends on private entrepreneurs and developers who are imposing their unrealistically high prices. Young families with lower incomes and the wider circle of the population in general can hardly afford an apartment under such conditions."

The study revealed that social housing, except for cases of acute need, is not a real topic on the agenda of local development in cities. Representatives agreed that the lack of resources in the city budgets would form a lasting obstacle to social housing development. For the time being, banks, which used to make huge profits in the housing market, are very reluctant to form partnerships with cities for the purpose of social housing programs. On the other hand, there is an apparent lack of pressure from local stakeholders to get cities to do something about social rental housing. The workshop participants recognized the potential of trade unions and the church to get social housing on the political agenda.

THE EFFICIENCY AND EFFECTIVENESS OF SOCIAL HOUSING

The lack of any real social housing strategy in Croatia recently can be explained through path dependence by very weak tradition of social rental housing in the past. Citizens learned about the abuse of public housing in the 1980s and 1990s and they have a firm conviction that everything in the housing sector must be private. In a country without reliable property records and with a large informal economy,[37] means-testing is a big challenge for policy implementation. In these circumstances citizens and local politicians do not trust the concept of social housing.

As explained in the preceding, Croatia's development was seriously affected by the war. The postwar reconstruction of the housing stock that was destroyed and the construction of housing for victims of the war served as a kind of substitute for social housing. Social housing in Croatia makes up about 2 percent of the housing stock, mostly unsold public housing built before 1990, under rent control regime. Rent regulation is applied to mostly poor households. Some newly built social housing is occupied by middle-income households. Consequently, social housing in Croatia can be evaluated as an effective form of help for needy households. However, low-income households in the new generations have little chance of getting this type of housing. The 'outsiders' (mostly young families, poor people, migrants, refugees, the Roma, and homeless people) are excluded from this kind of state aid.

Local authorities use different practices to set the rents in the newly built flats. Some local authorities set the rent in new social flats at a level four to five times higher than in the old social housing. However, the overwhelming majority of social housing was built before 1990 and the level of rent is very low there—so low that it is insufficient to cover even maintenance costs, which means that the system is financially unsustainable. From this point of view the social housing system in Croatia cannot be deemed efficient.

CONCLUSION

Croatian social housing policy, painfully affected by the war in the 1990s, is still floating around on the waves of liberal policy without any viable guidelines. No national program of social rental housing exists in Croatia. The problem was left to the local authorities, where in many cases it forms just a marginal part of local social care programs. Although the demand for social housing had been identified, only a small number of larger cities invest limited funds in social housing construction. Cost-ineffective rents make programs for the construction of social housing unsustainable, and as landlords the cities are increasingly selling flats from their current social housing stock in order to cover the budget deficit.

Croatian housing programs and tax incentives for housing, like in other transition countries (Hegedüs 2007a), mainly support higher-income households. The housing allowance program is ineffective and does not make housing more affordable or accessible for low-income households. Needy households that do not have a signed lease with a landlord are not eligible for the housing allowance and are socially excluded.

Social housing issues belong to the wider area of social policy, which in Croatia is currently a fragmented and marginalized area. On the other hand, the priorities of pension and health reform seem to question even the legitimacy of turning the discussion towards social housing. Relevant stakeholders do not care about social rental housing, and some of them are suspicious of its mission. The social capital necessary for the development of social rental housing does not exist.

The policy measure of selling social rental housing, which is increasingly supported by the cities, would further decrease the share of social housing in the housing stock. The universal principles of liberalization and privatization, which have deeply influenced the opinions of ordinary citizens, question the very idea of constructing housing that is not privately owned. The low level of trust and the inefficiency of the local institutional infrastructure dealing with housing issues are further obstacles to the development of social rental housing.

Possible resources for social housing construction could be found in the funds from the first sale of public housing during the 1990s. Launching such projects is primarily dependent on the political will of mayors. The new system of direct elections of mayors has put social rental housing issues on the agenda in more cities.

Empirical evidence suggests that the development of social renting housing in Croatia is making some progress. On the other hand, there are signs from the current economic crisis that this positive progress may be threatened.

NOTES

1. In the beginning of 1992 there were 550,000 displaced persons from different parts of Croatia and 150,000 refugees mainly from Bosnia (Puljiz 2008, 31). Croatia recorded 13,010 dead as a result of the war, and the official estimate of the cost of the war damage was 43 billion USD.
2. Croatia is a country of 4.4 million of people.
3. This innovation in housing was inspired by study visits made by public officials to Prague, Vienna, and the Netherlands. The officials learned about new developments in urbanism and design for social housing (Radovčić-Mahečić 2002; Bežovan 2008).
4. At that time there were 115 municipalities; today Croatia has 555 municipalities.
5. There were separate programs for privileged groups in society, like state and party officials, the military, and the police.
6. Housing cooperatives were self-governing units established by twenty citizens with housing needs, and some were established by state companies. In 1988 there were 165 housing cooperatives. They were able to obtain land for construction and loans under favorable conditions. As nonprofit organizations, they did not have to pay a profit tax or VAT on building materials (Bežovan and Dakić 1990). When the government canceled these provisions (1992) the coops became less competitive, and at present only a few of them still exist, now as normal private companies.
7. The programs were run locally. State subsidies were not so important for financing these programs because the main source of funding was contributions from employees and employers.
8. By *public housing* we mean housing stock owned by state companies; nationalized housing stock owned by municipalities; new housing built as municipal housing before the beginning of the 1970s; the small social housing stock (flats of solidarity), which was again in the hands of the local authorities; and housing stock that, as a part of ideology, met the needs of well-off families (called 'society housing').
9. Sitting tenants got price discounts calculated on the basis of the number of years in work, number of children, disabled family members, and whether a family member was a victim of the war.
10. The sale of public housing took a long period of time because of the war and because military flats were not intended for sale.

11. Even fifteen years later, journalists are still uncovering scandals of this kind.
12. About forty-five hundred housing units, with tenants who previously enjoyed the status of public housing tenant, have been part of restitution to the previous owners or their descendants. Former owners claimed their property back and could not accept low rents and, often, forced tenants to leave. Tenants in these housing units are at risk of social exclusion.
13. From 1992 to 2003, 126,297 housing units were renovated. International humanitarian organizations, the European Union, and government of developed countries made very visible contributions to that program.
14. The public views much of this program as part of clientelist style of governance that is in fact about buying the votes and political support of war veterans, who have a strong voice in political debates.
15. More details on the housing allowance will be given further on in this chapter.
16. 1 HRK = 0.17 U.S. dollar (winter 2011).
17. Four of the five housing savings banks are owned by foreign banks, and consequently they have a strong negotiating position and power. Although some voices and proposals have called for cuts to the elimination of state incentives for the housing savings scheme, in its antirecession measures in 2010 the government refused to do so.
18. When a new government came to power in 2003, the program ceased to be a political priority and consequently fewer and fewer housing units have been produced.
19. As a demonstration of political will, without adequate legal provision, the government announced the establishment of nonprofit housing organizations to be overseen by the local authorities. Three larger cities have such institutions and they now implement the government's program supporting first-time housing buyers in a more efficient way than the centrally implemented program.
20. Under pressure from the media, the government changed the legislation, and since 2007 housing units from this program cannot be sold for ten years.
21. This measure helps the most vulnerable young families, subtenants, who are renting flats in the open market.
22. According to estimates, housing prices decreased in Zagreb by 25–30 percent between 2008 and 2010.
23. Only seventy-seven housing units have been sold under this program. In February 2011 the government provided additional subsidies to sell housing units, and in June 2011 about one thousand housing units were sold.
24. *Housing with protected rent* is the official expression for social housing. The former expression is unknown to the general public—people and local authority representatives instead use the term *social housing*.
25. The ceiling can be seen here as a poverty line arbitrarily set up, and it is largely dependent on political will.
26. This part of social assistance is not connected to the general income adjustment program, which is the responsibility of the government and implemented through the Center for Social Care.
27. The government implemented this reform in order to help families living in municipalities, mostly villages. Local budget deficits make it impossible for the municipalities to have a housing allowance program.
28. Cities involved in the survey represent 48 percent of the total population in country.
29. The populations of these cities are: Zagreb—800,000; Velika Gorica—70,000; Varaždin—42,000; and Karlovac—60,000.

30. The cities, as the owners of social housing, old and newly built, can decide to sell them, but not under favorable conditions, as was the case in the 1990s. The value of each flat must be estimated by an official appraiser.
31. Under pressure from the trade unions, in 2007 the government set aside 11.5 million HRK (1.96 million USD) out of proceeds from the sale of public housing and allocated it to programs to provide housing for civil servants and employees (Bežovan 2008). Trade unions developing strategies of partnership with local authorities are also thinking about social and public housing construction.
32. Many suspicions are voiced in the media about such practices, labeling them as speculative and corrupt.
33. This program also provides support for first-time buyers and young families and offers affordable housing units in a less attractive location. 'Zagreb's model of house building', was in fact developed in opposition to the government's POS program.
34. Mayors from oppositional parties to the government see that they are not welcome in that program, or, as in the case of Zagreb, feel that they are strong enough to make it without "support", better to say patronage, from the state program.
35. On the priority lists households with more children and handicapped members have more chance to get social housing.
36. Waiting lists for elderly homes, operated by regional authorities, are very long and there are no more investments to increase number of places in this program. Due to the subventions cost of accommodation in this program is far below the market level. Recently, the first private investors invested into housing provision for the elderly.
37. The informal economy in Croatia is estimated to account for more than 20 percent of the GDP.

REFERENCES

Bakula-Anđelić, M. and Šostar, Z. 2006. "Beskućnici Grada Zagreba (Homeless in the City of Zagreb)." *Revija za socijalnu politiku (Journal of Social Policy)* 13: 399–412.

Bežovan, G. 2004. "Stambena prava u Hrvatskoj i problemi njihova ostvarivanja (Housing Rights in Croatia and the Problems of their Realization)." *Revija za socijalnu politiku (Journal of Social Policy)* 11: 89–106.

———. 2008. "Stanovanje i stambena politika (Housing and Housing Policy)." *Socijalna politka Hrvatske (Croatian Social Policy)*. Zagreb: Pravni fakultet.

Bežovan, G. and Dakić, S. 1990. *Alternativna stambena politika (Alternative Housing Policies)*. Zagreb: Radničke novine.

Družić, G. 2004. *Hrvatska obratnica (Croatia Capricorn)*. Zagreb: Golden marketing.

Hegedüs, J. 2007a. "Social Housing in Hungary." *Social Housing in Europe*. London: London School of Economics.

———. 2007b. "Social Housing in Transitional Countries." *Social Housing in Europe*. London: London School of Economics.

———. 2008. "Social Housing in Transitional Countries: The Case of Hungary." *Social Housing in Europe II: A Review of Policies and Outcomes*. London: London School of Economics.

Hegedüs, J., Mayo, S., and Tosics, I. 1996. "Transition of the Housing Sector in the East Central European Countries." *Review of Urban and Regional Development Studies* 8: 101–36.

Hegedüs, J. and Teller, N. 2005. "Development of the Housing Allowance Programs in Hungary in the Context of CEE Transitional Countries." *European Journal of Housing Policy* 5: 187–209.

Lux, M. 2003. "State and Local Government: How to Improve the Partnership: Local Government and Housing." *Housing Policy: An End or a New Beginning?* Budapest: Local Government and Public Service Reform Initiative, Open Society Institute.

Puljiz, V. 2008. "Socijalna politika Hrvatske (Povijest, zadanosti, usmjerenja)." *Socijalna politka Hrvatske (Croatian Social Policy)*. Zagreb: Pravni fakultet.

Radić, A. 2004. "Socijalna prava: prognanici, povratnici i izbjeglice (Social Rights: Displaced Persons, Returnees and Refugees)." *Revija za socijalnu politiku (Journal of Social Policy)* 11: 129–36.

Radovčić-Mahečić, D. 2002. *Socijalno stanovanje međuratnog Zagreba (Social Housing Inter-Zagreb)*. Zagreb: Horetzky.

Šikić-Mićanović, L. 2010. "Homelessness and Social Exclusion in Croatia." *European Journal of Homelessness* 4:45–64.

Tepuš, M. Mladen. 2005. *Modeli stambenog financiranja (Models of Housing Finance)*. Zagreb: Albatros media.

Tepuš, M. Mladen. 2006. "Analiza poslovanja stambenih štedionica: Rezultati drugoga HNB-ova projekta anketiranja stambenih štedionica (Performance Analysis of Housing Savings Banks: The Results of the Second CNB Project Survey of Housing Saving Banks)." *Pregledi (Views)*. Zagreb: Hrvatska narodna banka.

Tsenkova, S. 2003. "Housing Policy Matters: The Reform Path in Central and Eastern Europe." *Housing Change in East and Central Europe-Integration or Fragmentation*. Aldershot: Ashgate Publishing Limited.

World Bank. 2010. *Croatia—Social Impact of the Crisis and the Policy Response-An assessment*. Washington: World Bank.

9 The Czech Republic

Locked between Municipal and Social Housing

Martin Lux

INTRODUCTION

The goal of this chapter is to briefly describe the emergence and application of the social housing system in the Czech Republic after 1990. In this chapter, social housing is traditionally defined as housing offered at below-market rents and allocated to low-income and other vulnerable households. There are two specific features of the Czech housing system. The first is the scope of decentralization in housing policy (municipalities have the right to decide about the privatization of public housing). The second feature, a consequence of the first, is the slow pace of public (municipal) housing privatization in the Czech Republic. The early post-socialist governments decided to avoid introducing of right to buy policy in the Czech Republic. However, as I will demonstrate in this chapter, a larger share of public housing is no guarantee of more effective and efficient social housing policy. On the contrary, the overall policy in this field in the Czech Republic is evaluated in this chapter as ineffective and inefficient. Compared to other CEE countries, in the Czech Republic much of the urban housing stock expropriated by the state under the previous regime has been returned to the original owners or their descendants (about 7 percent of the total housing stock), and thus the quick emergence of the private rental sector is another distinguishing feature of the Czech housing system.

The first section of this chapter provides a broader context to social housing policy, including a brief description of its history to 1990. The next two sections discuss housing policy changes after 1990 and the post-socialist institutionalization of social housing. The subsequent section provides a partial evaluation of the effectiveness and efficiency of the social housing strategy applied over the past two decades and attempts to answer the questions of whether the latest system is capable of meeting the needs of low-income and vulnerable households and whether it is economically sustainable in the long term. The final section summarizes the main conclusions and challenges.

THE HISTORICAL CONTEXT OF HOUSING POLICY

Supply-side subsidies for the construction of rental housing designated for low-income households has a long tradition in the Czech Republic, going back to 1918 when the independent Czechoslovak Republic was established. The housing policy of the newly created state faced a postwar housing shortage by introducing several measures to increase housing output for low-income households. The state, for example, boosted housing construction by means of the following:

- *State guarantees* on mortgage loans were extended for the construction of small rental flats built by municipalities and nonprofit housing cooperatives.
- *Interest subsidies* covering the whole or part of the interest from mortgage loans were extended to municipalities and housing cooperatives for the construction of small flats.
- *Exemption from property tax* was granted for a period of twenty years for all new housing.
- *Grants* covering as much as 40 percent of the total costs of constructing apartment rental houses; these grants were offered in the years 1920 and 1921 to all builders (including private ones), as long as the building was situated in a town (above fifteen thousand inhabitants), contained at least four flats, the commercial area of the house did not exceed 30 percent of the total floor area, the construction costs were approved by the Ministry of Public Works, and the state received the first option.

The most effective incentive at that time was the exemption from property tax. Thanks to this indirect support and the exemption from rent control for newly built flats the housing boom (mostly provided by private investors) saturated the housing demand at the beginning of the 1930s.

After 1948 Czechoslovakia's economy shifted to central planning and housing construction began to be fully and centrally controlled by the state. The new regime introduced strong central state interventions directed at decommodifying housing—interventions that influenced the scope of housing production via extensive state financing, influenced the tenure structure through property expropriation, and influenced housing consumption through rent and price regulations.[1] Although the goal to make housing a pure public good remained basically unmet owing to the state's inability to finance housing output strictly out of public budgets, these interventions created a segment of mass public rental housing stock in which rents and utility prices were kept at a very low level.[2]

The official landlord of public housing was the state, but owing to strong tenure security, which guaranteed the occupancy title to relatives and descendants of the tenant, and owing to bureaucratic and ineffective housing management, many ownership rights were legally or illegally realized by tenants. No one spoke about 'renting', but about the 'personal use' of a flat. 'Personal use' became an institution separate from that of rental tenure—it could be inherited or transferred to relatives, or exchanged with some others holders of user rights. As Marcuse (1996) has shown, the tenancy title that existed under socialism was much like the title of ownership that existed in the West. In western countries the right of use is subordinated to the right of ownership, but in socialist countries the right of use was superior to the right of ownership, and the right of use "equalled or exceeded in many ways those conventionally associated with ownership and certainly were far stronger than those associated with conventional tenancy in United States" (Marcuse 1996, 135).

In the plan to liquidate private property state housing should eventually have replaced all other housing tenures. And because state housing was for everyone, the people who obtained it fastest (or obtained the best-quality housing) were recruited mainly from the regime's *nomenklatura* or those who used clientele networks or bribes—that is, people who would not usually rank among the neediest (Lux 2009).

Extensive state-financed housing construction increasingly had to contend with limited resources, so despite continued ideological declarations against the private sector, later other forms of housing construction and finance were also permitted—enterprise (state enterprise), cooperative (semi-state housing cooperative), and individual forms of housing. Individual housing construction primarily involved the construction of family houses; paid for with personal savings, contributions from local branches of state administration and long-term low-interest loans from state banks. When it existed, enterprise-based housing construction was financed partly by state enterprises, partly by the state, and partly with long-term bank loans. This system was, however, abolished in 1981.

Cooperative housing construction was first organized in 1958 and the costs were covered by contributions from the cooperative's members, state subsidies, and low-interest bank loans. Czechoslovak housing cooperatives differed from their counterparts in democratic countries. The prewar housing cooperatives were forcibly merged. New Building Housing Cooperatives were eventually managing as many as a few thousand flats. Cooperative statutes had to be uniform. Owing to the massive number of members of cooperatives, the initially democratic procedures were replaced with proceedings among 'delegates'. The 'nationalization' of the cooperative movement led to the destruction of the original idea behind cooperative associations as independent 'self-help' entities and extinguished individual initiative and cooperative democracy. Cooperative housing came to be perceived as simply a more expensive form of state rental housing.

Prefab technology and uniform residential development plans were also used to remedy the discord between the demand for flats and limited public resources. In 2001 (last census), 31 percent of the Czech population was still living in prefab flats, and in bigger towns the figure was as much as half the population. Ultimately, through huge state subsidies and adherence to the principles of mass prefab housing construction, the housing shortage was overcome just before 1989.

HOUSING POLICY REFORMS AFTER 1989

In 1989 the socialist system collapsed and the Czechoslovak Republic embarked on a path of numerous economic, political, and social changes. The core goals of this transformation process included the reintroduction of private property and the establishment of a market economy. Revenue subsidies for existing state rental dwellings and capital subsidies for new state rental housing construction almost disappeared entirely after the change of regime. The prices of construction materials were liberalized and quickly increased. These two factors led to a sharp decrease in the

Table 9.1 Number and Percentage of Started and Completed Municipal Housing Out of the Total Number of New Dwellings Built in 1990–2005

Year	Total no. started	Municipal no. started	Municipal %	Total no. finished	Municipal no. finished	Municipal %
1990	61,004	10,411	17.1	44,594	8,516	19.1
1991	10,899	1,524	14.0	41,719	9,610	23.0
1992	8,429	1,864	22.1	36,397	7,086	19.5
1993	7,454	1,920	2.6	31,509	6,213	19.7
1994	10,964	1,477	13.5	18,162	4,224	23.3
1995	16,548	3,015	18.2	12,662	1,689	13.3
1996	22,680	3,165	14.0	14,482	2,727	18.8
1997	33,152	4,123	12.4	16,757	2,835	16.9
1998	35,027	3,407	9.7	22,183	3,216	14.5
1999	32,900	3,246	9.9	23,734	2,925	12.3
2000	32,377	3,679	11.4	25,207	2,897	11.5
2001	28,983	2,585	8.9	24,759	2,686	10.8
2002	33,606	4,393	13.1	27,292	2,612	9.6
2003	36,496	3,782	10.4	27,127	2,605	9.6
2004	39,037	2,012	5.1	32,268	3,641	11.3
2005	40,381	1,968	5.4	32,863	2,430	8.4

Source: Czech Statistical Office.

volume of housing construction, which only began to grow again after 1996 and after 2002 (Table 9.1). Private capital became the dominant source of financing for the new housing supply and the share of municipal housing construction out of total housing starts steadily decreased. Nevertheless, when compared to other post-socialist states, the share of municipal housing construction remained relatively high, essentially reflecting the traditional attention the Czech state paid to supply-side subsidies for the construction of public housing.

In spite of the moderate scale of house construction, the number of permanently inhabited dwellings per one thousand inhabitants increased from 360 in 1991 to 372 in 2001. Other dwellings serve residential purposes, but their inhabitants do not have permanent residency there (they are mostly rented out or used for recreational purposes). If we count all habitable residential dwellings, the Czech Republic had 427 dwellings per one thousand inhabitants in 2001. In comparison with other developed and transition countries (Lux et al. 2005), this result indicates a relative housing sufficiency in the Czech Republic; the ratio was even higher than in some western EU member states.

CHANGES IN THE STRUCTURE OF HOUSING TENURE AFTER 1989

The first step in the transformation that affected housing tenure structure was the restitution of the housing stock. The process of property restitution began in April 1991, and it applied to that part of the housing stock that was expropriated between February 1948 and January 1990. According to the legislation, the original owner or his/her heirs were entitled to apply for the return of property. By 1993 most of the property transfers were completed; approximately 7 percent of the housing stock had been affected, although in the center of the capital city of Prague, for instance, as much as 70 percent of the housing stock was restituted (Sýkora and Šimoníčková 1994). The remaining state housing was transferred free of charge into the hands of the municipalities.

In the Czech Republic, right to buy legislation was not passed, and public housing privatization remained an option open to the municipalities to apply. However, the state decided to keep the original pre-1990 type of nontargeted regulation of rent (and to keep the pre-1990 form of tenure protection) and to allow only small and gradual rent increases.[3] Rent regulation was applied to all running tenancies, regardless of the type of tenure, that is, both to tenants in municipal housing and to tenants in the private rental sector that emerged out of the restitution of property. An amendment to the Civil Code in 1993 exempted from rent control only new leases signed on flats that had been vacated. Two extremely different regimes were applied to rental housing, with no regard to the type of landlord or the social situation of the tenant. Strict untargeted rent control with open-term contracts and strong tenant protection for running tenancies were combined with an extremely liberal system of rent setting, with no restrictions on the terms of the contract and no effective tenant protection for new tenancies. The rental market became deeply segmented and a variety of tensions and conflicts emerged (Lux and Sunega 2010).

Municipalities in the Czech Republic, although not obliged to sell their newly acquired housing, were unable to introduce any effective way of managing this housing stock that could free them from subsidizing it. With their hands tied by rent control, they opted to privatize their housing. The flats were mostly sold to sitting tenants at a low price, although price conditions (and the scale and speed of the sale) varied from one municipality to the next. It is estimated that by the end of 2009, 74 percent of the municipal housing stock transferred into municipal ownership in 1991 had been sold to sitting tenants. According to a survey conducted by the Institute for Regional Development among selected municipalities in 2009, the municipalities plan to continue this course of privatization. It is estimated that ultimately 80 percent of the 1991 stock of municipal housing will be privatized, in which case the share of municipal housing would decrease to below 10 percent of the total housing stock.

Table 9.2 shows the marked increase in the homeownership rate in the Czech Republic (by more than ten percentage points) between 1991 and 2001 and, conversely, the reduction in the share of rental flats by almost eleven percentage points. Estimates based on the EU-SILC 2008 survey indicate a further increase in the homeownership rate (especially in flat ownership) offset by a drop in the share of rental housing—these estimates can only be verified once data from the 2011 census become available.

Privatization also had a significant effect on the cooperative housing sector. The basic objective of the Transformation Act from 1992 was to

Table 9.2 Changes in Tenure Structure

	1991		2001		Estimates for 2008
	abs.	%	**abs.**	%	%
Own detached house	1,367,027	36.9	1,371,684	35.8	39.0
Own flat	31,164	0.8	421,654	11.0	21.6
Rental housing	1,465,231	39.5	1,092,950	28.6	23.2
Cooperative housing	697,829	18.8	548,812	14.3	12.4
Tenants cooperative	-	-	103,216	2.7	3.8
Others	144,430	3.9	289,362	7.6	
Total	**3,705,681**	**100.0**	**3,827,678**	**100.0**	**100.0**

Source: Census 1991, Census 2001, SILC 2008, Czech Statistical Office.

increase the ownership entitlement of cooperative members to use cooperative flats. Cooperative members occupying cooperative flats, unlike occupants of municipal flats, acquired the right to 'sell' their flats (in reality, to transfer the cooperative ownership share together with the right to occupy the flat) on the free market and in particular the right to the free-of-charge transfer of a cooperative flat to their full ownership. Cooperative housing thus in essence became homeownership tenure although it formally remained a part of the rental sector.

INEQUALITIES IN HOUSING AFFORDABILITY AND THE RESPONSE OF THE CENTRAL ADMINISTRATION

After 1989 economic and political reforms were given precedence over reforms in the field of social policy (Krebs et al. 2005). Social policy remained embedded in the past and highly redistributive, with an especially high redistributive burden put on the middle classes (Večerník and Matějů 1998). This helped to achieve the necessary economic reform changes, but at the same time it strengthened the inherited false social norm of people's heavy dependence on the state. Možný (1994) wrote that the new political elite inherited the misfortune of the previous elite: social peace is no less important to the feasibility of economic transition than it was in the decades of 'building socialism' to the maintenance of the communist regime.

Thanks to public revenue from the privatization of former state enterprises the state could afford such a generous social policy at the beginning of the transition. However, later on, when the well of privatization revenue had dried up, such 'generous gifts' were necessarily beginning to be distributed unequally and the state budget deficit began to swell. This does not mean that the state's generous social policy was all negative. The Czech Republic has the second lowest at-risk-of-poverty rate in the EU-25, people enjoy free university education and largely improved health care services, and the problem of social segregation and exclusion remained for a long time more of a potential threat than a reality (Večerník 2009).

Lux and Sunega (2006) described in detail how housing affordability evolved over the course of the economic transformation, both for individual groups of households and for segments of the housing market. Their study indicates that not only was there a significant increase in the level of the housing expenditure burden (which is the logical result of the socialist era's cheap housing policy being abandoned), but inequalities in this area grew. However, the growth of social inequalities was specific, as it was mainly determined by state interventions and state housing policy, and less by influence of the free market. Rent regulation caused the rental housing market to cleave into two segments—'privileged' housing (with strong protections and low, regulated rents) and 'nonprivileged' housing (with no protections and leased for market rents).

The housing expenditures-to-income ratio differed substantially between segments. Whereas many 'rich' households profited from rent regulation or giveaway housing privatization (Lux and Sunega 2004), many young and vulnerable households had to pay for housing of comparable quality at several times higher market rent or price. Despite this situation, social housing and not-for-profit housing are still not legally defined in the Czech Republic even today.[4] There is no housing law, nor is there a law on housing intended for households with low income or other priority groups of households. The application of any social housing principles was left to the municipalities and was only marginally shaped by new state subsidies.

Responsibility for formulating and implementing the national housing policy is shared by three ministries in the Czech Republic: the Ministry for Regional Development (MRD),[5] the Ministry of Finance (MF), and the Ministry for Labour and Social Affairs (MLSA). Housing allowances remain the responsibility of the MLSA under its general social policy and the most important programs supporting owner-occupied housing (state premium to housing savings, tax relief) remain the responsibility of the MF. Although officially the MRD is responsible for state housing policy, its authority is weakened by the interests of the other two ministries. Of all three ministries the MRD allocates the least portion of public housing expenditures. If we compare the levels of state subsidies according to their target housing tenure, public expenditure in support of owner-occupied housing has clearly dominated recent Czech housing policy (Lux 2009). The weak power of the MRD and the preference for owner-occupied housing reinforced by Czech politicians are the primary factors explaining the lack of any central (legal) social housing strategy.

THE ROLE OF THE MUNICIPALITIES: PUBLIC HOUSING

Municipal housing now makes up 10 percent of the housing stock and includes both prewar brick buildings and postwar prefab buildings. Information about the quality or stratification of this housing stock is not, however, currently available.[6] With the exception of one, albeit important, restriction on their right to dispose of the property—that is, rent regulation—Czech municipalities are free to manage and allocate housing as they see fit. There is no state or regional regulatory framework on public housing management, no regulations on the scale or form of public housing privatization, and no regulation of public housing allocation (no rules biding municipalities to allocate municipal housing to specific target groups).

Only a few municipal flats become vacant annually. Some of these vacated municipal flats are leased for market rents (to the highest bid), and others are leased for a regulated rent to those in housing need. For the latter case, municipalities have passed their own local housing policies and introduced different scoring systems to assess housing need. However, it is impossible to estimate how many such flats there are or obtain an overall picture of allocation schemes. Each municipality incorporates into its strategy its own interests and needs; for example, towns in declining regions losing the young population often have specific 'start-up' housing programs targeting young families.

The decentralization of power in this field is truly substantial. For example, the capital city of Prague (with a population of approximately 1,200,000 of inhabitants) is divided into twenty-two administrative districts and fifty-seven independent 'municipalities'. Each of the fifty-seven 'municipalities' (in fact, city districts or neighborhoods) has its own elected council, board, and mayor. Legislation enacted in 1991 transferred state housing stock to the ownership of the city of Prague. But in conformity with the Act on the Capital City of Prague the overwhelming majority of the housing stock is managed independently by the city's 'municipalities' (which make decisions about privatization, rent setting, allocation criteria, etc.). Consequently, within one city there is a variety of housing policies (and social housing strategies). And the same applies across the territory of the Czech Republic, which is divided into more than six thousand independent municipalities. In relation to the size of the population (about ten million inhabitants), the Czech Republic is one of the most decentralized countries in Europe. This enormous fragmentation makes any generalization or firm evaluation impossible—things are too diverse and change too quickly.

This high level of decentralization is clearly another factor explaining the lack of any consistent central social housing strategy. The number of small and financially weak municipalities is large, and they are effectively resistant to any kind of central government intervention, by pleading a lack of municipal resources. All attempts to draw up a universal social housing strategy or strengthen the legislative responsibility of municipalities for providing housing to their poor citizens have been unsuccessful. The municipalities will only accept state-prepared strategies if there are financial motives to do so, but state budget resources are also limited owing to the growing public deficit. The municipalities often argue that social transfers (including social housing) are primarily the responsibility of the state and should consequently mostly be financed out of the state budget; even if this financing arrangement were set up the municipalities still want to be free to decide whether to participate in the financing arrangement or not. There was also an attempt to introduce a cofinancing principle into the housing allowance scheme (cofinancing the total allowance due from municipal budgets), but the resistance from the municipalities was so strong that it was never introduced. Lobbying from the municipalities has been effective because many MPs are former mayors.

THE ROLE OF NGOS: CRISIS SHELTER

NGOs (private not-for-profit organizations) are engaged in housing provision for vulnerable and low-income households only in the form of providing temporary 'crisis' housing for people in acute housing need (asylum housing, lodging housing, halfway housing). Their activities are mostly financed by the MLSA under the provision of social services. Each year NGOs apply to the MLSA for funding through a grant procedure, which means that NGOs have no long-term income and have to seek new funding for their projects each year.[7]

The current system does not take much account of the need to provide social housing. There is no social service that is directly responsible for the provision and management of social housing. Moreover, the form of financing does not guarantee that the NGOs will be able to work in this field long term; they do not even know whether they will be able to offer asylum housing in the next year. Their activities are sometimes also financially supported by municipalities, but municipal contributions, in the opinion of NGOs, are marginal and again usually for just one year.

Despite the fact that no incentives are created for nonprofit organizations to be engaged in long-term social housing provision, no law prohibits NGOs from owning a housing fund. NGOs are now thinking more about deeper involvement in the provision of social housing. However, only some of them back this new perspective (shifting from the provision of temporary social services to long-term social housing), and there is an ongoing discussion on this topic nowadays. Currently, they have no ownership share in the permanent housing stock, but they have about a 70 percent share in the total stock of temporary 'crisis' housing (the remaining 30 percent is operated by municipalities).

STATE SUPPORT FOR SOCIAL HOUSING CONSTRUCTION

The state retained only an indirect influence on local social housing strategies, through the allocation of specific, and relatively marginal, state housing subsidies. The subsidy programs were drawn up by the MRD and passed by the Government. In 2010, there were basically two programs.

The Supported Housing Program

Introduced in 2003, the supported housing program aims to promote the construction of *supported (protected) municipal rental flats* for people with disadvantages in access to housing owing to health reasons (people with disabilities) or age (the elderly). Supported flats include protected flats for citizens with disabilities, flats in buildings with social care services for the elderly (over the age of seventy), and flats in halfway houses (for citizens living in a conflict situation, risky environment, or other special circumstances). The program also supports the construction of *start-up municipal rental flats* for citizens who, having tried all other social means, still find housing unattainable, young people who left institutional care, people undergoing resocializing programs in halfway houses or shelters, people with refugee status, and so on.

Under this program a capital subsidy is allocated in the form of a grant (equivalent to 30,100 U.S. dollars for a supported flat; 28,380 U.S. dollars for a start-up flat). The recipient of the subsidy is a municipality or group of municipalities. The rent is regulated at the level of cost rent, and supported housing allocation is subject to household income ceiling. Table 9.3 shows the number of flats built under this program in the past four years: it is clear that the volume of housing construction is very small.

The government backed the construction of new public rental housing even before 2003 (since 1995) through grants amounting to equivalent of 20,640 U.S. dollars (using current exchange rate) per housing unit built (in the late 1990s that was equal to around one-third of the cost of construction a housing unit). This subsidized housing construction formed a sizable portion of new housing output between 1995 and 2002; in total, around seventy thousand state-supported flats were built in this period.

Because there was no income ceiling (or other targeting) on dwelling allocation and above all because the program was legally transformed in a way where co-op form substituted public renting and, consequently, allowed speculation and abuse, it was heavily criticized and ultimately amended in 2003. The program allowed for the formation of housing cooperatives between the municipality and participants (future 'tenants'): a municipality, with the help of commercial developers, often did nothing more than secure the state subsidy and the remaining costs of construction were covered by down payments made by future 'tenants' and commercial mortgage loans taken by co-ops. Many co-op flats constructed under this program were consequently soon sold or rented out by participants who

Table 9.3 Number of Flats Built under the Program of Supported Housing, 2006–2009

Year	Subsidy (thousands U.S. dollars)			Number of flats		
	Total	Start-up flats	Supported flats	Total	Start-up flats	Supported flats
2006	2,672	8	26,710	698	4	694
2007	3,851	64	3,210	179	11	168
2008	6,023	4,698	1,354	210	156	54
2009	6,301	3,952	2,349	230	149	81

Source: Ministry for Regional Development, exchange rate as of January 2012

had profited from state subsidies. Moreover, some flats built under the program were actually secondary homes, and some were built as luxurious dwellings.

The abuse of the original system was criticized by the Supreme Audit Office, and it was discovered that high-ranking political representatives had also benefited from the program. Although some flats continued to serve as municipal rental housing, most of them were transformed into co-ops and can no longer be labeled social or public housing. As mentioned in the preceding, co-op housing is close to homeownership recently. Moreover, there is a pressure from co-op members to become full homeowners sooner than it is allowed by the program (i.e., after twenty years from the year of dwelling completion). Since 2003 the co-op form has been banned, cost and income ceilings have been introduced, and the level of subsidy has been increased. However, the volume of new subsidized housing construction sharply decreased.

Introduced in 2009, the social housing program allocates grants from the SFHD for the construction of *social rental flats* to all investors. The construction is supported with a grant of a maximum of 32,250 U.S. dollars per dwelling. Additionally, an investor may receive a grant of 2,580 U.S. dollars if the flat is accessible to people with disabilities (or can easily be converted into such a flat). The social dwelling must retain the status of social rental housing for a period of ten years; again the principle of cost rent applies and there are incomes caps on qualifying for allocation of a flat under the program. However, only a small number of social dwellings have been constructed under this program to date. Because the grant is relatively small (in relation to the low rent ceiling), private investors, and even NGOs, are not interested in it.

THE EFFECTIVENESS AND EFFICIENCY OF SOCIAL HOUSING STRATEGY

Property restitution, the segmentation of the rental market (as a result of rent regulation), and the giveaway privatization of municipal housing generated a variety of inequalities in housing accessibility and affordability. Tenants in restituted flats suddenly found themselves in a position different from that of tenants in flats owned by the state (later transferred to municipal authorities). Although their rents were regulated, restitution denied private tenants the opportunity that some public tenants later received—the option to buy their flats at a very advantageous price as part of public housing privatization. In addition, owing to a substantial decrease in the supply of public housing and the low tenancy turnover in rent-regulated housing, new households (young families) were restricted to securing housing in the public sector. This meant they had to find their housing in the private sector and pay a market rent several times higher than the rent paid for comparable housing in the regulated sector (Mikeszová, Lux, and Morisseau 2009).

Despite these inequalities the state did not introduce any central social housing strategy and instead came up with fragmented and indirect forms of interventions; specifically the two subsidy programs supporting new social housing construction. These have sparked little interest among investors because the grants were so small. Social housing is consequently still just a scattered collection of various approaches set independently by Czech municipalities, and it is almost impossible to make any overall systemic comparison and evaluation.

Social housing often takes the form of public housing operated under a specific rent control regime; such housing currently accounts for up to 10 percent of Czech housing stock. According to an analysis of rent-controlled housing made in 2002, rent regulation was almost equally applied to both 'rich' and 'poor' households (Lux and Sunega 2004). If the difference between market (equilibrium) and regulated rent is computed as an example of an implicit public economic subsidy, in 2002 higher-income households and middle-income households were the main recipients of this subsidy, whereas the lowest-income households benefited from this subsidy relatively the least. The overall stock of 'inherited' public housing under the rent regulation regime in the Czech Republic could therefore hardly be evaluated as effective help to those in need; on the contrary, it gave higher benefits to those who did not need it. New low-income households had very limited chances of getting into this type of housing unless they were in a position to benefit from the intergenerational transfer.

Under a stricter definition of social housing as public housing with controlled (regulated) rents allocated administratively according to the social situation of the applicant, the only cases that qualify are the municipal housing vacated and rented out again during the transition for regulated rent to those in need as part of a municipal social housing strategy, new municipal housing built since 2003 when the MRD's program was reformed, supported housing, social housing, and housing with social care built under the programs of the MRD. In this case the total social housing stock would make up an estimated 1–2 percent of the Czech housing stock. The difference from the figure cited earlier (10 percent) shows how ineffective the Czech national housing policy has been in the area of real supply-side subsidies targeting those in need. *Public housing* is not actually always a synonym for *social housing*. Growing spatial and social segregation in the past decade is a clear sign of how Czech housing policy has failed to better target public housing expenditures.

The total amount of the economic subsidy allocated to households living in rent-regulated housing is difficult to calculate, but it was estimated at 0.39 billion U.S. dollars in 2002 (Lux et al. 2004). If estimated correctly, this could be one of the largest housing subsidies in the Czech Republic. It has already been demonstrated that much of this subsidy could have been saved because it was going to households that did not need it. Moreover, rent regulation in one housing market segment can have a substantial impact on rent prices in another market segment where rents are negotiated freely. This theoretical argument has been verified in the Czech environment by econometric simulations (Lux and Sunega 2004). According to these simulations, in Prague equilibrium market rents in 2002 would have been about one-third lower than the skewed 'market' rents that existed then if rent control had been immediately abolished. People with no access to 'privileged' housing paid in this way a substantial part of the bill for hidden economic subsidies to tenants of rent-regulated housing.

I also mentioned in the preceding how the state subsidy program for the construction of 'municipal' housing was abused. Here again the state distributed public expenditures among many households that did not need it. The substantial amount of these subsidies went to the construction of dwellings for high-income occupants or even to the construction of luxurious or secondary housing. Consequently, the Czech state's social housing policy can hardly be evaluated as efficient.

It is impossible to make a final conclusion owing to the unprecedented level of decentralization in housing policy. In some cities with an active local government the supply of social dwellings from both the existing and new municipal housing stock may be sufficient, but it seems that in most cities, and especially in the main centers of employment, the demand for social housing far exceeds the supply. The lack of social rental housing is partially substituted by the intergenerational transfer of wealth and 'privilege', but this does not really apply to the most vulnerable households. The whole system is unsustainable in the long term as it produces inequalities in housing accessibility and affordability. 'Insiders' (including both low- and high-income households) are well protected, but 'outsiders' (including again both low- and high-income households and especially young families, poor people with no chance of inheriting privileged housing, and migrants) have almost no protection and little chance of getting any supported housing. Homeless people have to rely on temporary housing provisions provided mostly by NGOs or private landlords. The road back to affordable rental housing is extremely difficult for them, in part owing to the unwillingness of municipalities to cooperate with NGOs on this issue.

CONCLUSION

The segment of social housing in the Czech Republic is small, mainly owing to the following facts: a substantial portion of the existing public housing does not serve people in need; the central government has consistently failed to introduce any social housing legislation or long-term social housing strategy; and there is very little new construction of real (well-targeted) social housing subsidized by *ad hoc* government programs. Almost all social housing is owned by the municipalities. Due to the decentralization of power the municipalities are free to pass their own local social housing strategies. NGOs play a role only in the temporary provision of 'crisis' housing, but this situation may change in the near future.

The main factors for the lack of any central (state) social housing strategy are: disconnected nature of housing policy, overseen by three ministries; the preference of MPs to support owner-occupied housing than rental housing; the decentralization of power among numerous small and financially weak municipalities; and very effective lobbying on the part of municipalities to resist any uniform social housing strategy or any legislative change that would increase the responsibility of municipalities in this area. The Czech state's path-dependent housing policy, promoting public housing construction with poor or even no targeting, is also a factor. The Czech state was traditionally generous in subsidization of new public housing construction, but under the new market reality of growing income inequalities since 1990 the lack of clear targeting made this policy ineffective.

Extending the part of socialist legacy by conserving various 'privileges' for sitting public tenants (through regulated rent and low purchase prices during privatization) had the effect of compensating for the lack of social housing in the early phase of the post-1989 transition as 'privileges' were transferred between generations. However, the consequences of this untargeted policy, such as inequalities in housing affordability and accessibility, show that such an approach is neither effective nor sustainable in the long term. Spatial segregation, almost unknown until 1990, has surfaced and intensified in recent years and has especially affected households of ethnic minorities and households in a difficult financial situation. The long-term and centrally framed social housing strategy is needed. It seems that even politicians, who until now favored growing homeownership, understand the new reality, and proposals on social housing have a better chance of being introduced in practice recently.

NOTES

1. Most private residential buildings were expropriated and became the property of the state. Private landlords were forced to sell their buildings to the state for extremely low prices or received no compensation at all.
2. For example, between 1965 and 1990 there was no change in the level of rent.
3. The deregulation of controlled rents started in 1992 allowing landlords to introduce a onetime, 100 percent rent increase. In the following years the maximum regulated rent was set in relevant government decrees. However, since 1999 the maximum ceased rising in real terms and since 2002 also in nominal terms (a decrease in real regulated rents occurred). The process of rent deregulation was not restarted until 2007.
4. With the exception of Law on Value Added Tax No. 235/2004, §48a.—which defines social housing for the purpose of keeping a lower VAT tax rate on new housing construction and as such represents only a formal issue

of how to cope with the EU requirements on VAT—almost all new housing construction is included into the 'social housing' category there.

5. Additionally, the State Fund for Housing Development (SFHD) executes some programs prepared by the MRD.
6. Due to dynamic privatization processes after 2001, the 2001 Census is not suitable for qualitative description of the stock and recent information will be released only after the 2011 Census.
7. The other possibility to finance activities of NGOs in the field of temporal (asylum, halfway) social housing provision is the grant from the European Social Fund, respectively from structural funds of the EU. The main program in this field is the Operational Program: Human Sources and Employment. The grants allocated through the MLSA may be, in this case, used also on long-term projects (such as three-year projects), covering both personal and investment costs and not limited to types of social services defined by the Law on Social Services.

REFERENCES

Hegedüs, J. and Tosics, I. 1998. "Rent Reform—Issues for Countries of Eastern Europe and the Newly Independent States." *Housing Studies* 13:657–58.

Krebs, V.,, Durdisová, J., Kotýnková, M., Mertl, J., Poláková, O., Žižková, J., Vlček, M., Vychová, M. 2005. *Sociální politika (Social Policy).* Prague: ASPI.

Lux, M. 2009. *Housing Policy and Housing Finance in the Czech Republic during Transition.* Amsterdam: Delft University Press.

Lux, M. and Sunega, P. 2004. "Modelování rovnovážné úrovně nájemného a důsledků aplikace vybraných nástrojů bytové politiky (Modeling Equilibrium Market Rents and the Impact of Selected Housing Policy Tools)." *Finance a úvěr* 53:31–59.

———. 2006. "Vývoj finanční dostupnosti nájemního a vlastnického bydlení v průběhu hospodářské transformace v České republice (1991–2003) (Trends in the Affordability of Rental and Owner-Occupied Housing in the Course of the Transformation in the Czech Republic [1991–2003])." *Sociologický časopis/Czech Sociological Review* 42:851–81.

———. 2010. "Private Rental Housing in the Czech Republic: Growth and . . . ?" *Czech Sociological Review* 46:349–73.

Lux, M., Sunega, P., Kostelecký, T., Čermák, D., and Košinár, P. 2004. *Standardy bydlení 2003/2004: Bytová politika v ČR: efektivněji a cíleněji (Housing Standards 2003/2004: Housing policy in the Czech Republic: More Effective and More Efficient).* Prague: Institute of Sociology.

Lux, M., Sunega, P., Kostelecký, T., Čermák, D., and Montag, J. 2005. *Standardy bydlení 2004/05 (Housing Standards 2004/05).* Prague: Institute of Sociology.

Marcuse, P. 1996. "Privatization and Its Discontents: Property Rights in Land and Housing in the Transition in Eastern Europe." *Cities after Socialism.* Cambridge: Blackwell Publisher.

Mikeszová, M., Lux, M., and Morisseau A. 2009. "Potenciální finanční nedostupnost nájemního bydlení po deregulaci nájemného—regionální perspektiva (The Potential Unaffordability of Rental Housing after Rent Deregulation in Regional Perspective)." *Sociologický časopis/Czech Sociological Review* 45:315–43.

Možný, I. 1994. "Pokus o mimoekonomické vysvětlení současné plné zaměstnanosti v České republice (An Attempt at a Noneconomic Explanation for Full Employment in the Czech Republic)." *Sociologický časopis/Czech Sociological Review* 30:463–74.

Sýkora, L. and Šimoníčková, I. 1994. "From Totalitarian Urban Managerialism to a Liberalized Real Estate Market: Prague's Transformations in the Early 1990s." *Development and administration of Prague*. Amsterdam: University of Amsterdam.

Večerník, J. 2009. *Czech Society in the 2000s: A Report on Socio-Economic Policies and Structures*. Prague: Academia.

Večerník, J. and Matějů, P., eds. 1998. *Zpráva o vývoji české společnosti 1989–1998 (Report on the Development of Czech Society 1989–1998)*. Prague: Academia.

10 Estonia

Residualization of Social Housing and the New Programs*

Anneli Kährik and Jüri Kõre

INTRODUCTION

The transition from a communist to a post-communist society ushered in major changes in the housing system in Estonia. Processes and reforms connected with the decentralization of power, housing, and land privatization appeared in all Central and Eastern European (CEE) countries but each country (group of countries) has had its own specific features throughout the reform process and its own specific outcomes determined by the path dependence of specific policies and cultural patterns (Hegedüs and Tosics 1998; Pichler-Milanovich 2001). The communist system treated housing as a public asset that is not part of the market and to which every citizen should have access (Hegedüs and Tosics 1996; Kornai 1992). The principles of the system aimed at ensuring egalitarian living standards for all (Smith 1996). The extensive nationalization of private housing was launched in Estonia in 1941 soon after its incorporation into the Soviet Union. At the end of the socialist period, two-thirds of the housing stock belonged to the state. The communist system did not use term *social housing* because state-owned dwellings were in principle accessible to all.

After 1990, privatization was carried out at a faster pace and on a broader scale than in the other CEE countries (Lux 2003). Modifications in tenure concepts based on occupancy rights and obligations were altered as well. Reforms were based on neoliberal policy, that is, housing relations were determined mainly by market principles and according to filtration theory (Bourne 1981). However, like in the communist period, social housing did not become a clearly defined concept in post-1990 Estonia. Consequently, in this chapter we simply consider all residual public housing owned recently by municipalities as social housing because it has features characteristic of social housing in developed societies: subsidized rent, eligibility criteria, and more favorable disposal rights than in the private rental sector.

In this chapter we aim to analyze the impact of the extensive reform of public housing tenure in Estonia from two main perspectives—first, its impact on the concept of social housing and, second, its impact on spatial distribution patterns and the physical conditions of social housing. We also provide an assessment of the new municipal housing construction program applied in Tallinn. The analyses are based on legal documents, aggregated data from the Population and Housing Census 2000 (Statistics Estonia), data on new social housing construction initiated by the Municipality of Tallinn[1], and data from the Survey on Municipal Housing (SMH) 2005 (Ministry of Social Affairs 2005).[2] We apply the capital city of Tallinn as a case study area to analyze intraurban differentiation in social housing.

EVOLUTION OF THE CONCEPT OF SOCIAL HOUSING

The Communist Period

Estonian housing policy lacks long-term continuity. Radical shifts in housing policy were introduced in 1940. The policy based on the prevalence of owner-occupied housing until 1940 was replaced by a 'state-owned housing system', where the financing, construction, and allocation of housing were subordinated to central planning (Kõre et al. 1996; Szelényi 1996). The nationalized pre-1941 housing stock contributed to public housing, but so did new construction, peaking in the prefabricated housing construction between 1958 and 1985 to house large numbers of labor immigrants from other parts of the Soviet Union. To a much lower extent, semipublic cooperatives (5 percent of total stock) and private (semi)detached housing (13 percent of total stock) were also built (Ibid). The private rental sector took the form of a 'black market'.

Soviet enterprises, ministries, and local administrations played the main role in public housing allocation during the socialist period (Tammaru 2001). Despite declarative goals of equal housing distribution and universal access to public housing, inequalities existed in the allocation of public housing: advantaged groups were often members of the 'nomenklatura', that is, the political and economic elite, and selectively also people working in creative industry and top researchers. In addition to social capital, human capital also mattered, as people with a university degree enjoyed the best housing conditions (Gentile and Tammaru 2006; Kulu 2003), so residential segregation in public housing existed by age, education, occupation, and ethnic origin (Raitviir 1990). The pre-Soviet housing stock suffered from a lack of maintenance and was inhabited mostly by lower social status groups (Szelényi 1996; Ruoppila and Kährik 2003). The good availability of housing amenities and infrastructure and high state subsidies encouraged an overall preference for newly built public flats in prefabricated buildings (Kährik and Tammaru 2010; Temelová et al. 2010).

Rents in public housing were below replacement costs, covering about 20 percent of cost rent. Once the dwelling was allotted, public housing tenants enjoyed almost unlimited occupancy rights for their dwellings, similar to owner-occupation under market conditions: open-term leases, the right to inherit property, the right to carry out maintenance work, and so on. Although no official system for exchanging or subletting public rental flats existed, in reality tenants could also sublet flats or exchange them on the black market. Good lease terms and occupancy rights made public housing the preferred housing among the public.

Housing Reforms after 1990

In 1991 the prewar housing system began to be restored. Housing policy reforms contrasted with the objectives of the communist regime, aiming at the quick expansion of owner-occupied housing and the withdrawal of government from housing maintenance. Whereas prior to ownership reform in 1994, 64 percent of dwellings in Estonia belonged to the state (44 percent in rural and 72 percent in urban areas), by 2002 the share of privately owned dwellings had increased to 96 percent.

The ownership reform in Estonia, like in many other CEE countries (Lux et al. 2012; Clapham and Kintrea 1996), was grounded in a discourse based on ideology (i.e., redressing the injustices caused by the communist regime and a belief in markets and individual responsibility) and pragmatism (reducing public expenditure and increasing economic efficiency). Ownership reform involved restoring the pre-1940 ownership structure (i.e., restitution) and the privatization of the housing stock. Restitution affected about 3 percent of the housing stock, and all of the affected properties had sitting tenants. Special housing policy measures later targeted tenants in restituted properties (for more, see Kährik et al. 2003; Lux et al. 2012). However, rent regulation stipulating upper rent limits in restituted dwellings was abolished in 2004 and the sector now functions like the free private sector.

Large-scale housing privatization started in 1994 and had two stages: state-owned dwellings were transferred to municipal ownership and then they were privatized to tenants. Due to strong pressure for privatization by tenants and the heavy burden social dwellings put on municipal budgets, municipalities seldom used their right to retain certain dwellings as social housing. No consideration was given to future needs at that time. National capital vouchers (NCVs) were used for privatization and the direct financial costs of purchase were very low. Altogether 98 percent of the apartment housing stock was privatized through NCVs to sitting tenants. Because public tenants under the communist regime enjoyed a status similar to homeowners in market economies, former tenants got almost no additional disposal rights from privatization, except for the legal right to sell or exchange the dwelling in the housing market. Consequently, privatization did not cause any change in social status. Vertical mobility in status could only appear when selling/renting out the property for profit.

Social Housing Today

The basic legal instruments and principles regulating housing relations changed after 1991, when Estonia regained its independence. The country's social housing policy derives from basic laws and directives and from individual political initiatives tabled by central or LAs. The implementation of social housing policy is mainly delegated to the level of the LAs, yet their strategies and actions depend on the political orientation and financial resources of each LA. The capital city of Tallinn is the only LA in Estonia that applied the two new social housing programs created in the post-1990 era: the Residential Construction Program 5,000 Dwellings for Tallinn in 2002 (RCP-1 2002) and the 2nd Residential Construction Program for Tallinn in 2008 (RCP-2 2008).

Table 10.1 shows that the provision of social housing is the main supply-side public measure targeting lower-income groups, whereas the only demand-side measure is the subsistence benefit system (tenure neutral). The share of households receiving the benefit declined between 1998 and 2009

Table 10.1 Main Housing Policy Measures in Estonia in the Post-Transition Period, 2000s

Type of means	Policy measures	Target groups
Supply side	Allocation of subsidized (existing, new) social housing	Low income/less than average income
	State/LA subsidy for constructing new social housing	Low income
	Allocation of municipal sites and provision of infrastructure for the construction of social housing/ private housing	Low income, average income
	State/ LA renovation grants for apartment blocks	All
Demand side	Tax deduction on home mortgage interest	Average, upper income
	Housing loan guarantees to eligible groups	Average
	Special housing loan schemes/ other measures aimed at sitting tenants in restituted housing	Low income, average income
	Subsistence benefits (including compensation for housing and utilities costs)	Low income, average income

(from 13.9 percent to 3.3 percent) as a result of improving socioeconomic conditions and the creation of other social welfare benefits (Ministry of Social Affairs 2011).

The Social Welfare Act (1995) established the right to state assistance in case of need, which requires LAs in such a case to provide appropriate housing (see also Kährik et al. 2003). The criteria of eligibility are set the by LAs, but there are two principal ways in which dwelling allocation is handled. In most cases dwellings are allocated according to a priority list. According to SMH the following households have priority: families whose dwellings have been destroyed in an accident, catastrophe, or by demolition; orphans; disabled people or people with special needs; and former tenants in restituted housing. In other cases, each applicant is assessed individually using multiple evaluation criteria, for example, applicants' current housing situation and his/her socioeconomic status.

In some LAs a distinction is made between specific social housing, which means housing that is allotted to social welfare clients, and other municipal housing, which is the residual (unprivatized) public housing with sitting tenants, or dwellings allotted to other households. In reality the difference between social and other municipal dwellings is vague. According to SMH, most social housing in Estonia is in the direct ownership and administration of LAs; in 83 percent of cases the regular housing management is also implemented by LAs or LA-owned companies. In Tallinn, public–private partnership (PPP) schemes have been developed in the field of social housing (see the following).

Over 90 percent of LAs subsidize rent to cover the costs of the housing (SMH). Recent rents in social housing are estimated to cover on average one-third of total costs. The bases of rent setting vary between LAs, but are most often related to the physical conditions of dwellings, location, and the tenants' socioeconomic status. Only one-quarter of LAs have applied the same rent level to all social dwellings. Despite subsidies, rent arrears form a wide-scale problem in social dwellings: in total, 7 percent of social tenants have had rent arrears lasting more than three months (Kõre et al. 1996). A part of the problem of rising debt is the lack of coordination between the provision of social subsistence benefits (operated by the Ministry of Social Affairs) and rent payments in social housing.

The standard (prescribed) duration of a lease is five years, after which the tenant normally has a right to prolong the lease for another five-year period. This generally applies to sitting tenants in the residual social housing left after privatization. The same law provides landlords with an opportunity to sign leases that terminate after one year, after which the tenant is obliged to leave. New leases for social housing clients most often fall into the latter category. In the case of justified need the lease is prolonged for another year. Short-term leases are preferred because social housing has recently come to be considered a temporary form of housing, especially in larger municipalities.

The survey conducted among municipalities (SMH) reveals that the need for social housing exceeds the existing supply in most LAs in Estonia. On average, the existing supply covers 80 percent of the need, and the need for social housing is estimated as higher in larger cities, where the existing stock covers two-thirds of the estimated need. The LAs regard the eligibility criteria for social housing as mostly adequate: the majority of LA representatives agreed that there is no need to extend the target group, and just a minor share of LAs suggested allocation housing also to young families and labor immigrants.

The low political priority accorded to formulating a social housing strategy, the lack of finance, the policy of treating social housing as a temporary form of housing, the unstable political environment, and the minimum criteria on social housing standards all help to explain the relatively poor status of social housing recently and the insecurity of such tenure today.

NEW SOCIAL HOUSING CONSTRUCTION IN TALLINN

An Overview

Tallinn is the largest city in Estonia, with a population of 400,800 in 2000 (399,400 in 2010) (Statistics Estonia). It has 172,800 dwellings, and per capita floor space is equal to 23 square meters (in 2000). The housing market is largely made up of Soviet high-rise housing estates, which is where most of the city's residents live. About 12 percent of apartment dwellings were built before 1946. In total 91 percent of citizens live in apartment buildings.

In an atmosphere of general apathy towards social housing, the municipality of Tallinn stands out with its new policy to significantly increase the social housing sector. The Residential Construction Program adopted in 2002 (RCP-1 2002) envisioned the construction of two thousand municipal dwellings and three thousand private dwellings (PPPs) between 2003 and 2007, with the aim of addressing the problem of the lack of affordable modern living space in the city and decelerating the rapid inflation of housing prices over that same period. Social dwellings were to be established under direct LA ownership or as PPPs in the form of long-term lease of dwellings built and owned by private developers to the LA. In the PPP projects, it was planned that the LA would participate on construction costs by providing municipal land and technical infrastructure (RCP-1 2002; Interim Report of the RCP-1 2007). The main criteria for choosing potential locations for social housing developments were the following: (a) the land is available to the municipality or is owned by the municipality; (b) the areas are not attractive to private sector developments and cannot be regenerated without public support. The planned budget for the five-year period of the project was 75.4 million U.S. dollars, with a state contribution of 25 percent or 19.5 million U.S. dollars and a contribution from Tallinn's LA of 45.9 million U.S. dollars.

The main target groups were, however, tenants in restituted housing: thirty-five hundred out of the five thousand applicants registered on the waiting list in 2002 were tenants in restituted housing. The rent that was to be paid by tenants was regulated at a level of 1.7 U.S. dollars per square meter per month and 1 U.S. dollar per square meter per month for regular expenses, that is, on average 166.4 U.S. dollars per month per dwelling. In addition to the social housing program, the municipality of Tallinn also aimed to implement owner-occupied housing construction projects as PPPs targeting former tenants in restituted housing and young families. The plans were to build around one thousand dwellings between 2002 and 2007 as detached, semidetached, or apartment housing, with a total estimated investment of 93.6 million U.S. dollars, of which the municipality would cover 15.6 million U.S. dollars.

Compared to the social housing program passed in 2002, the RCP-2 program passed in 2008 broadened its ambit: it planned to support more the labor force the city relies on ('key workers') and improve the housing conditions of young families. The program also aimed to create a stable (in terms of prices), adequately sized and secure rental sector. The term *key workers* refers to public sector professionals with below-average income, such as people working in educational institutions, social welfare services, health services, police officers, and rescue services. Nevertheless, the document states (RCP-2 2008) that in the future the definition of the key workers eligible for social housing will broaden in scope. A 'young family' here is a family or single parent with at least one child under the age of sixteen. This program envisioned the construction of around one thousand dwellings.

Thus, the main difference between the program passed in 2008 and the previous program is that a shift occurred away from specifically targeted social housing tenure to much broader eligibility criteria, with the quite ambitious goal of integrating social rental housing in the overall housing market. The principles for implementing the program were similar to those in the RCP-1: a part of the housing would to be built under the direct ownership of the LA and the rest as PPPs. It was estimated that the rent would be around two-thirds of cost rent and half of market rent in new flats built in the private sector (RCP-2 2008). The rent was to be differentiated according to target groups: two-thirds of cost rent for the 'key workers' and five-sixths of cost rent for 'young families'; this was 6.5 U.S. dollars per square meter per month on average. The rule implemented was that rent could increase by 5 percent per year, which meant shifting the actual rent to cost rent level over a seven- to ten-year period.

Outcomes and Estimated Impacts on Equity and Efficiency

As an outcome of the RCP-1, 914 housing units were built in LA ownership and 680 as PPPs between 2003 and 2008. Most of them are five- and eight-story apartment buildings and they are rented to tenants for a period up to five years. As a result of the RCP-2, 1,214 social housing units were built as PPPs by private developers between 2009 and 2011; these are concentrated in three fifteen-story tower buildings. Thus, two RCP programs added almost three thousand new social dwellings, or nearly 2 percent of the total housing stock of Tallinn, with one-third of them in the direct ownership of the LA. All of the newly built dwellings are located in buildings with 100 percent social dwellings.

Of the new social housing units built between 2000 and 2011, 63 percent were allocated to tenants in restituted housing, 20 percent to social welfare clients, and 17 percent to young families or 'key workers'. Nearly 2 percent of all households in Tallinn got an apartment in new social housing between 2000 and 2011. Due to the high demand for social housing, the eligible households were selected on the basis of an evaluation form (the sum of points assigned to each applicant household) that took into consideration factors such as the applicant's existing housing conditions, socioeconomic situation, number of children in the household, and other criteria (Tallinn City Government 2009a, b).

In 2009, coinciding with the bottom of the economic regression cycle, which had some severe social consequences, we noticed an important turn in the neoliberal housing policy that had existed in Estonia: there was an effort to encompass a broader range of population groups in the allocation of social housing. Therefore, between 2009 and 2011, 45 percent of newly built social housing units were allocated to young families and key workers. Moreover, there is a plan to extend eligibility also to other below-average income groups in the future (RCP-2 2008).

The three different methods for providing social dwellings in Tallinn are following:

1. social dwellings in LA ownership: with a rent of 2 U.S. dollars per square meter per month intended to cover the management and maintenance costs, but not construction costs;
2. dwellings built and owned by private developers and leased to LA (PPPs), where LA substantially participated on construction costs (providing land and infrastructure free of charge): with a rent of 9 U.S. dollars per square meter per month, of which 2.3 U.S. dollars per square meter per month (26 percent) is paid by the tenant and the rest by the LA;
3. dwellings built and owned by private developers and leased to LA (PPPs) with minor public participation on construction costs (built on private land): with a rent of 11.7 U.S. dollars per square meter per month, of which 2.5 (2) U.S. dollars per square meter per month is paid by the tenant (i.e., 21 percent/18 percent of the total rent) and the rest by the LA.

Consequently, even in the last category of social housing where the largest client group is formed by young families or 'key workers', four-fifths of the rent is directly subsidized by the LA and only one-fifth is paid by the tenant. Considering the high level of subsidization, methods 2 and 3 can be considered as economically ineffective and with the side effect of subsidizing private developers and paying them high profits at the expense of city taxpayers. Considering the rent arrears among occupants (long-term debtors make up 5 percent of tenants), the financial burden on the municipal budget is very heavy. In addition, the contracts that were made between the LA and private developers at a time of a real estate boom (2007) were concluded for a twenty-year period. However, from 2007 to 2011, rents in the private market decreased from 9 U.S. dollars spent per square meter per month (2007) to 5.2 U.S. dollars per square meter per month (2011) in the same area (see http://spot.city24.ee, page visited 10.10.2011).

The implementation of policy also diverged from the initial plans. Instead of building dwellings in LA ownership or providing municipal land to reduce the cost of housing, the path taken led to long-term lease flats from a private developer that were built on private land, with an agreed fixed rent much higher than originally assumed. In view of the fact that these social dwellings were built with the public sector's participation in the form of providing infrastructure, the rent paid by the LA to the private developer is unreasonably high. Another departure from the initial plan was the agreed rent paid by tenants: contrary to initial plans it is ultimately more subsidized and is further below the level of cost rent. Consequently, there is a large gap between the established goal of gradually adjusting cost rent and the real situation: this housing was subsidized in the same extent as public housing under the communist regime.

SPATIAL DISTRIBUTION AND THE CONDITIONS OF SOCIAL HOUSING

Methodology

To examine analytical questions of the physical patterns of social housing distribution, we used mainly Census 2000 data (next to the SMH 2005 data described in the preceding). The year 2000 is a good year for analyses because by that time the new housing construction programs had not yet been launched and the pattern in evidence is the one most directly resulting from housing privatization and the Soviet housing construction/allocation policy. We used aggregated data to analyze the spatial distribution of 'old' social housing (residual public housing after privatization), where data on dwellings is aggregated by 0.25 km^2 spatial units (cells). Census data on 'old' social housing are complemented by data on new social housing built in Tallinn between 2000 and 2011 under programs described in the preceding.

Our hypothesis was that significant intraurban differences in spatial distribution of social housing existed in following building-related variables: (a) type of building (categories: single-family/apartment) and (b) time of building construction (categories: before 1946 and after 1946). We also aimed to study other spatial regularities outside the spatial distribution of these variables, including whether a higher concentration of social dwellings can be found in large housing estates. We used the socioeconomic variables of different city subdistricts and other local characteristics identified in previous studies as background variables to explain spatial variations in social housing.

To study the regularities of spatial patterns, we applied a statistical general linear model (Model 1), with binary coding 0:1 of the dependent variable: social dwellings not available/available in the subarea. The independent variables were the following: (a) dwelling type and (b) the age structure of dwellings by spatial units. The respective types were classified into 2-by-3 classes (e.g., prevailingly single-family areas/mixed type areas/apartment-dominated areas). But we also used a visual comparison of maps to explore regularities in social housing distribution in 2000 and the locations of new social dwellings in relation to the existing social housing pattern.

The Physical Conditions of Social Housing in Estonia

The supply of social housing is mostly made up of 'old' unprivatized public housing. A residual share of public dwellings was not privatized for two main reasons: the conditions of the dwellings were very poor and tenants lacked resources for privatization (NCVs, money) (Kährik 2000). Also, with the departure from Estonia of military and other migrants returning to the former Soviet republics in the early 1990s, a number of municipal dwellings were vacated, many of them in areas that are not attractive enough for them to sell well in public auctions.

The Census 2000 data give the best overview of the results of ownership reform, which reflect regional differences in the number of social dwellings. On average, half of all social dwellings are located in buildings that contain 100 percent social housing (SMH). The overall physical conditions of social dwellings are poor and reveal the need for substantial investment (Census 2000). Compared to owner-occupied housing, the share of social dwellings that lack modern amenities (running water, sewerage, bath/shower, indoor toilet) is high; for example, 57 percent of social dwellings have a bath/shower whereas in the private sector the figure is 84 percent (Kährik et al. 2003, 208). According to the SMH, the share of social dwellings that lack modern amenities ranges between 46 percent and 57 percent in different settlement types. The rest are apartments in high-rise housing built during the 1960s–1980s. These are full-amenity flats, but without modern renovations.

The Case Study of Tallinn

Figure 10.1 portrays the spatial distribution of the total housing stock. There are four districts with large socialist high-rise housing estates: the densely built high-rise subarea in North-Tallinn (built in the 1950s–1960s; now the most depreciated housing stock relative to other estates); Mustamäe (built in the 1960s); subarea of Haabersti ('Õismäe' built in the 1970s, with relatively good-quality and good-size apartments); and Lasnamäe (built in the 1980s, the largest and most densely built estate, with one hundred thousand inhabitants or 25 percent of the city's entire population). The dense central city is surrounded by old historical quarters consisting mostly of smaller-scale, wooden apartment buildings from the nineteenth century. However, the quality and attractiveness of these historical dwellings vary. Nõmme, Pirita, and parts of Haabersti are the districts dominated by single-family housing (Figure 10.1).

The final model presented in Table 10.2 gives the following results. First, it shows a significant correlation between the share of apartments by subareas and the availability of social dwellings. Importantly, the mixed-housing areas (25–75 percent apartments) have the highest (relative) share of social dwellings. Areas dominated by detached housing contain very few social dwellings (see Figure 10.2). The share of pre-1946 dwellings in subareas (both areas dominated by prewar housing stock or areas with housing of mixed age) became a significant factor explaining higher share of social housing only in interaction with the type of dwelling structure in subareas.

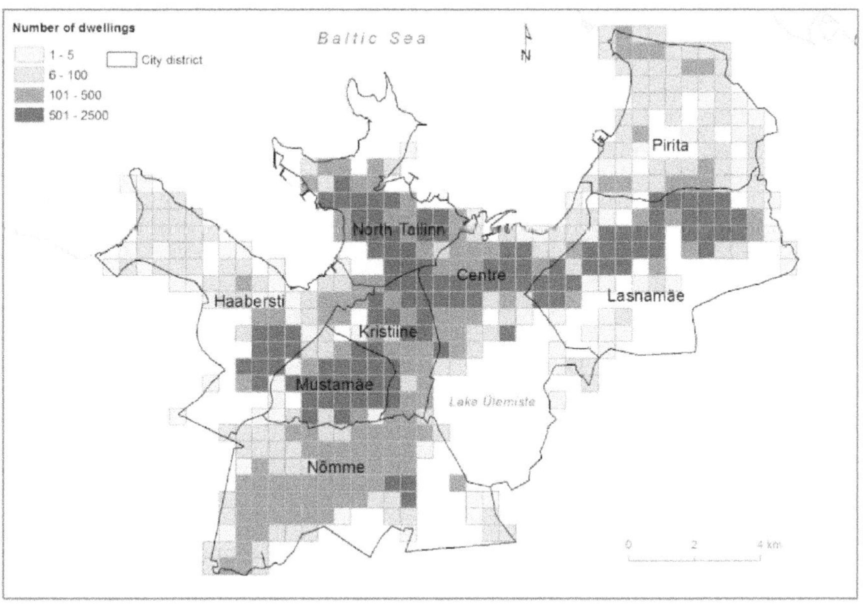

Figure 10.1 Distribution of dwelling units in Tallinn in 2000 by spatial units (0.25 km^2 cells) (number of dwellings).

Table 10.2 Impact of Housing Type Structure in an Area on the Presence of Social Housing Units (Model 1). Parameter Estimates; No Social Housing = 0; Social Housing Exists = 1

Parameter	B	t	Sig.
Housing types in area (ref = single-family housing with less than 25% flats)			
Mixed (25–75% flats)	0.276	2.750	0.006 **
Apartment area (75%+ flats)	0.285	5.172	0.000 ***
Period of construction (ref=1946–1991, with less than 25% in pre-1946 dwellings)			
Mixed (25–75% in pre-1946 dwellings)	0.104	1.279	0.202
Old (75%+ in pre-1946 dwellings)	-0.098	-1.073	0.284
Interactions			
Mixed dwelling types* Mixed age	0.059	0.352	0.725
Mixed dwelling types*old housing	0.331	1.925	0.055
Flat area*mixed age	0.302	2.211	0.028 ***
Flat area*old housing	0.513	3.909	0.000 ***
Intercept	1.133	27.158	0.000 ***

Note: R Squared = 0.219 (Adjusted R Squared = 0.203).

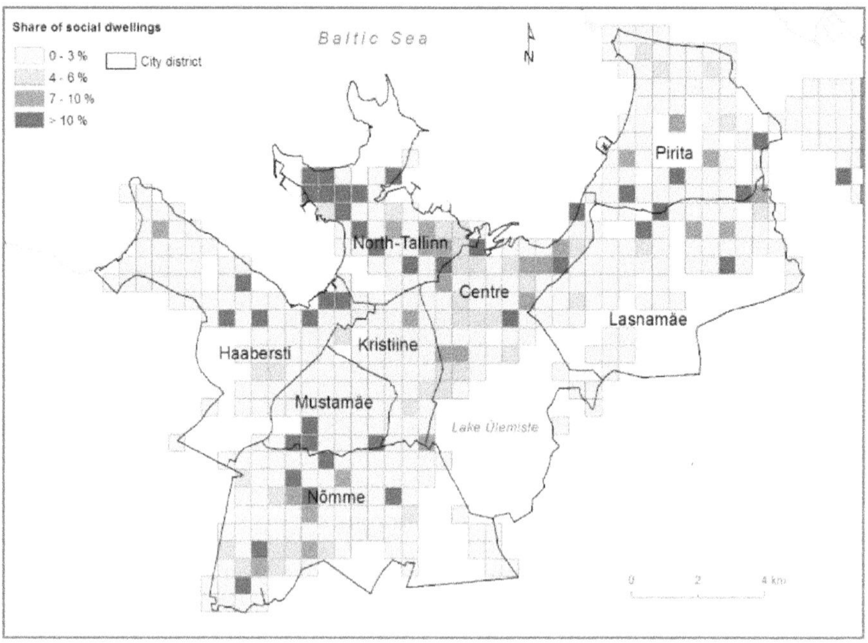

Figure 10.2 Percentage of social housing units in Tallinn in 2000 by spatial units (0.25 km² cells).

We did not find a general correlation between the share of social dwellings and socialist high-rise housing estates by comparing maps. Two estates in particular (Mustamäe and Õismäe) have a tenant structure with higher socioeconomic status, have better physical surroundings (Ruoppila and Kährik 2003; Kährik and Tammaru 2010), and have a relatively low share of social dwellings, except a few social dwelling hostels on the edges of Mustamäe (Figure 10.2). Yet, some locations with a high concentration of social dwellings were found in Lasnamäe and North-Tallinn: the estate with the highest share of industrial workers and lower-educated groups. In total 24 percent of social dwellings in the city of Tallinn are located in North-Tallinn, compared to 12 percent of private housing, which is the highest over-representation of social housing in the city. We can thus confirm that high-rise estates in general do not represent concentrations of social dwellings, but the tenant structure with lower socioeconomic status and worse physical conditions in certain locations increases the likelihood of a concentration of social flats.

Figure 10.3 maps the locations of new social housing construction in Tallinn and analyzes the spatial patterns of new social housing relative to existing social housing. In total, 3,259 new social dwellings were built between 2000 and 2010: 40 percent in municipal ownership and 60 percent as PPPs. Figure 10.3 shows that 75 percent of new social dwellings

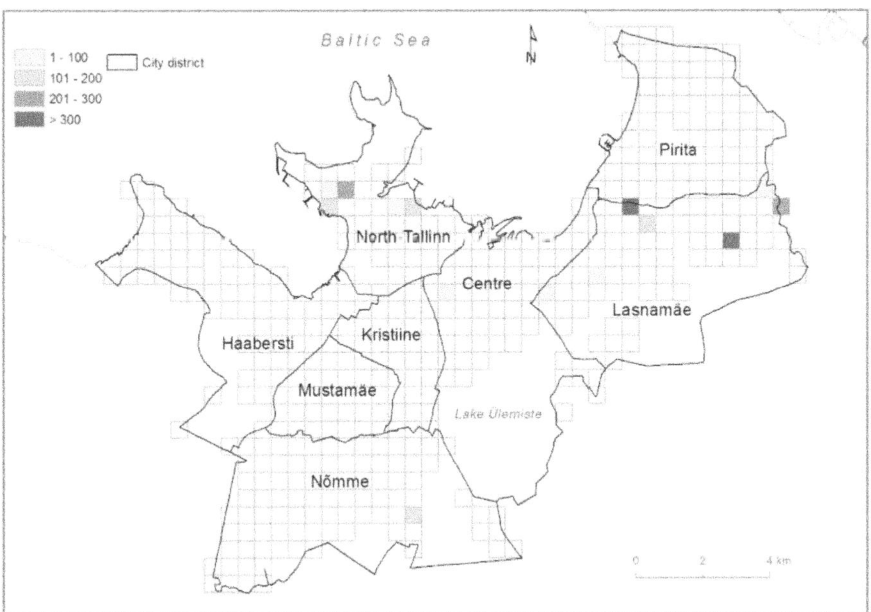

Figure 10.3 Number of new social housing units built in 2000–2010 by spatial units (0.25 km² cells).

were constructed in Lasnamäe and about 20 percent in North-Tallinn. The pattern of new housing locations is very concentrated. Although the new housing is equipped with all modern amenities and is of relatively good standards, its high concentration in certain areas is likely to have severe consequences, most notably the further spatial segregation of lower social-status groups in the urban space (because the social status of the two districts is already among the lowest in Tallinn).

CONCLUSION

This chapter analyzed the evolution of the concept of social housing from the time of the communist regime to the post-transition era and investigated the impacts of housing privatization and new social housing policies on the spatial patterns of social housing distribution during the 2000s. Whereas public housing in Soviet Estonia was a universal type of housing and a highly subsidized tenure, in the post-transition era only selected groups of the neediest families had access to 'old' public housing that remained after giveaway privatization. Compared to the communist era the terms on which social dwellings are leased have generally become less favorable for tenants and the tenure less secure. Yet, the rent is still mostly subsidized by the LAs. Despite this, rent arrears are a common problem due to the low income of tenants, resulting in low economic efficiency and difficulties in property management. The marginal size of social housing in Estonia today means that it is not an integrated part of the housing market in direct competition with other tenures. For this same reason the effect of social housing on social equality is slight. However, despite its inflexibility and problems, social housing plays a modest role in eliminating housing market deficiencies and enabling housing access for the most needy.

Ownership reform and the strong pressure for privatizing on the part of both citizens and the LAs were the factors most responsible for reducing the number of public dwellings to just a marginal share of the housing stock and relegating this form of tenure to housing with much poorer conditions than in the privatized sector. Our analyses revealed a highly spatially segregated pattern of social dwellings on the intraurban level in Tallinn, with the highest concentration of social housing in certain inner-urban neighborhoods made up of poor quality pre-1946 housing. The distribution of social housing follows the more general patterns of disadvantaged areas in Tallinn in 2000, although in some older areas now gentrification takes place as well. We can thus see a certain trajectory of path dependence here, because these tenancies were the least attractive for privatization, and tenants with lower social, human, and financial capital at the end of the communist era had fewer chances to participate in privatization.

Based on socio-spatial dialectics, we can argue that the vulnerability of social housing clients is reinforced by the lower-status location of their residence, which affects their lives and future prospects. The concentration of social housing and lower-social-status tenants, however, also makes it harder for the locality to improve itself.

The new policies in most LAs have had minor effects on the redistribution of social dwellings. In Tallinn the stock of social housing almost doubled during the 2000s, but that was the only city in which this occurred. The spatial patterns of new social housing investments reinforced the differences inherited from the 1990s. Beyond the positive effect on improving access to housing for eligible groups, the impact of increased segregation levels of social housing in certain subareas is likely to have severe side effects. Such segregation is reinforced by the concentration of social housing in large multifamily buildings containing 100 percent social dwellings.

The current situation and the pattern of social housing in Estonia are thus the outcomes of path dependence from the communist regime and of ownership reform and the subsequent policy paradigms: the paradigm of neoliberalism, and the paradigm of the efficiency of property management, according to which management and service provision is more effective if social dwellings are concentrated in buildings specially targeted as social housing. Housing policy is mainly seen as just one dimension of the overall neoliberal political environment, reproducing social relations applicable to this system. The housing market will thus also remain vulnerable to economic cycles and associated social risks. Although the main approach affirms the described role of social housing as a form of social assistance and not an integrated part of housing market, the new directions of social housing policy in the city of Tallinn have marked an interesting turning point in the previous approach. It remains to be seen whether this will lead to broader changes in defining the new role for social housing in Estonian society.

NOTES

* This chapter was prepared with the support of research grant No. 7588 of the Estonian Science Foundation, and the target funding project No. SF0180052s07 of the Ministry of Education and Science Estonia. The authors would also like to acknowledge PhD Siiri Silm for cartographic help.

1. The database of new social housing dwellings constructed in Tallinn contained the data on all new buildings and dwellings constructed during the period 2000–2011, with the basic information provided for each building.
2. The SMH was carried out by the Ministry of Social Affairs as a Web-based survey in 2005 among professionals working in the field of local housing policy for local authorities (LAs). The sample covered all 240 LAs in Estonia with a response rate of 62 percent; the results were weighted according to the size of the LAs.

REFERENCES

Bourne, L. S. 1981. *The Geography of Housing*. New York: Silver Spring.

Clapham, D. and Kintrea, K. 1996. "Analyzing Housing Privatization." *Housing Privatization in Eastern Europe* 117:1–13.

Gentile, M. and Tammaru, T. 2006. "Housing and Ethnicity in the Post-Soviet City: Ust-Kamenogorsk, Kazakhstan." *Urban Studies* 43 (10): 1757–78.

Hegedüs, J. and Tosics, I. 1996. "The Disintegration of the East European Housing Model." *Housing Privatization in Eastern Europe.* Westport, CT: Greenwood Press.

———. 1998. "Rent Reform—Issues for Countries of Eastern Europe and the Newly Independent States." *Housing Studies* 13:657–58.

Interim Report of the RCP-1. 2007. *Tallinna elamuehitusprogrammi. "5,000 eluaset Tallinnasse" täitmise vahearuanne (Tallinn's Residential Construction Program. "5,000 Dwellings in Tallinn").* Tallinn: Tallinna Linnavalitsus.

Kährik, A. 2000. Housing privatisation in the transformation of the housing system. The case of Tartu, Estonia. *Norsk Geografisk Tidsskrift—Norwegian Journal of Geography* 54:2—11.

Kährik, A., Kõre, J., Hendrikson, M., and Allsaar, I. 2003. "From a State Controlled to a Laissez Faire Housing System." *Housing Policy: An End or a New Beginning?.* Budapest: Open Society Institute.

Kährik, A. and Tammaru, T. 2010. "Soviet Prefabricated Panel Housing Estates: Areas of Continued Social Mix or Decline? The Case of Tallinn." *Housing Studies* 25 (2):201–19.

Kährik, A., Tiit, E.-M., Kõre, J., and Ruoppila, S. 2003. *Access to Housing for Vulnerable Groups in Estonia.* Report Financed by the European Commission within the Community Action Program on Combating Poverty and Social Exclusion, PRAXIS Working Paper No. 10, Tallinn.

Kõre, J., Ainsaar, M., and Hendrikson, M. 1996. "Eluasemepoliitika Eestis 1918–1995 (Housing Policy in Estonia 1918–1995)." *Akadeemia* 10:2133–63.

Kornai, J. 1992. *The Socialist System. The Political Economy of Communism.* Oxford: Clarendon Press.

Kulu, H. 2003. "Housing Differences in the Late Soviet City: The Case of Tartu, Estonia." *International Journal of Urban and Regional Research* 27 (4): 897–911.

Lux, M., ed. 2003. *Housing Policy: An End or a New Beginning.* Budapest: OSI/LGI.

Lux, M., Kährik, A., and Sunega, P. 2012. "Housing Restitution and Privatization: Both Catalysts and Obstacles to the Formation of Private Rental Housing in the Czech Republic and Estonia." *International Journal of Housing Policy* 12 (2): 137—158, DOI:10.1080/14616718.2012.681574.

Ministry of Social Affairs 2005. *Munitsipaaleluruumide vajaduse uuring. Kokkuvõte uuringu tulemustest. (Survey of the Need for Municipal Housing).* Tallinn: Sotsiaalministeerium.

Ministry of Social Affairs. 2011. Statistics on subsistence benefits. http://www.sm.ee/meie/statistika/sotsiaalvaldkond/sotsiaalhoolekanne/toimetulekutoetus.html accessed on 11.10.2011

Pichler-Milanovich, N. 2001. "Urban Housing Markets in Central and Eastern Europe: Convergence, Divergence or Policy 'Collapse'." *European Journal of Housing Policy* 1:145–87.

Raitviir, T. 1990. *Linna sisestruktuurid, faktorökoloogiline lähendus (Structures of the City, a Factor-Ecological Approach).* Tallinn: Tallinna Linnauurimise Instituut.

RCP-1 2002. *Tallinna elamuehitusprogramm "5,000 eluaset Tallinnasse."* (Residential Construction Program "5,000 Dwellings to Tallinn"). Tallinn: Tallinna Linnavalitsus. RCP-2 2008. *Tallinna teine elamuehitusprogramm.*

(The 2nd Residential Construction Program for Tallinn). Tallinn: Tallinna Linnavalitsus.

Ruoppila, S. and Kährik, A. 2003. "Socio-Economic Residential Differentiation in Post-Socialist Tallinn." *Journal of Housing and the Built Environment* 18:49–73.

Smith, D. M. 1996. "The Socialist City." *Cities after Socialism*. Oxford: Blackwell.

Szelényi, I. 1996. "Cities under Socialism—and After." *Cities after Socialism*. Oxford: Blackwell.

Tallinn City Government. 2009a. Guideline for Assessing the Housing Need. Tallinn City Government 26.08.2009, order number 1376 https://oigusaktid.tallinn.ee/?id=3002&aktid=115100 accessed October 11, 2011.

———. 2009b. Regulation Act No 66 on Tenancy Agreements by the Tallinn City Government. 19.08.2009. https://oigusaktid.tallinn.ee/?id=3002&aktid=115022 accessed October 11, 2011.

Tammaru, T. 2001. *Linnastumine ja Linnade Kasv Eestis Nõukogude Aastatel (Urbanization and Urban Growth in Estonia during the Soviet Period). Dissertationes Geographicae Universitatis Tartuensis, 13*. Tartu: Tartu University Press.

Temelová, J., Novák, J., Ouředníček, M., Puldová, P. 2011. "Housing Estates in the Czech Republic after Socialism: Various Trajectories and Inner Differentiation." *Urban Studies* 48 (9): 1811–1834.

11 Hungary

Ideas and Plans without Political Will

József Hegedüs

In Hungary, the social housing problem changed after the transition as a consequence of political decentralization and privatization. With the collapse of the Eastern European Housing Model (EEHM), affordability—the ability to pay housing-related costs for a socially accepted level of housing consumption—became the key element of social housing. As a consequence of the emerging income inequality and increasing housing costs (both "operational" and access costs), more and more households had to face serious hardships to achieve a socially accepted level of housing consumption. The social housing sector was formed as an interaction between the strategies and behavior of households and the following three areas of the housing and welfare sector: (a) the social rental sector, (b) housing allowances and income benefit programs, and (c) low-cost housing opportunities. There was no consistent strategy for social housing policy after 1989, as policies were set according to the interventions of fragmented public and private institutions of different sectors (energy, water, construction, social care, etc.) and the decentralized local governments. After a brief introduction concerning the main macroeconomic changes in the background, the Hungarian case study will describe the developments in these policy areas.

MAIN MACROECONOMIC AND SOCIAL FACTORS

The political transition had an enormous effect on macroeconomic trends. As a result of the transitional recession, GDP fell by 15 percent in the first part of the 1990s. Structural reforms (privatization and bank reform) were complemented with a strong fiscal stabilization package (1995–1998) and the maintenance of sound macroeconomic policies.

In the 1990s, changes in the labor market due to the closing of many previously state-owned companies and to the restructuring of the production sector led to a dramatic decrease in the employment rate—almost one million employees left the job market, many of whom were forced into early retirement or became "entrepreneurs" (forced entrepreneurship).

During the 1990s poverty became one of the most important social issues. Whereas the average income decreased, income inequalities increased dramatically in the first part of the 1990s and remained stable over the last decade. The ratio of average income in the lowest percentile to the average in the highest percentile increased from 4.6 in 1987 to 7.6 in 2004 (Keszthelyiné Rédei and Szabó 2006). Economic recession associated with the transition increased regional inequalities in the country: the eastern part of Hungary was hit much more by the economic decline than other areas. The net income per capita is 50 percent higher in the most developed region than in the two least developed regions.

Tax evasion became a typical strategy for households to manage hardships caused by the transitional recession. Informal economy was estimated to be as large as 25–33 percent of GDP between 1990 and 1997 (Laczkó 2000). Informal transactions have been widely accepted by the population: consumers pay and accept payments for service without invoices (VAT tax evasion); employers pay wages or part of the wages directly into the employees' 'pocket' (income tax evasion). According to a recent study, 25 percent of all jobs are affected by these types of transactions (Semjén et al. 2008). We know little about the income effect of the informal economy, but most studies support the hypothesis that it increases income inequalities and poverty (Rosser et al. 2000).

However, households that have no access to either the formal or the informal economy (for example, "closed" marginalized settlements in underdeveloped regions) sink into deep poverty because of the low level of income benefit payments. Intergenerational (interfamily) transfers are a widely used option for helping households or household members in economic hardship. According to empirical research, 44 percent of families with children engage in intergenerational transfers (Medgyesi 2003), and these transfers tend to help poorer households more (Bócz and Medgyesi 2004). The role of the family in Hungary can be as important as in the Southern European welfare regimes, and it is especially important in the housing system (Hegedüs and Teller 2007). In the housing system, intergenerational transfer fosters inequity in household wealth and household income, although within households there is a trend to help family members in difficulty (Hegedüs and Szemző 2009). Consequently, households that have no access to the informal economy and no family support face the highest risk of poverty, because loss of employment, health problems, and family problems (for example, divorce) may force them into huge financial difficulty.

Hungary's population has been constantly decreasing since the early 1980s. Its population today is slightly above ten million. The average household size has been stable around 2.65, which is slightly larger than the European average (around 2.53). Total fertility decreased from 1.92 in 1980 to 1.32 in 2007, which is among the lowest in Europe and exacerbates the aging of the Hungarian society to a large extent. Since the 1990s there has been no significant demographic pressure on the housing market; the quantitative shortage of housing had ceased to exist by the end of the 1980s. Urbanization slowed down and inner migration trends did not increase the demand for housing substantially.

Before the change of the regime, Hungarian housing policy discussed housing questions in terms of the 'quantitative and qualitative housing shortage' paradigm. Demographic circumstances and the size and composition of housing investments determine the quantitative indicators of housing conditions. The number of housing units grew from 3.5 million to 4.3 million between 1980 and 2008, whereas the urban population only increased by 4 percent (from 65 percent to 69 percent). Urbanization thus put only moderate pressure on the urban housing market.

The qualitative problems with the housing stock are clearly indicated by the fact that 40 percent of all housing units in 1980 had no bathroom, and 27 percent had only one room. Although quantitative growth between 1980 and 1990 was significant, even if less so than in the previous decade, qualitative changes dominated in the following twenty years. The number of people per room decreased from 1.6 to 1.1 between 1980 and 1990. The process of qualitative improvement slowed down in the 1990s, but piped gas availability grew from 40 percent to 70 percent, the ratio of housing units connected to the communal sewer system grew from 43.8 percent to 57.2 percent, and the proportion of housing units with flush toilets and bathrooms also increased.

AN OVERVIEW OF HOUSING POLICY PROGRAMS UP TO 2009[1]

We can differentiate four periods in Hungarian housing policy after 1990.

In the *first period* (1989–1994) the Hungarian government tried to manage the housing crisis related to the economic decline and the unsustainable subsidy system of the socialist period. The government 'moved out of the housing sector' by diminishing its direct role and decreasing subsidies. Decentralization was part of this process, as local governments were assigned to manage housing allowance programs partly financed from their own resources. The housing policy of this period could basically be characterized as crisis management: the two major programs consisted of the privatization of the state rental sector and the consolidation of the 'old loans'. Both measures had a regressive social effect: the financial gains of privatization and early repayment of the loans were proportional to the households' wealth. Low-income households were thus trapped in the residualized social rental sector or were unable to pay back their mortgage at a discount price.

In the *second period* (1995–2000) new institutions were set up and the legal framework was improved. Meanwhile, the level of subsidies gradually decreased as a consequence of the decreasing housing output. Two basic institutions for housing finance were established: contract savings banks and mortgage banks. The law on contract savings banks was very controversial, as the subsidies given to savers made the housing subsidy system even more regressive, and there was no direct relation between the subsidies and the increase in housing investments. The subsidy system was changed to compensate for the big cuts in 1994, and this had a temporary effect on housing output. Starting in 1998 (when a new right-wing government stepped into office), a new rhetoric was introduced in housing policy, expressing the need to support middle-income households, but for two years nothing important happened. In spite of a different approach in housing policy papers, no real changes in the subsidy system and housing programs took effect in the period.

The *third period* started after 2000, when the Hungarian government launched a new housing program enabled by positive macroeconomic changes. The government housing program of 2000 targeted three housing areas: (a) emergence of the mortgage market, (b) expansion of local government-provided social housing, and (c) renewal of the housing stock (especially the urban housing estates built in the 1970s and 1980s). A new subsidy system was introduced for housing mortgages ("dual" interest rate subsidy, tax exemption after mortgage payment, and so on), which resulted in an unprecedented increase of housing loans starting in 2001. A grant program was initiated to support social housing investment by local governments, which covered 75 percent of the costs for social housing investment. Preferential loans were offered for the renovation of housing estates. Because of the fiscal cost of the program, the new socialist-liberal government in 2002 tried to slow these programs down, but it took almost three years to make radical changes in the subsidy schemes.

The *fourth period* started when the Hungarian housing market was hit by the 2008 financial crisis. Borrowing stopped, the quality of loans deteriorated, mortgage payment arrears appeared, and so on. In 2009 most housing subsidies were suspended. The government initiated a program to help the most affected households. But it is yet to be seen how deep the crisis will be and how effective the government assistance package will turn out to be.

RENTAL SECTOR PROGRAMS

In Hungary 88 percent of households have owner-occupied tenure status; social housing ("below market rent") makes up only 4 percent, and the remaining 8 percent is private rental (market rent and "rent-free"). This, by European comparison, extreme tenure structure is the result of privatization after 1990 and the lack of a social housing program in the last two decades. At the beginning of 1990, 721,000 housing units were municipally owned, 85 percent of which were privatized to sitting tenants. In the following seventeen years, municipalities bought or built no more than a

Table 11.1 Municipally Owned Housing Stock, 1990–2007

		Municipal housing, thousand apartments	Source of Information
Housing stock, beginning of 1990		721.3	1991 Census
Sales	1990–2007	605.6	CSO regular housing statistics
Housing construction		12.7	
Housing demolition		10.8	
Purchases		23.8	CSO estimate
Housing stock, end of 2007		140.9	CSO municipal real estate asset statistics

Source: Central Statistical Office.

total of thirty-six thousand housing units. Taking housing demolition into account, there were barely 140,000 housing units in the public rental housing stock at the end of 2007 in Hungary (see Table 11.1).

Public rental housing is concentrated in the cities: 69 percent of the stock is to be found in Budapest and in cities with county rights.[2] There is next to no rental housing in villages, with only 1 percent of that housing stock owned by the municipality.

After the housing stock was privatized, the units that remained the property of local governments were overwhelmingly in a bad state of repair, concentrated in the poorest parts of the city, and inhabited by low-income households. The allocation system also contributed to the residential segregation of disadvantaged households.

According to the framework of the Housing Law, the owner (in this case, the municipality) has the right to set the rent; that is, no rent control exists in Hungary. The law also allows local authorities to define allocation procedures—whether to use waiting lists or case-by-case tenders for vacant units—and decide on the organizational form of the housing maintenance company. Most municipalities determine the rent separately for each apartment according to local ordinances, which generally contain a modifying factor taking the apartment's condition, location within the building, the building's facilities, and so on, into account. Public housing rents are much lower than in the private sector, usually reaching 20–40 percent of private rents. This ratio varies from settlement to settlement.

As a result of giveaway privatization, the percentage of the housing stock in the public rental sector fell from 20 percent in 1989 to 4 percent in 2003. Households trapped in the public sector were typically the neediest, and could not afford to pay even the discounted sum or did not consider it worthwhile to buy their apartments because they were of such low quality. In cities with more than fifty thousand inhabitants, the proportion of dwellings owned by local governments is between 4–10 percent. In total, 58 percent of municipal flats are in cities with a population over one hundred thousand, whereas only 20 percent are in towns with a population of less than fifty thousand inhabitants.

Municipalities employ a variety of methods to allocate social housing; the two main techniques are waiting lists and special bidding systems. There is generally an income criterion, which is offset by various other criteria (no private assets owned by the applicant, minimum period of stay in municipality, etc.). In the bidding systems, solvency is the most important criterion, and solvent applicants are generally at an advantage.

Local authorities can choose which type of rental contract to use—fixed or open term; social or cost rent or market rent. After 2001 they could also freely decide when and whether to sell dwellings. Public sector rents are very low, and they cover approximately 30–40 percent of actual costs. Moreover, the vast majority of tenants have difficulty paying even these rents, and many are in arrears. According to a 2003 housing survey, 22 percent of households in the public sector were in arrears, whereas in the private sector the figure was 5 percent. Due to financial disincentives and their own limited resources, local governments have underinvested in the maintenance of their housing stock, which continues to deteriorate. The public housing sector requires an estimated 1.5 billion U.S. dollars for renewal and rehabilitation of the stock—thirty times the yearly rent revenue of 2004. Local governments can only allocate vacated and newly built rental units, which represents no more than 4–5 percent of all housing market transactions, including buying and renting. The need for social housing is high; according to our need assessment study of 2001 based on Census data, the stock of potential unmet demand for rental housing is around 750,000 units, including about five hundred thousand social units—approximately two and a half times the stock at the time (Hegedüs et al. 2010).

The housing policy launched in 2000 included a grant program for local authorities supporting five housing areas: the rental sector, energy-saving renewal, rehabilitation, land development, and renovation of housing owned by churches. The most important element was support for the public rental sector. Local authorities were eligible for a grant of up to 75 percent of the cost of investments for social rental, cost-based rental (see the following), housing for young families, and retirement homes. Between 2000 and 2004, several hundred local governments took part in the program. The total investment amounted to 0.3 billion U.S. dollars and close to 12,800 units were established (eighty-nine hundred rental units and thirty-nine hundred special accommodation units in retirement homes, assisted living homes, and temporary homes for young couples). A cost-based option was introduced to ensure long-term cost recovery in the sector, with rent levels higher than existing social rents but lower than market rents. The regulations set the minimum annual rent at 2 percent of the construction cost. Although this cost rent approach did not guarantee long-term cost recovery, in the first years the actual operational and maintenance cost of the units was considered to be lower than the rent. The cost rent was about 40–60 percent of the market rent. The high level of interest in the rental sector program is an indication of the commitment of local authorities to solving the housing problem. Before the launch of the program, the Hungarian government's Housing Policy Committee was concerned that local authorities would not be able to participate because most of them would not be able to afford the 25 percent own contribution required, but the demand for the fund exceeded the budget resources, and, in fact, only 45 percent of the amount requested by local authorities was funded.

The program had several weaknesses. Average costs were considered to be very high, although one of the most important selection criteria was the average cost per square meter. Allocation criteria for new tenancies were not regulated, and local politics played a role in discretionary allocation. The cost rent was considered too high for poor people but not enough for long-term cost recovery. Moreover, during the period of operation of the scheme, the privatization process continued; thus, local authorities privatized twenty-five thousand units, but built, bought, or renewed only eighty-nine hundred rental units.

In 2004, the government stopped the social rental program because of fiscal pressure, citing the high cost per unit as the reason. The government proposed a rent allowance program as a substitute for the budget-financed rental program. According to the proposal, local governments would have entered into long-term contracts with private investors to use newly built rental units for social purposes. The central and local governments would have jointly provided a rent subsidy to bridge the gap between affordable and market rent—cost plus profit. The proposal failed because the guaranteed rent level required by investors was unacceptably high—twice the actual market rent, because of the high construction cost. However, the importance of the social rental sector was never questioned in government documents. In 2005 a new rent allowance program was finally introduced, which aimed to use the private rental sector for social purposes. Local governments could apply for rent allowance for low-income families with children who had private rental contracts. The central government would pay a maximum of 30 percent of the rent or 22 U.S. dollars per month,[3] and the local government would also contribute at least as much. The program was a failure: very few local authorities put forward a proposal. One reason for this was that the program required that landlords be registered with the Tax Authority. The majority of private landlords do not pay tax, and they did not change their approach for the sake of participating in this program. A second problem was that the income limit, under about 140 U.S. dollars per capita per month, was so low that eligible households were not able to pay the rent. In 2006, another new loan program was launched, giving local governments access to subsidized loans from the Hungarian Development Bank for investment in the public rental sector. However, the interest by local governments was very limited.

The cost of maintaining the municipal rental stock is not supported from the central budget. The maintenance of social housing is thus costly for the municipalities, as rents do not cover their expenses. This does not in itself have to be a problem if municipalities acknowledge the demand for social rental housing. However, many municipalities would like to get rid of their social rentals and the social problems posed by typically poor tenants. Some municipalities are more open to dealing with social problems and attempt to treat the social rental housing question rationally. One method of doing so is to introduce specific local rental subsidy systems, which increase the targeting of support systems (Szombathely, Nyíregyháza, Debrecen, and so on). Demand for social rental housing is, according to conservative estimates, around three hundred thousand to four hundred thousand apartments (8–10 percent of the housing stock); that is, the living conditions of this many households would justify living in social rentals. The current social housing stock is less than half of this, and neither the municipal nor the government housing policy is moving towards expansion, although many people face a multitude of problems with high social costs (being in arrears and debt, lack of mobility, segregation), which could be countered by a modern rental sector.

HOUSING ALLOWANCES

Of total household expenditures, housing-related expenditures increased from 9 percent to 20 percent in the first ten years of the transition, whereas income disparity increased from 4.7 percent to 7.3 percent. Paying for housing-related expenditures poses a serious problem for 14–18 percent of households, which leads to a growing number of arrears. Energy-related expenditures represent the biggest segment of housing cost: in 2007, they constituted almost 70 percent of housing-related expenditures. (CSO 2007).

The Social Law (1993) introduced a housing allowance scheme financed through the local governments' discretionary budgets. Local governments had wide autonomy to set the eligibility rules and the amount of the allowance. However, local governments only used this program on a limited scale, because it was financed exclusively out of their budget, unlike other income benefit programs (such as support for permanently unemployed persons), where the central (70–90 percent) and local governments (30–10 percent) shared the burden. In 2004, the government introduced a new housing allowance program, which received 90 percent of its financing from the central budget. The eligibility rules were also set centrally. This new system provided an incentive for local governments to increase their housing allowance programs. The total cost of the two programs accordingly grew from 15.5 million U.S. dollars (2003) to 88 million (2009). In 2009, the main part of the total, 80 percent, was spent on the new housing allowances. Housing allowances financed through the municipalities' own resources made up 20 percent of the whole subsidy, 15 million U.S. dollars.

The introduction of the centralized housing allowance was aimed to ensure that it would reach the lowest-income groups, thus broadening the group of recipients. Around 8 percent of households received support in 2005 as compared to 4 percent in 2003. Even so, support reached only a narrow group of eligible people, especially considering that 13 percent of households (around five hundred thousand) were in arrears with housing costs (estimate based on a 2003 survey[4]). According to the 2007 Household Budget Survey, around 10 percent of households are not able to pay their housing costs and a further 10 percent cannot enter the housing market. The design of the subsidy system cannot guarantee that low-income households can pay their housing costs after providing for their basic needs. Analyses have identified two basic deficiencies in the system. Firstly, due to the low income limit (one and a half times the minimum pension), the proportion of individuals whose housing expenses exceed 25 percent of their income is higher among groups with an income somewhat over this limit than in groups having a lower income but receiving the allowance. If we look at groups with equivalent incomes (weighted according to household composition as well as size), the difference is even greater.[5] The second deficiency is that the centralized housing allowance does not take into account differences in specific costs due to actual living conditions. The monthly housing allowance (housing unit size defined in terms of number of inhabitants multiplied by cost per square meter) differs significantly from the actual housing costs of households in different housing conditions. Specific expenses differ due to the following three factors: (a) useful floor area, (b) type of housing unit, and (c) type of heating. Expenses per square meter in a housing unit under 40 square meters are twice as much as expenses in housing units over 70 square meters. The second factor, which also explains differences between settlement types, is the housing unit type. Concerning heating, the expenses associated with district heating (2.7 U.S. dollars per square meter per month) are nearly twice as expensive as in a traditional family house or row house.

To sum up, subsidies only cover a small proportion of housing cost, which poses a further problem. Despite positive changes, the housing allowance system is not yet effective enough either with regard to the range of recipients or with regard to the degree of support.

The accumulation of housing-related debts since the beginning of the 1990s has posed a serious problem for a significant proportion of households. Debts are related to utility costs and mortgages (particularly loans from before 1989 and from between 1989–1993). Due to unpaid utility costs, five hundred thousand households (13 percent) have over three months' worth of debt, and three hundred thousand households owe one to two months of utility costs. In order to deal with debts systematically, a debt management service was included in the welfare system in 2003. An estimated fifteen to twenty thousand families participated in the program between 2003–2005, which involved only a small share of households in arrears and only helped with smaller debts. For those with a very low income, new debts accumulate constantly. This fact also shows that the debt management system can only have a real effect in conjunction with the housing allowance system.

The household energy consumption subsidy has existed in its current form since January 1, 2007. It cost 581.24 million U.S. dollars in 2007, which made up around 83 percent of all housing support. The reduced support foreseen for 2008—450 million U.S. dollars—also represented around 80 percent of housing support. A further reduction in the energy consumption subsidy is to be expected.

HOMEOWNERSHIP OPPORTUNITIES: EMERGING MORTGAGE MARKET AND HOUSING REHABILITATION

From 1990 to 1998 housing construction dropped to twenty thousand units/year (25 percent of the construction rate of the 1980s), and house prices also decreased in real value by 40 percent. However, as most state subsidies were cut, access to housing became less affordable. The only exception was a cash grant for new construction, the housing construction allowance.

The *housing construction allowance* was first introduced in 1971, and its function changed several times. It is a cash grant that helps with the down payment of homebuyers. The size of the subsidy depends on the number of children in the household, it is not a means-tested grant, and only buyers of newly built homes or 'self-builders'—households who themselves build or organize the building—are eligible. Further criteria are that applicants do not own a dwelling of their own at the time when they apply, and the standard of the new home is according to centrally decided standard size and cost limit. In 1995 the amount of the grant was increased in the case of families with two and three children, which made it possible for low-income households to build new "low-cost" housing without substantial savings or loans. Interestingly enough, although this was not the intention of policymakers, this subsidy scheme was used by large poor families (for example, Roma families) with the help of intermediaries (builders, lawyers, contractors, and Roma NGOs). It was particularly significant in less-developed regions, where the grant covered almost the total cost of the construction. Private developers emerged who specialized in using the advantages of this scheme (Zolnay 2002). The program had several negative effects. Many of the homes built in this manner were of bad quality. Furthermore, much of the construction took place in less-developed regions with higher unemployment rates. According to some estimates, ten thousand homes were built using the allowance between 1995 and 1997, which was the largest, albeit unintentional, Roma housing program after 1990 (Hegedüs 2004).

The right-wing government (1998–2002) introduced major changes in housing policy in 2000. The most significant element of the program was the support to housing mortgages. Interest rate subsidies and an income tax mortgage payment allowance were introduced. This was the most expensive housing program between 2000 and 2004, which not only caused an extremely large burden for the budget, but also contributed to social inequality, as 60 percent of the subsidy went to the highest 20 percent income group. As the program was fiscally unsustainable, mortgage subsidies were cut in 2004 and opened the way for unsubsidized foreign exchange loans with a high exchange rate risk carried by the borrower.

Housing credit grew very quickly in Hungary between 2000 and 2004, and the cut in subsidies did not halt the expansion of the market, because foreign exchange–dominated (FX) loans with variable rates successfully replaced the subsidized HUF loans. Their share went from close to zero in 2004 to 90 percent in 2008. There were no direct fiscal burdens in relation to the loans issued in FX. The availability of cheap funds and the exceptionally high spread gave a high motivation for the banks and mortgage brokers to expand the market to the consumer loans.

The rehabilitation program (under the housing policy objective to improve housing quality) became important after 2004, especially the 'panel program', the program to rehabilitate buildings built using prefabricated technology. This was a politically popular program as it reached wide strata of society and was relatively cheap from a fiscal point of view. A constant expansion of the 'panel program' has taken place since 2004, as a result of which 25 percent of this stock (190,000 housing units) were renovated to some degree by 2009. There are more serious social problem areas in segregated housing estates and run-down urban areas with a high share of Roma population, which require more social attention and fiscal resources. Some programs were started in 2005, but mostly on a pilot scale. Urban rehabilitation programs were started slowly after 1990 under the control and support of the local governments, but in most cases the urban poor were forced to move out of the renewed neighborhoods. The first urban rehabilitation program aimed at improving the living conditions of the 'sitting poor' was started in 2006.

The economic crisis in late 2008 hit the mortgage market. The weakening Hungarian currency (HUF) caused a 31–41 percent increase of the mortgage repayment for borrowers of FX loans, which—together with increasing unemployment—has led to an increase of mortgage defaults. The stock of the nonperforming mortgage loan portfolio (overdue more than ninety days) has increased to 6.3 percent of the total stock from 2.6 percent between 2008 and 2009.

The government cut housing subsidies drastically as part of the fiscal adjustment program, under which both the interest subsidy and the homeownership down payment grants were abolished. The government also introduced several mortgage rescue programs. One of them was the establishment of a crisis fund, to which well-off individuals and companies could contribute. The crisis management fund would provide one-off assistance to some thirty thousand of Hungary's most disadvantaged families, whose members had lost their job after October 1, 2008, or for whom loan repayment installments had increased by more than 20 percent.

The Hungarian government also launched a mortgage-to-rent scheme that offers preferential loans to local governments so that they can buy repossessed homes and let the original owner remain as a tenant in the property. However, many local governments have refused to participate in this scheme because there is no long-term guarantee that the central government is going to continue to support this newly created rental stock. The new government, installed after the May 2010 parliamentary elections, introduced further restrictions: a complete ban on foreign currency mortgage loans and a strict regulation of bank borrowing practices, such as securing the option for borrowers to extend their loan repayment period by five years without incurring a penalty. In 2010 there were already more than ninety thousand households in default. The new government promised to set up an institution to help them avoid the foreclosure procedure and the loss of their homes through a Property Fund, which would buy the bad loans and rent the property out to the borrowers. However, this plan had not been realized until the end of 2011.

CONCLUSION: EVALUATION OF THE SOCIAL EFFECT OF THE HOUSING POLICY

Despite the rhetoric of the housing policy white papers of various governments, there was no consequent social housing policy to systematically help households that could not afford their housing consumption (to pay the access and the operation costs of a socially accepted level of housing). There were programs that directly increased social inequality among different income groups, such as housing privatization that transferred 20 percent of the housing assets in a regressive way to the households, or the 2002–2004 mortgage program, during the course of which 60 percent of the subsidies went to the upper 20 percent of the households, as measured by household income. The social rental program targeted at vulnerable groups was limited in size, and it was discontinued after three years, in 2004. The housing allowance program did not provide enough help to guarantee that a household could stay out of debt, and it was not successful in targeting the neediest. Moreover, some programs that offered direct help to relatively poor households (for example, the "low-cost housing programs" or the financial compensation of poor people in the area of urban rehabilitation) contributed to the marginalization of low-income households in the mainstream labor market, public infrastructure, and so on.

First of all, the affordability problem is not determined exclusively by income disparities, but also by the "behavior" of different actors in the specific sectors (local governments, service providers, interest representation bodies, etc.). For instance, it is in the service providers' economic interest to use their facilities at maximum capacity, which makes them reluctant to help consumers reduce their consumption (i.e., by installing water meters or modernizing insulation and heating systems). Furthermore, central and local governments have a dual (partly conflicting) function: as the owners of service providers or as tax levy authorities, they are interested in increasing housing service fees, because these fees can be considered indirect taxes, but they simultaneously have to guarantee the financial security of the households with income benefit programs.

The affordability problem can be dealt with in two ways: either by increasing housing incomes, or by decreasing housing expenditures. We concluded that scarce central and local resources did not offer low-income households enough support, which forced them to increase their income from the informal economy. The reluctance of social policy towards means-tested targeted social assistance further deepened the gap between the incomes and the expenditures of the needy population. Furthermore, the lack of trust between the different sectors and actors resulted in a totally incoherent system of housing allowances.

The magnitude of the informal economy is partly the reason for, but also the consequence of, underfinancing. The welfare system could be far more efficient if social benefits were means-tested. Otherwise, those in a relatively good financial position due to their income from the informal economy are also eligible for these benefits. On the other hand, those dropping out of the labor market have no other choice than to enter the informal market in order to sustain their living on an acceptable level.

The other way of handling the affordability problem is to decrease housing costs. One option is social migration, when households struggling with unaffordable housing costs move to a smaller housing unit with lower housing expenses. This tendency can be very problematic, especially when, as a consequence of downward mobility, households lose their chance to enter the labor market, education system, and health system, and lose access to other welfare benefits.

Poverty is not merely a consequence of the income disparity–generating effect of the market economy—it is also due to the failure of the welfare system, because the informal economy limits the degree to which the tax burden can be shared, and scarce resources are thus split into programs that cannot guarantee the affordability of housing costs. The study does not justify the theories that hold local governments responsible for discrepancies in the benefit system.

From a housing policy perspective, the study concludes that the lack of social housing, which could provide real help for struggling households, is one of the causes of impoverishment. The estimated need for social housing is three hundred thousand units (minimum double the size of the existing stock). But even for those living in social housing, housing expenditures are barely affordable, due to very high energy costs. This is an area that would require cooperation between housing policy and social policy.

The Hungarian public rental sector is still in transition. Local governments and their housing companies are the most important social landlords and enjoy broad autonomy. The privatization drive seems to be over, but even now some local governments see this as the most preferable option. One of the richest district governments in Budapest sold twenty-eight thousand units after 1990, and in 2006 they sold an additional five hundred of the two thousand remaining units. From time to time, politicians declare privatization to be a mistake, but when in power they are eventually forced to support privatization under pressure from the sitting tenants and due to financial incentives.

What are the chances that a stable public rental sector will develop in the transitional countries, and how will it affect the forming welfare regimes?

First of all, if the institutional structure of the public rental sector has not been developed; the social housing programs—if there are any—have to support access of the needy households to owner-occupied housing. This is a second-best option, but could be justified either in rural areas or with respect to the lower-middle class, who only need minor help to get or to remain in the owner-occupied market. These could be good social programs, but would compete with the rental programs, as the Hungarian example showed.

Second, are there real political and business interests behind social rental programs? Any models that are not supported by real political and social forces are transient. Several donor agency programs in the region have had to face the fact that their programs are missing support and are therefore not sustainable.

NOTES

1. This section draws on Hegedüs (2010).
2. Cities with a population exceeding fifty thousand and county capitals enjoy a special legal status in Hungary.
3. In 2005 1 U.S. dollar was equal to 186 HUF.
4. In December 2003, the Social Ministry conducted a survey on arrears exceeding three months for electricity, gas, and district heating bills, as well as outstanding debts on so-called loans taken out from the OTP Bank before 1993.
5. Based on 2006 Household Budget Survey data, 11 percent of households had housing expenses (not including rent) that exceeded 25 percent of household income. As a result of the housing allowance, in a second group of households making up 7.6 percent of the total (where income per person is one to one and a half times the minimum pension) the proportion of households with high housing costs is reduced from 37 percent to 14 percent. In the third group of families (where income per person is one and a half to two times the minimum pension) 16 percent spend over 25 percent of household income on housing expenses.

REFERENCES

Bócz, J. and Medgyesi, M. 2004. *Characteristics of Households' Cooperation II (A háztartások közötti együttműködés jellemzői II)*. Budapest: CSO.

CSO 2007. *Statistics on income and living conditions in Hungary, 2007* Budapest: CSO.

Hegedüs, J. 2004. "The Housing Market and Residential Regional Mobility in the 1990s—The Case of Hungary." *Hungarian Labor Market, Review and Analysis 2004.* Budapest: Institute of Economics, HAS Hungarian Employment Foundation.

———. 2010. "Towards a New Housing System in Transitional Countries: The Case of Hungary." *Housing Market Challenges in Europe and the United States.* Basingstoke: Palgrave Macmillan.

Hegedüs, J., Eszenyi, O., and Teller, N. 2010. *Housing Needs in Hungary.* MRI. http://www.habitat.org/eurasia/pdf/MRI_housing_needs_hungary_study.pdf accessed May 12, 2012.

Hegedüs, J. and Szemző, H. 2009. *Households' Perception of Old Age and Housing Equity: The Case of Hungary.* WP2 Report of the DEMHOW Project.

Hegedüs, J. and Teller, N. 2007. "Hungary: Escape into Homeownership' Homeownership beyond Asset and Security." *Housing and Urban Policy Studies.* IOS Press, Delft.

Keszthelyiné Rédei, M. and Szabó, Zs. 2006. "The Level and Distribution of Incomes in the Last One and Half Decades in Hungary (A jövedelmek színvonalának és elosztásának alakulása Magyarországon az elmúlt másfél évtizedben)." *Incomes and Income Distribution, 2004 (Selected Studies).* Budapest: Central Statistical Office.

Laczkó, M. 2000. *(Egy rázós szektor: a rejtett gazdaság és hatásai a poszt-szocialista országokban a háztartási áramfogyasztásra épülő becslések alapján. Elemzés a rejtett gazdaság magyarországi szerepéről. MTA KTK és Tárki közös kutatási program). The Hidden Economy and Its Effect on Post-Socialist Economy on the Basis of Household Energy Consumption. An Analysis of the Role of the Hidden Economy in Hungary. Joint research program of Economic Institute of Hungarian Academy of Science and TARKI).* Budapest: TÁRKI.

Medgyesi, M. 2003. "Flow of Domestic Income and Assets—Research Results Based on Hungarian Data (Családon belüli jövedelem és vagyonáramlás—kutatási eredmények Magyar adatokon)." *Apák és fiúk és unokák (Jövedelemáramlás együtt élő korosztályok között.* Osiris, Budapest.

Rosser, J., Jr., Rosser, M., and Ehsan, A. 2000. "Income Inequality and the Informal Economy in Transition Economies." *Journal of Comparative Economics* 28 (1): 156–71.

Semjén, A., Tóth, I. J., Medgyesi, M., and Czibik, Á. 2008. "Tax Evasion and Corruption: Population Involvement and Acceptance (Adócsalás és korrupció: lakossági érintettség és elfogadottság)." *Discussion Papers Institute of Economics, Hungarian Academy of Sciences. 2008/13.* Hungarian Academy of Science, Budapest.

Zolnay, J. 2002. *A Housing Program of the Social Housing PBC set up by the Nation-Wide Roma Self Government.* http://www.romaweb.hu/romaweb/cikk.jsp?p=7 accessed May 12, 2012.

12 Poland

Old Problems and New Dilemmas

Alina Muzioł-Węcławowicz

NEED FOR SOCIAL HOUSING IN POLAND

The Housing Shortage and Social Housing Needs in Poland

Poland comes last in Europe in terms of housing rates. At present there are only 348.5 apartments per one thousand inhabitants (384.9 in cities and 291.7 in the countryside), which means that an average of 2.87 persons live together in one apartment and the average amount of space per person is 24.6 square meters. This housing shortage is one of the country's most important social and economic problem, which is partly rooted in the pre-transition period (shortage of dwellings, low standards of old stock) and partly in a lack of efficient housing policy after 1989.

The statistic shortage of apartments in 2002 was estimated at 1.7 million units, according to data from the National Census. About 950,000 apartments were built between 2003 and 2009, but the number of households also increased by circa 1.1 million. The actual shortage is calculated to reach around 1.4–1.5 million apartments if one takes estimates of the rental black market and real estate statistics shortcomings into account (Ministry of Infrastructure [MI] 2010). Independent experts have estimated that if the aims of deficit liquidation and managing current demographic needs are to be met, 2.6 million apartments must be built in Poland by the end of 2013 (HRF 2007). This is unachievable (see Figure 12.1). In 2010, Social Building Associations (TBSs in Poland) completed thirty-one hundred new apartments (2.3 percent of the total output) and local governments built thirty-four hundred, that is, 2.5 percent of total production (Central Statistical Office of Poland [GUS] 2011).[1] The shortage mainly concerns the sector of available housing, both rental and privately owned apartments, and encompasses the entire territory of Poland, with big cities and attractive labor markets particularly strongly affected. According to the Institute of Urban Development (Instytut Rozwoju Miast [IRM]), Poland desperately needed more than 215,000 rental apartments, including ninety thousand TBS apartments (see definition later), seventy-five thousand other social apartments, and fifty thousand council apartments in 2008 (IRM 2009, 17).

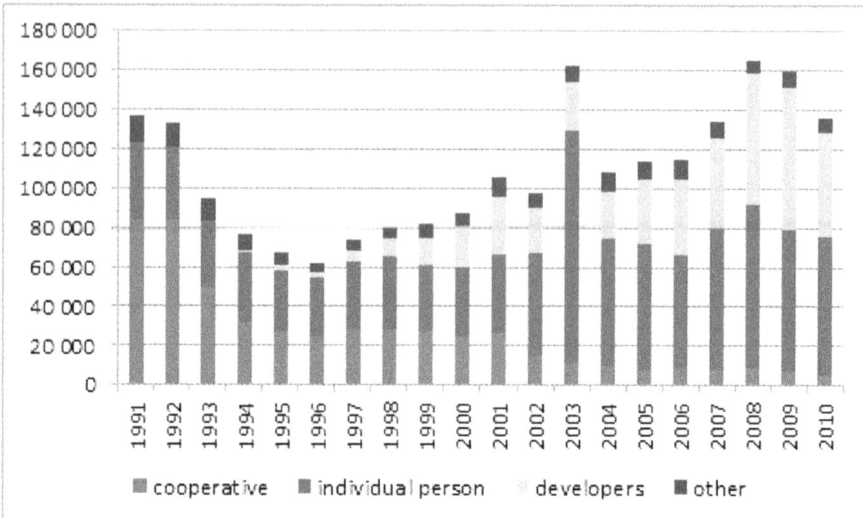

Figure 12.1 Housing construction, 1991–2010.
Source: The Central Statistical Office

Considering the scale of poverty and particularly unfavorable affordability conditions in housing investments from the consumers' perspective (high house price to income ratio, low level of savings, banks' conservative credit policies), the view that the majority (up to 70 percent) of the population is incapable of meeting their housing needs without public support is accurate. It also seems that the claim to keep circa 30 percent of apartments in the social housing sector is a minimum requirement.

A profound lack of renovation and modernization of the existing stock poses an additional issue for Polish housing. As the IRM analyses indicate (Korniłowicz and Żelawski 2006), spending for the renovation of apartment blocks in cities in 2000–2005 hardly reached 35–40 percent of necessary maintenance spending in council properties, 33–52 percent in condominiums, 66–89 percent in housing cooperatives, and 14–39 percent in private rental properties.

Tenure Structure in the Polish Housing System

By the end of 2009 there were 13.2 million apartments in Poland (Table 12.1). The dominant form of housing in rural areas, small towns and on the outskirts of large cities is one- or two-family houses as well as detached houses. The centers of large cities are made up of apartment blocks with a diversified ownership structure.

The majority of apartments, circa 70 percent of the total, are privately owned by natural persons. These properties differ greatly in terms of

Table 12.1 Housing Stock by Ownership, 2009

dwellings	in thous.	in %
communal	1 062,8	8,0
housing cooperatives	2 583,3	19,4
in it: owner-occupied	*2 150,6*	*16,1*
tennement	*432,7*	*3,3*
companies	132,5	1,0
State Treasure	57,4	0,4
Social Building Associtions	79,3	0,6
other entities	26,7	0,2
natural persons	9 360,5	70,4
in it: in housing condominiums	*1 986,8*	*15,0*
single family houses[2]	*7 373,7*	*55,4*
TOTAL	**13 302,5**	**100,0**
in it: in cities	*8 959,2*	*67.3*
in villages	*4 343,3*	*32,7*

Source: Gospodarka mieszkaniowa w 2009 r. (The housing economy of 2009).

quality and location. In the private sector, apartments are rented out or sublet without government control. Additionally, the sector wrestles with ownership claims from those who lost their property during the socialist era because of nationalization. An estimated 10 percent of all privately owned apartments (8 percent of the total number of apartments) are rented out, the majority of which are let informally, without taxation.

Currently, 83.3 percent of the 2.6 million cooperative apartments in Poland are practically privately owned on the basis of cooperative ownership (owner-cooperatives) and a mere 16.7 percent can be considered rental-cooperatives (Table 12.1). Around 5 percent of cooperative apartments are private rentals.

The State Treasury's housing stock comprises mostly tied accommodation for the needs of the army or the judiciary. The apartments belonging to state-owned companies typically date back to the postwar period. The tenants of these apartments are now buying the apartments through the privatization process. In the beginning of the transformation period there was a program to transfer the state-owned companies' housing stock to other public landlords, such as local governments, which were not entitled to reject the transfer of these housing units. Presently these housing sectors (stock owned by the State Treasury and state companies) are utterly marginal.

A state program established TBSs in Poland in 1996. Their statutory goal is to build and manage social rental apartments. These apartments are meant for tenants who are financially stable but have a defined maximum per capita income, and who are generally expected to occupy the apartment until they raise the means to purchase an apartment. Because old public housing in Poland was of extremely low quality, the idea was that new, high-quality, and energy-efficient buildings should be constructed to ensure cheaper maintenance costs. The main policy goal was to induce upward mobility so that low-standard public housing could be freed up for social use.

Currently, there are around eighty thousand apartments in the social rental sector. This includes 63,800 constructed using preferential loans by the public associations and 12,400 by private ones. Less than 1 percent of the total number of apartments have been constructed by TBSs, and these are located almost exclusively in cities. However, they play an important role in the local housing market in many urban areas.

There are only rough estimates concerning the proportion of rental units in the Polish housing market. There is very little information available concerning the private rental market, which has very little government oversight. The classification of housing cooperatives, especially cooperative rental housing, is also unclear. Housing cooperatives are part of the private sector, and their members enjoy rights that are similar to ownership rights. For this reason, this analysis treats cooperative housing as a privately owned sector. Rental properties in the private and public sector are estimated to make up around 19.5 percent of the total number of apartments. The public rental sector accounts for 10.5 percent; these apartments are owned by local governments, TBSs, state-owned companies, and the State Treasury. The private rental sector is mainly composed of individual apartments owned by natural persons.

Ambiguities in the Term of Social Housing

The social policy of socialist ideology claimed to meet collective needs (including housing needs) under the condition of maintaining citizens' incomes at a relatively low level. In Poland, the state never fully attempted or succeeded in meeting housing needs due to its low political priority, the inefficiency of the political system, and high costs. The processes of industrialization and urbanization amplified the need for housing. In the 1980s, the waiting time for a cooperative apartment (the most typical form of housing with state support at that time) could exceed ten years, even if housing cooperative members complied with all formal and financial requirements, including down payments. One of the famous twenty-one demands of the 1980 "Solidarity" labor union strikes was to shorten this waiting time.

The term *social housing* was never clarified after the transition, and its meaning depends on the context.[3] Traditionally, social housing is assumed to comprise apartments that enjoy public funding for construction and/or maintenance, clear allocation criteria (usually some sort of means-testing), cost supervision (rents among others), and being under the control of public agencies responsible for satisfying the housing needs of society. In Poland, the term *social housing* is broadly defined, including all sorts of housing that receive financial support from the state and local governments. For example, a lower VAT rate applies to building materials and services, which is justified as a part of 'social housing programs'. This approach is highly controversial, as housing needs are poorly met overall and direct budget spending on housing is low, slightly exceeding 330 million U.S. dollars per year in recent years. By comparison, the preferential VAT rate—which applies equally to luxury housing—is estimated to cause a 3.3 billion U.S. dollars decrease in tax preferences and revenues. This state of affairs reflects the power of the construction lobby, and it should not be described as a program that helps citizens meet their basic housing needs.

An additional program for "privately owned social housing" offers a refund for around 50 percent of mortgage interests for the first eight years of repayment. Families and single parents who purchase a moderately priced apartment or house of small floor area are eligible to participate in the program. The aim of the program was to create conditions in which families can flourish and to raise the birthrate, so it defines no income limits for the beneficiaries.[4]

The rest of this analysis will focus on the sector of rental apartments that receive partial public funding, and are available in limited numbers. This sector is composed of three subsectors: local government units (council and social); units under the control of TBSs, funded with preferential loans; and apartments rented out by state-owned companies or the State Treasury. The first two are important and a subject of governmental and local housing policy.

From a legal perspective, the obligations of public authorities regarding housing in Poland are high. The Polish constitution obliges public authorities to pursue policies conducive to "satisfying the housing needs of citizens, in particular combating homelessness, promoting the development of low-income housing and supporting activities aimed at acquisition of a home by each citizen" (Article 75). A March 8, 1990, act concerning local governments points out that it is the local government's task to satisfy the collective needs of a community, including local housing.

Local governments have a great deal of freedom to pursue economic and housing policy. There are no government grants to local governments for housing. However, there are some government policy programs, such as the social rental housing program, the energy saving ("thermomodernization") program, and the social housing subsidy program, financed from a special central fund (Fundusz Dopłat), which assists local governments in carrying out their tasks. The common characteristics of these programs are their brief duration and low budgets, much lower than the needs reported by local governments. A decentralization of responsibility for social housing took place throughout the transformation period, but the central government delegated tasks to the local governments without providing adequate financial support.

In daily practice, local governments are responsible for providing social accommodation for the citizens with the lowest incomes who live in poverty and for those who are evicted, when the court decrees the right to shelter.

Social council apartments form a category of their own. These are apartments meant for the impoverished or people/families with eviction verdicts. Local governments are legally obliged to designate a part of their rental properties as social apartments. Rent in these units is very low, up to 50 percent of council rents, housing allowances do not apply here and the apartments are rented for a fixed period. They can be of low quality (but have to be suitable for habitation), the minimal floor area is 5 square meters per person in a numerous household and 10 square meters in a single-person one. However, when it comes to newly constructed social accommodations, apartments have to comply with modern construction standards. Therefore, the only opportunities to lower the construction costs of new social apartments are smaller floor areas and cheaper building materials. Presently in Poland there are 61,400 social apartments (5.8 percent of council apartments) and the average floor area of an apartment is 31.6 square meters.

THE SOCIAL HOUSING STRATEGY IN TRANSITION PERIOD

Privatization and Restitution

Housing privatization must be discussed in the context of housing cooperatives and the so-called public housing stock (council, company, State Treasury, and TBS properties).

The privatization of council apartments has a complex history. Postwar nationalization mainly affected industrial facilities and large farms, not housing. Housing estates of Warsaw were communalized and subsequently nationalized because the heavily damaged capital city stood in need of large-scale redevelopment. A promise of compensation in return for the expropriation remained unfulfilled for many decades. Ex-owners now find it difficult to document their titles, and, due to lasting transformations of individual properties such as the sale of apartments to their tenants, the present legal status of Warsaw's prewar rental properties is a hindrance to direct reprivatization. In other cities after World War II, rental units were subject to public administration of the stock, which meant that private owners were limited in their right to maintain and dispose of their property.

Regardless of the question of privatization and ownership, private rental properties, located in city centers, are often responsible for the negative image of cities and lead to the escalation of urban decay.[5] Many prestigious council investments have been suspended because of the unregulated legal status of the properties, or because they were privatized in violation of the prewar owners' interests. These facts limit the possibilities for a reasonable modernization policy of old tenement houses. The famous *Hutten-Czapska v. Poland* case in the European Court of Human Rights, which concerned the title to manage a prewar tenement house, exemplifies management problems with this type of property. In 2006 the court decided that the state of Poland had violated the regulation of the Convention for the Protection of Human Rights and Fundamental Freedoms by limiting the owner's right to raise the rent and to issue notices to quit the lease.[6]

The present liberal regulations for establishing rent rates are incapable of generating financial flows for thorough renovations of such neglected properties. In spite of the fact that the tenants are typically immobile (elderly or low-income) people, the state does not significantly support the process of gaining control over this sector.

In 1990 there were 1,980,300 council rental apartments. Of these, 144,400 had already been sold to the sitting tenants during that year; 7.2 percent of the council stock was privatized before the transformation. The selling price before 1990 was set based on value assessment, taking the rate of depreciation into consideration, and there were considerable discounts for those who paid cash up front.

Until 1994, local governments were not entitled to sell properties below their assessed value, which slightly slowed down the privatization of council rental apartments. However, getting rid of such council properties was a priority for many local governments, because the rents did not cover the maintenance and management costs, thus resulting in severe budget losses. The relevant regulations were soon changed, and local governments are now free to set their own prices when selling council apartments to sitting tenants.

In these transformation processes, apartments of the poorest quality, which are unattractive and/or occupied by economically weaker tenants, usually remain in public management. This means that local governments are left with the most difficult cases. Rent arrears statistics provide evidence of this trend, as 44.5 percent of council rental tenants are in arrears. These arrears are caused not only by the poverty of tenants, but also by a lack of serious sanctions.

By the end of 2009 the council sector consisted of 1.1 million apartments. All local governments are obliged to design long-term programs (at least for five years) to manage their own properties, in which they publish renovation plans, rental as well as privatization policy, and local regulations for access to council rental apartments. But individual cities implement different policies. Some dispose of their contributions in condominiums, aiming to mix various social groups; others sustain dispersion of council ownership. As a rule, local governments divide their properties between public and social housing.

Rent Regulation and the Housing Allowance

In the first years of the transformation, the central government made all the decisions concerning rent regulations. The frequency and scale of increases depended on political factors. This was a period when housing investment declined and the political priority of housing was pushed back in government policy. Energy and council service prices were liberalized. Following these changes, household budgets could not bear an economically rational scale of rent increases. Furthermore, unemployment in this period was consistently very high. There was also a special tax penalizing public companies where salary raises were too high.

A 1992 state program, the New Housing Deal (Nowy Ład Mieszkaniowy), became the foundation for reform in the housing sector. A 1994 act on the rent of apartments and apartment allowances launched a rental reform. Due to social factors, reform was gradual:

- Until the end of 2004, the rent increase rate was capped at 3 percent of the renovated apartment value for all properties previously under public housing management.[7]
- Property owners decide the rent rate, raises and reductions of the base rate with regard to the characteristics of a given property.
- Apartment allowances were introduced for low-income citizens living in small apartments.

Public property rents were to be liberalized starting from the beginning of 2005. According to the observations of the IRM,[8] in 2001, after seven years of decentralized rent policy in council rental properties, rents covered approximately 68 percent of maintenance costs (excluding such council services as water supplies). With an acceptable limit at 3 percent of reconstruction cost, average rents barely reached 1.3 percent, and local governments that implemented more aggressive rent policies were in the minority. As with the central government, rent increases were politically difficult to implement.

Since 2005, all rents have been liberalized. However, public owners have a legal obligation to justify a rent increase if it approaches 3 percent of the reconstruction cost.

The law regulates a maximum rent rate for TBS properties in a different way. At the time when tenants move into a property, the maximum rent is 4 percent of reconstruction cost per year. Customarily, the rent in TBS properties follow average construction cost increases.

Before 2005, there were numerous attempts by the government to limit rent increases by setting a ceiling for a possible proportional increase ratio. However, the Constitutional Tribunal consistently took the view that the law may allow for statutory limits to rent increases, but the rent revenues cannot fall lower than the necessary spending for property maintenance. And this was precisely the case in Poland. From a legal perspective, it is even acceptable for the public owner to obtain decent profits.

The new legal concept of "occasional rental" was introduced in January 2010 in order to pull private rental transactions out of the black market. An apartment owner who is not an entrepreneur living off rental services and who wants to obtain additional, legal income can make use of certain new rights: to define a given period of renting, to oblige the tenant to move out on the owner's demand with no legal procedures, and to take advantage of an attractive preferential flat-rate income tax. The primary goal of this legislation is to persuade people to formalize rental contracts and pay taxes—even if scarce—on business income. Apartment owners' worries concerning irresponsible tenants, protected by tenants' rights, should not impede apartment usage. The latest amendment, dated August 2011, aims at diminishing the local government's burden to provide a shelter for evicted people. Depending on the cause of the eviction, evicted persons can be allocated to a temporary shelter or a homeless shelter (in case of violent behavior) directly.

However, central and local level politicians still frequently present a pro-social (pro-tenant) attitude that is passive towards a number of challenges concerning apartment rentals. Decision-makers, terrified at the scale of necessary changes to the council rental sector, have made no wide-ranging attempts to rationalize property management. Thus, a standard lease is not limited in time. It is unpopular to resettle tenants who cannot pay the rent in smaller and/or cheaper apartments. It remains socially accepted in public rentals not to pay the rent on time. Analyses indicate that people are more likely to pay their phone or TV bills punctually, because media companies are quicker to sanction arrears. Council property managers, who have very limited budgets, are incapable of improving living conditions in a significant way or of influencing tenants to change their attitude. However, expected changes to rental regulations will limit the scale of tenant protections: for example, it has been proposed that new leases in council stocks will be for a fixed period.

Recent data on rent levels demonstrate that rent increases in local government units accelerated slightly, mainly due to large rent increase programs in the biggest cities. In 2009 the average council rent increase was 14 percent (IRM 2010). Nonetheless, in relation to the average level of recovery, rent in council properties is still around 1.2–1.3 percent of recovery value.

The evolution of the housing allowances program comprises three phases: the launching of the program in 1995, an attempt to modify it in 2001 and a change of financing in 2004. The 1994 Tenants Protection Act, part of the rent reform, introduced apartment allowances as a form of support to meet housing needs.[9] In 2001 a separate act concerning apartment allowances was introduced, slightly changing particular criteria.

Housing allowances are meant for those who simultaneously meet the three following conditions:

- They have a legal title to the occupied apartment.
- The average monthly income per household member does not exceed a certain level (defined as the lowest old-age pension category).
- The property is not too big considering the number of occupants, that is, the floor area of the apartment does not exceed the need standard.

The housing allowance is the difference between housing expenses per standard floor area of the occupied apartment and the real expenses incurred by the person who receives the allowance. The types of housing expenses that constitute the basis for calculating apartment allowances comprise practically all apartment usage costs, such as rent, energy, water, and waste disposal bills.

Floor area standards show that the allowances were meant to stimulate cross-sector migration of people and apartment exchange. The wide range of entitlement to the allowances has not changed until now. In the beginning, 50 percent of the funding for the allowances came directly from the local governments, and 50 percent came from state subsidies to the local governments. The local government then transferred the money to the program participants. The central government raised budget subsidies for the allowances in 2001 in order to encourage local governments to increase rents, but this regulation was quickly dismissed by the subsequent government. The public finances act was finally changed before Poland joined the European Union. As a result, local governments came to receive more of the taxes generated in their area, but had to fully finance apartment allowances out of their increased budget.

Such a solution weakens local governments' motivation to rationalize their policies, as part of the profit from rents has to be spent on allowances. According to the IRM data, allowances were paid to circa 4.0 percent of households in 2008, and 3.9 percent in 2009 (IRM 2010). The housing allowance system has been positively evaluated from the perspective of income and floor area eligibility criteria. Planned reform of the housing allowance system aimed at excluding homeowners from the system.

Social Building Association—An Innovation

A specific solution that has occasioned both interest and controversy is the government program for supporting rental sector housing addressed to those who are able to pay cost rents. The social rental housing program has been realized by TBSs since 1996 based on a special 1995 law.

The concept of using public financing to construct rental housing that could subsequently sustain itself from rental income, based on the French HLM model, aroused broad interest. This solution was unique for Eastern and Central Europe, and was frequently described in the literature (Donner 2006; ECE 2006; Muzioł-Węcławowicz 2007; Kierzenkowski 2008; Brzeski et al. 2009). In practice, local governments use TBSs in various ways. In many cities, some of them large, no such entity was established. In other cities, they serve as a major public institution—they build new apartments, frequently directly for the local government and with its considerable financial support, and often run their own investment programs based on preferential loans and on the contribution of the beneficiaries (future tenants). TBSs frequently manage local government-owned housing and serve as a public housing developer. There are many possibilities of cooperation between TBSs and local governments, which makes TBS apartments available to economically weaker tenants who meet the conditions for getting a council apartment. For instance, a local government may subsidize a TBS so that it can have a smaller loan quota (50–30 percent of costs), which allows it to establish a lower rent rate. The income from the rents is used by TBSs to pay off their loans. Local governments can appoint candidates for TBS tenants. They are also able to rent apartments from TBSs at standard TBS rates and sublet them to those who are waiting for council or even social apartments. The difference in rent rate is then paid by the local government. However, this is not a large expense in relation to the direct costs of the investment. A considerable advantage of TBS apartments is that, due to high thermal insulation parameters that exceed standard construction norms, the total maintenance costs of TBS apartments do not diverge in any meaningful way from the maintenance costs in an apartment of similar floor area in other properties and are much cheaper than on the private rental market.

The program had the following phases:

1. There was the initial activity (1996–1999) when TBSs were created, first investments were launched, and preferential financing was easily available.
2. There was intensive growth (2000–2003) when the demand for loans was the highest; the program received significant contributions from the BGK (Bank Gospodarstwa Krajowego—the Bank of National Economy).[10] The bank used a loan from international financial institutions supplemented with a budget subsidy.
3. There was stagnation (2004–2008) when initially, in 2004–2006, local governments interested in EU funds reduced TBS investments; a commercial housing market was developing, rising prices in construction impeded the realization of the social rental housing program; and contributions to the National Housing Fund (Krajowy Fundusz Mieszkaniowy) from public means were limited. In 2007–2008 the fund was only insignificantly supported from the budget, despite the fact that interest in social rental housing was growing, due to more restrictive loan policies in banks after the Lehman Brothers bankruptcy,
4. There was decline (since 2009) after the dissolution of the fund, the bank received only 7 million PLN for its further activity, and taking over preferential crediting is not beneficial for the BGK. What is more, further development of the program demands new legal regulations. The National Housing Fund was established to finance the program in the structures of the BGK. It was financially separated from the bank but operated according to bank norms and standards. In 2009 the National Housing Fund went into liquidation and its assets were included into the capital of the BGK. The last applications for

> preferential loans were accepted in 2009. The government is working on defining new financial and legal principles for the program of building apartments to rent with moderate rent rates.

The fifteen-year period of the social rental housing program did not manage to visibly influence development in the rental sector. The primary reason, at times unperceived by program critics, is the inadequacy of public means directed to the program in relation to the demand on the part of investors. This is dramatically shown by data concerning loan applications inflow in 2009. TBSs reported demand for preferential loans for circa 3,330 million U.S. dollars.[11] In the meantime the bank could fund as little as 9 million U.S. dollars credit. Practically speaking, since the end of the first phase of the program, that is, since 2000, refusals regarding crediting of a large portion of projects were common due to means shortages. Thus there are few TBS properties. From a technical point of view, the properties are of good quality, were built under strict discipline to warrant energy efficiency, minimal floor areas were defined, and so on. A certain deficiency of the program is that the financial contribution of the future tenants was a necessary element of the financial package because of a shortage in the central and local budgets. Nevertheless, the consequences are problematic—such participation in financing triggers a justification for privatization claims.

In August 2011 the Parliament adopted amendments to the law on TBSs, that is, the law on certain forms of supporting housing construction that, in essence, allow tenants who have participated in construction costs to become the owners, given prior consent of TBS or housing cooperative owners. Apartments will then be sold at market prices and the association will have to repay the part of debt corresponding with the particular unit to BGK. Any financial surplus generated by the TBS will have to be returned to the Surcharge Fund in order to finance governmental housing programs. The expectations of a number of investors were met with a positive reaction from the politicians. The latter perceive privatization as a 'market approach' and an opportunity to regain a part of invested means to allot for further social rental housing financing. The agreement to repurchase apartments from TBSs was not supported by detailed economic analyses (with the exception of a report from the World Bank; see Brzeski et al. 2009). The supporters drew on opinion polls carried out among tenants, who are usually satisfied with the apartments' quality and willing to repurchase. Furthermore, these attitudes are founded in a long-lasting practice of apartment privatization with considerable discounts. Arguments against privatization, indicating the scale of unmet needs in this sector and the possibility that wealthier tenants would have a better chance to move to the homeownership sector, do not draw the politicians' attention.

Until the end of 2010, within the social rental housing program, the BGK granted loans of 366 million U.S. dollars to housing cooperatives, which allowed them to build 17,100 cooperative apartments. TBSs received loans of 1,471 million U.S. dollars and completed 75,600 apartments. A couple of thousand apartments are currently under construction.

Conclusion: Limits of the Social Housing Policy

Sociological research indicates that it is essential to citizens that their housing needs are met and that housing conditions improve. Polish people do not feel financially secure: they do not expect stability, although their views are fairly positive. Traditionally, they do not trust the state, and in matters of housing often rely on their own initiative. This is why so many houses are built in the individual system (52 percent in 2010). This also provides the basis for the informal housing sector.

Around two million mainly young people emigrated just after Poland joined the EU. Although their labor market position in the 'old' European Union countries is well documented, it is difficult to find analyses concerning their housing situation. In many instances, a chance of obtaining a good-quality individual apartment in the public sector is an essential factor in the decision to settle abroad permanently, especially among emigrants who are in stable relationships and have children.

The low priority of housing issues in government policy has a long history. The state housing policy has been changed frequently and inconsistently. Governments always issued policy documents dealing with social housing, but most of them remained on paper. The major criticisms of the post-1990 housing system are:

- the briefness of individual programs and concept instability
- insufficient financing for housing policy programs

It seems that each subsequent government wanted to leave its mark on housing policy, in spite of the fact that housing issues were not a priority. The first and easy step was to denigrate the predecessors' work; it was more difficult to work out a new program. The only housing policy programs that maintained their position over a longer period of time were the social rental housing program and the energy efficiency support program (thermomodernization).

In effect it is difficult to present long-term tendencies in government housing policy. When the governments had to choose between improving the standards of the existing housing stock and developing new housing, the second option attracted more attention. This is why the social rental housing program, which made more apartments available for target groups and simultaneously soothed the housing market perturbations, is favorably evaluated.

Whether housing should be decentralized, that is, whether local governments should be responsible for housing policy, is a subject of permanent debate and critical evaluation. Local governments inherited the shortages and problems from the previous socioeconomic system. Local governments took on more and more responsibility for housing over time, but without receiving adequate financial support from the central budget.

There are many examples of cities implementing advanced housing programs, of the kind that introduce local instruments of housing support and make it possible to use the public housing stock effectively. Nonetheless, highly effective tenants' rights protection, excessive renovation needs, and an increasing number of low-income families eligible for social housing all created permanent obstacles to cities being able to realize their obligatory tasks.

A shortage in population income statistics is an essential concern in Poland. Social policy relies on categories such as the lowest pension or the lowest or median salary. In this situation it is difficult to responsibly set precise income limits according to which citizens can be placed in the social housing system.

No formal housing policy programs operated that could be understood as national government programs after 2003. Implementing housing policy was limited to working out detailed legal regulations and annual budget allocations for subsequent statutory tasks. The high budget deficit became a rationale for the government not to base the program on any forecasts and financial prognoses. In an extensive recent housing policy document (MI 2010), only the social housing and energy saving programs were promised high governmental priority.

NOTES

1. Construction by local governments, TBSs according to data presented in Figure 12.1 fall into the "other" category, along with companies and other small investors.
2. The idea is to contrast private dwellings in multifamily buildings, i.e. housing condominiums and single family, two-family, detached units, i.e. individual buildings where in majority cases one house equals one apartment.
3. In Polish the term *social* has several meanings, as far as housing is concerned, it may mean "public housing" as well as housing for very vulnerable groups (council social apartments).
4. Recent legal amendments of that program, dated July 2011, introduced stricter price limits. The program became accessible to single persons and will be closed down by the end of 2012.
5. Paradoxically, the present acknowledgment of ownership obliges courts to refuse local governments the right to subsidize, for instance, the renovation of a private house located on a main street under a local urban regeneration program because it does not belong to the local government's tasks to contribute to the "rise in private property worth" or to "act for the sake of improving the image of the local government" (quotation from the explanation of the sentence of the Superior Administrative Court).
6. The subsequent settlement of the plaintiff with the state of Poland deterred further complaints of the type. The settlement defined individual compensation and the representative of the state of Poland recognized the necessity to establish a general compensation form for tenement house owners.

7. The regulation also concerned those private rental properties that were previously under public housing management—until the end of 2004 rents here were set by local governments.
8. Earlier a branch of the institute dealing with housing operated under the name of the Institute of Housing Management (Instytut Gospodarki Mieszkaniowej) with its headquarters in Warsaw.
9. Before that, certain forms of social support existed related to one's inability to pay rent, although they were unsystematic.
10. In 2003 TBSs put into use 6.5 percent of the total number of new apartments and 23.7 percent of apartments built by economic and social subjects (excluding individual building).
11. That demand came from applicants who provided formally proper documents and were verified as creditworthy.

REFERENCES

Brzeski, W., J. Chiquier, L., Dübel, H. J., and Taffin, C. 2009. *"Residential Rental Market in Poland."* TBS Review/Final Report. World Bank http://bip.transport.gov.pl/pl/bip/programy_i_strategie/budownictwo/reforma_bud_spolecz/px_poland_fi nal_report_july_1.pdf accessed June 10, 2011.

Central Statistical Office of Poland. 2010. *Gospodarka mieszkaniowa w 2009 r. (The Housing Economy of 2009)*. Warsaw: CSO.

———. 2011. *Budownictwo—wyniki działalności w 2010 r. (Construction—Effects of Activity in 2010)*. Warsaw: CSO.

Donner, Christian. 2006. *Housing Policies in Central Eastern Europe*. Published by Christian Donner, Vienna.

ECE. 2006. *Guidelines on Social Housing*. New York: United Nations Economic Commission for Europe.

HRF. 2007. *Raport 2006 o naprawie sytuacji mieszkaniowej (The Housing Reform Report 2006)*. Unpublished manuscript, Warsaw.

Instytut Rozwoju Miast. 2009. *Informacje o mieszkalnictwie. Wyniki monitoringu za 2008 r. (Information on Housing. The Results of Monitoring for 2008)*. Published by IRM. Kraków.

———. 2010. *Informacje o mieszkalnictwie. Wyniki monitoringu za 2009 r. (Information on Housing. The Results of Monitoring for 2009)*. Kraków: IRM.

Kierzenkowski, R. 2008. *Bridging the Housing Gap in Poland*. OECD Economics Department Working Papers No. 639.

Korniłowicz, J. and Żelawski, T. 2006. *Analiza i ocena gospodarki remontowej oraz szacunek potrzeb remontowych w ujęciu wartościowym w wielorodzinnych zasobach mieszkaniowych (Analysis and Evaluation of the Housing Renovation Economics and Estimation of the Renovation Needs in Multifamily Properties)*. Kraków: Instytut Rozwoju Miast.

Ministry of Infrastructure. 2010. *Główne problemy, cele i kierunki programu wspierania rozwoju budownictwa mieszkaniowego do 2020 roku (The Major Problems, Goals and Directions for the Program of Housing Construction Development Support until Year 2020)*. Warsaw.

Muzioł-Węcławowicz, A. 2007. *Perspektywy rozwoju społecznego budownictwa czynszowego (Possibilities of Development of Social Rental Housing)*. Finansowane Nieruchomości. Kwartalnik Związku Banków Polskich. Zeszyt 4/2006: 2–12, Warsaw.

13 Romania

The National Housing Agency—A Key Stakeholder in Housing Policy

Wolfgang Amann, Ioan Bejan, and Alexis Mundt

In this overview we present information on the housing market in Romania and in particular on the role social housing has played within it since the transition. An analysis of the policy stages of social housing support in Romania shows that it is only in the period of 1997 to 2007 that there was a tendency to increase social rental construction. After these years the stock declined considerably from the extensive privatization after 1990.

With the support of international financing institutions a National Housing Agency (ANL) was established in 1999 to finance and create affordable rental housing. Yet, much public support was directed into the new construction of subsidized owner-occupied dwellings. In general, rental housing, not just social but also market rental, is clearly on the defense in Romania. There is a strong and prevailing 'ownership ideology'. When the funds for new social rental housing programs were cut in the aftermath of the financial crises, new housing construction was financed out of the earnings through the sell-off of existing social dwellings to tenants at prices lower than the replacement value. Moreover, there is no long-term social housing policy framework; social housing projects have instead been conceived as part of day-to-day political initiatives.

When trying to evaluate the current system in terms of equality of treatment and effectiveness of housing the poor and vulnerable households, we will show that for most programs the basics for such an evaluation are missing: There is no monitoring and documentation of the various, frequently changing social housing programs dispersed among the local authorities. We have little information on the beneficiaries.

In addition we will show that the main obstacles to the establishment of a social rental housing sector are: the lack of a long-term social housing policy and frequent political changes, the absence of civil society and policymakers committed to the task, the lack of a clear legal framework under which a social housing system could operate, and the tendency to cut back on social rental housing expenses in times of fiscal austerity.

THE MAIN MACROECONOMIC AND SOCIAL FACTORS

Population and Incomes

With its 21.46 million inhabitants (2010) Romania is the largest country of Southeast Europe. The economy and population are strongly concentrated in the capital, Bucharest, which has two million inhabitants. Next in size is a group of cities with almost the same number of inhabitants at around three hundred thousand, namely, Cluj-Napoca, Braşov, Timişoara, Constanţa, and Iaşi. Romania suffers from strong emigration. Since 1990 the population has decreased by 1.7 million (National Statistical Office of Romania, further on referred to as INSSE). A further decrease is expected, but in a smaller scale than previously forecasted (Eurostat). Migration flows to the metropolitan areas face limitations in the labor market and heavy deficits in affordable housing provision.

The dynamic economic development in Romania since the early 2000s has caused incomes to rise. But during the economic crisis incomes stagnated while inflation remained high. Hence, household incomes in real terms decreased. Average gross monthly incomes are 565 U.S. dollars (2009), which is only a fraction of the EU average. In purchasing power, GDP per capita is 46 percent of the EU average (Eurostat data for 2009). Income inequality has grown substantially in recent years. An inequality of income ratio of 7.2 (2009; the ratio between the highest and the lowest income quintile) is one of the highest in all Europe. Together with Bulgaria, Romania has the highest share of households at risk of poverty and social exclusion within the EU and all candidate states. Around 43 percent (2009) of the population or almost twice the average in the EU can be regarded as poor. A large part of the population has difficulty affording everyday commodities, such as accommodation (Eurostat data based on EU-SILC).

The Housing Supply

Romania has a housing stock of 8.43 million units (2010). This is around 390 dwellings per one thousand inhabitants. The average useable floor space per capita is 24.5 square meters (INSSE). This is one-third below the EU-27 average of 38 square meters (OTB 2010). Romania is a 'super' homeownership state (Stephens 2005), with an ownership rate of no less than 96.5 percent (EU-SILC data). Even before the transition period, two-thirds of the housing stock were private property. After the transition, some 2.2 million formerly public rental dwellings have been privatized, which represents 27 percent of the total housing stock (see the following; Tsenkova 2009; PRC Bouwcentrum International 2005).

Today, only 2.2 percent of the housing stock is social rental housing (less than two hundred thousand units, three-quarters of them in a few big cities), and an additional 1.3 percent is private rental housing. The housing stock in the capital city of Bucharest is just under eight hundred thousand dwellings, again only 2.3 percent of which are social rental dwellings (INSSE). Many dwellings are rented out individually without written contracts. However, there are no official statistics on the number. Estimates reach as high as one million units, which would represent 12 percent of the total housing stock (IIBW 2008). In absence of any rent regulation in Romania, this form of tenancy conforms to the requirements of the civil code, and in many cases there is no written lease at all.

Romanian households spend 25 percent of their disposable incomes on housing, which is slightly more than the EU average (EU-SILC data for 2009; in 2008 the figure was 28 percent). Also, 16 percent of households report a housing cost overburden, compared to 12 percent on average in the EU.

Housing mobility in Romania is very low. Many households live in apartments that were privatized at below-market prices and have very low running costs, so they are unlikely to move to places where affordable housing options are scarce. In the old housing stock, maintenance and management are still underdeveloped; tenants pay almost no upkeep costs while their buildings deteriorate. On the other hand, energy prices are internationally influenced and thus are a much higher burden on Romanian households compared to higher-income Western countries. The situation is quite different for those households that have bought or newly signed leases on rental apartments in recent years. The situation is very serious in the small rental sector, as 27 percent of tenants in social rental dwellings and as much as 57 percent in market rental dwellings suffer from housing cost overburden (the EU average is 12 percent and 26 percent, respectively, 2009).

Market prices for new owner-occupied apartments skyrocketed between the early 2000s and 2007, when prices in Bucharest and other bigger cities reached the level of many Western European countries at around as much as 3,900 U.S. dollars per square meter. With the economic crisis and the breakdown of retail mortgage financing, prices in the housing market tumbled. Today, it is possible to buy a new apartment in Bucharest for around 1,300 U.S. dollars per square meter. Market rents used to be around 6 to 13 U.S. dollars per square meter per month. However, the downturn in this market segment was not as bad as in the condominium market (IIBW 2008).

Housing Construction

Housing construction has increased considerably over the years, peaking in 2008 with the construction of sixty-seven thousand units in Romania as a whole, then decreasing to forty-nine thousand units in 2010 (2.3 per one thousand inhabitants). Many less economically dynamic or smaller cities or villages still have very little new construction. The vast majority of new construction is in the form of single-family houses and condominiums. More than 90 percent of new construction is realized by private persons or companies, and around one-quarter of this by foreign companies (INSSE; Nae and Turnock 2011).

It is quite difficult to identify a benchmark for real housing demand. Although there has been a slight decrease in the size of the Romanian population, the number of households has been increasing and so has the demand for affordable housing options. The average floor space per capita is far below the EU average. Much of the existing housing stock is in poor condition and requires substantial renovation. Romania's economic development depends on further urbanization and thus the existence of affordable housing options in urban areas. Housing construction that would match the EU average of some 5.0 new units per one thousand inhabitants would mean a yearly production of one hundred thousand units, which is two times the volume built in Romania in 2010. Previous construction projects in many cases missed the demand in terms of location and affordability. Increasing the volume of construction only makes sense if there is substantial improvement in its targeting to meet demand by location and affordability.

Social Housing Construction

Social housing is regulated under the Romanian Housing Act (Act No. 114/1996), which has been amended more than ten times since 1996. The definition of all kinds of existing dwellings in Romania can be found in Article 2 of the Romanian Housing Act. *Social housing* is defined as dwellings with a subsidized lease, allocated to individuals or families whose financial position would not otherwise allow them access to housing leased on the market. It is the public property of the local authorities. 'Emergency dwellings' are intended as temporary accommodation provided after a natural disaster or accident, or in the case where homes have been demolished to permit the construction of public utilities or have been vacated to permit the performance of rehabilitation work that cannot be undertaken while homes are occupied. In this overview we include all the models of subsidized housing included in the definition of social housing (see the following and Table 13.2); therefore, we include subsidized owner-occupied housing as well as social rental housing. The key point is that they have rent levels or selling prices below market value.

Social housing construction in Romania is quite volatile. The public used to be responsible for not less than 88 percent of new construction in 1990. This diminished to only 5 percent in 2000. Public funds were used for only 6 percent of new construction in 2010, which is the lowest level since 2001 (see Table 13.1). With the establishment of the National Housing Agency (Agentia Nationala pentru Locuinte [ANL]; see the following), the share of social housing construction again rose to 24 percent of all construction in 2003, but decreased thereafter to the present level. The most important segment of social housing construction is the ANL program Rental Housing for Young People with up to five thousand new units built per year (2003;

Table 13.1 Macroeconomic and Housing Indicators

	1990	1995	2000	2005	2008	2010
Population (1,000)	23,211	22,712	22,455	21,659	21,529	21,462
Households (1,000)	7,289	n.a.	7,656	7,360	7,500	7,400
GDP per capita (index, PPS, Ø EU 27=100)	n.a.	n.a.	26	35	47	46
Gross monthly income in industry (USD*)	224	166	186	333	621	534
Consumer prices (HCPI, 2005=100)	n.a.	5.0	43.2	100.0	120.7	135.5
HCPI Housing (2005 = 100)	n.a.	2.1	31.5	100.0	138.4	155.1
Housing stock (1,000)	8,006	7,782	7,908	8,202	8,329	8,430
Housing stock Bucharest (1,000)	950	777	783	784	790	793
Ø size of apartments (useable floor space, m²)	47	52	54	61	63	63
Useable floor space per capita (m²)	16	18	19	23	4.3	15.7
Ownership rate (%)	67.0%	n.a.	95.2%	n.a.	96.5%	96.5%
Social rent (below market level, %)	33.0%	n.a.	n.a.	n.a.	2.1%	2.2%
Market rent (%) official figures	n.a.	n.a.	n.a.	n.a.	1.4%	1.3%
Housing completions total (1,000)	49	36	26	33	67	49
of which with public funds	88%	25%	6%	16%	9%	6%
Housing completions (per 1,000 inhab.)	2.1	1.6	1.3	1.5	3.1	2.3
Housing completions Bucharest (per 1,000 inhab.)	n.a.	1.9	0.6	1.1	1.6	1.5

Source: IIBW, INSSE, Eurostat, EU-SILC, Buildecon, Tsenkova (2009), *exchange rate as of January 2012

see Table 13.2). The level of social housing construction in Romania in the current decade is close to the EU average, but far below the share of social housing construction in some Western and Northern European countries (INSSE; OTB 2010).

THE CHANGE IN SOCIAL HOUSING POLICY DURING THE TRANSITION PERIOD

The development of the economy during the transformation period also led to changes in housing policy. Three important processes impacted development:

- Privatization contributed to the reinforcement of ownership rights, but caused a drastic decrease in the public housing stock and led to the emergence of some major social problems related to satisfying housing demand and social cohesion (Dübel et al. 2006; Tsenkova 2009).
- Decentralization encouraged the emergence and development of the private sector, but at the same time caused a dramatic decrease in public funds invested in housing construction and infrastructure. Usually decentralization involved transferring additional tasks to the local authorities without providing them with the necessary additional financial resources (UNECE 2001, 52). Most municipalities are consequently practically incapable of independently dealing with the housing problems of socially disadvantaged groups.
- Restitution of the formerly nationalized stock, like in other countries in the region, meant compensating the former owners in kind. This process is still under way in the courts and has caused numerous problems, mainly as a result of corrupt practices and a shortage of affordable housing for compensation (Dawidson 2004, 2005).

After the political changes in 1990, various initiatives were carried out to transform the Romanian housing sector. For an analysis it is helpful to distinguish four phases with changing priorities.

1990–1996: Privatization and Replacement of State Role

In the first stage of the transition (1990–1996) the housing reform focused on strengthening market forces and minimizing state intervention in the housing system. The policies promoted deregulation, increased the role of private sector institutions and reduced public expenses. Reform during this period also involved the privatization of the public rental stock and of state construction companies.

Government Decree No. 61/1990 enabled the privatization of housing units built with state funds through their sale to sitting tenants, who could make a down payment and sign the purchase contract backed by a loan. Persons not citizens of Romania and wishing to settle in Romania could purchase a housing unit with foreign currency. Legally, repatriated Romanian citizens got priority if they purchased a dwelling with foreign currency. Altogether 27 percent of the total housing stock was privatized in

Romania, leaving just a very marginal share of social housing (PRC Bouwcentrum International 2005).

The terms of sale to sitting tenants were that they put down a minimum partial payment of 10–30 percent of the official price and sign an installment plan with the CEC (State Savings Bank) for the remaining amount at a 2–4 percent rate of interest over twenty-five to thirty years. However, many chose to pay in full in cash or pay back the loan as quickly as possible. The high levels of inflation during this period would otherwise have fully dissipated the real value of these debts.

After privatization, the 'maneuvering space' formerly offered by social housing was lost. This was harmful, especially for young households (which did not benefit from privatization), for migrants to the cities, and of course for low-income households.

After the general withdrawal of the state from the housing sector and the privatization of the state rental stock, there were no significant interventions until 1994, when the state started to provide support for the completion of projects initiated prior to 1989 but left unfinished. Shortly thereafter, the state intervened to provide a limited number of low-interest housing loans through the CEC, the state savings bank.

The special 'unfinished houses' program came with two subsidies: one was a discount to the buyers of these houses of 30 percent of construction costs, the second was a below-market interest rate. In total, some ten thousand dwellings were completed in this way.

A second CEC scheme targeting young households up to the age of thirty-five was introduced. Young households were offered local currency loans at a 15 percent interest rate. Although not that low in absolute terms, this interest rate was still very low relative to inflation.

1997–2002: More State Involvement and the National Housing Agency (ANL)

In the second period of the transition (1997–2002), new institutions were set up and the legal framework for housing policy was improved. In 1996 the Romanian Housing Act (Act No. 114/1996) was introduced, modeled on the French housing act and regulating, among other things, social housing construction, the general conditions of condominium housing, and housing management. Although it has been amended more than ten times since 1996, the main principles of this law still apply today, as shown in the following.

In 1999, the government made a policy decision to end the subsidy scheme through the CEC and focus on social housing provision through a new state-owned enterprise, the ANL. This entity would work with local governments, which had to provide the building land and infrastructure, to build and finance affordable housing, that is, low-rent dwellings for young people, owner-occupied dwellings, and single-family homes for first-time buyers.

Initially, the ANL focused on 'pioneering' the use of mortgage lending under the terms of the Mortgage Act adopted in 1999. It offered long-term loans with interest rates of 7–9 percent, depending on the age of the borrower. These loans were, in principle, usable for any kind of housing, but after 2002 restricted to new construction funded by ANL and to first-time buyers. Given the free provision of land and utilities by local governments and the other indirect subsidies enjoyed by ANL, these dwellings were offered (for sale) at around 50 percent below their market prices or even lower.

After introducing the necessary legislation in October 2002, Romania adopted a system of separate contract-savings banks for (the construction/purchase of) housing that is much like the German and Austrian 'Bausparkassen'. These institutions are designed to collect deposits at a below-market rate and recycle these funds into low-rate housing loans. To attract funds, the banks offer a yearly premium and the interest is tax deductible. The first contract-savings bank in Romania was set up in 2004 (Raiffeisen Banca pentru Locuinte) and the second in 2005 (HVB Banca pentru Locuinte).

2003–2008: Rental Housing for the Young and the Mortgage Market

After 2003, backed by positive macroeconomic developments, the Romanian government launched an intensive program focusing on three housing-related areas: (a) developing a mortgage market, (b) expanding the program of Rental Housing for Young People, and (c) energy-efficient refurbishing of the housing stock.

Following the formation of a new public–private partnership (PPP) between ANL and several banks in 2003, ANL stopped its housing lending activities, as it was felt that its pilot program had fulfilled its catalyst function. The banks started to grant mortgage loans to eligible applicants who were registered in the ANL database as qualified beneficiaries. However, in 2005 subsidies for the construction of new privately owned housing were canceled for interfering with market principles. To make up for this, a new law was passed for providing a subsidy of up to 20 percent of the housing value (up to 10,000 euros). In 2006 another program was launched to encourage young people to take mortgage loans for the construction of new homes. This involved a 30 percent subsidy of construction costs (up to 15,000 euros) for first-time builders, if the construction was carried out by a developer and with the use of a mortgage loan. These programs were clearly focused on promoting owner-occupied housing.

The ANL program of Rental Housing for Young People, which was launched in the early 2000s, is still the main housing policy program in the country today. Under this program, within almost one decade more than twenty-six thousand (rental) housing units were built all over the country (Table 13.2). With this program the government tried to put the focus of housing policy on the population group that had not benefited from large-scale privatization and had difficulty affording rental housing in the private market.

In 2007 the Romanian government decided to amend the legislation governing this program to allow sitting tenants (in this new housing) to buy their apartments, after a minimum lease period of just one year, for a price well below market value. The revenue from these sales had then to be redirected into the construction of new social housing. The sale could be initiated only at the tenant's request. The sales revenues are insufficient to finance the construction of a similar number of new social dwellings. Moreover, this right to buy scheme was not as popular as expected. Considering the very low rent in this housing, the open-term contracts, and the tenure security, for many beneficiary households it is economically rational to continue renting instead of buying.

In 2003 a thermal refurbishment program was initiated with funds provided by the Romanian government and Swiss development aid. To date the program has produced unsatisfactory results owing to the very frequent changes to the legal framework governing housing, the ineffectiveness of homeowners' associations, and the banks' reluctance to loan money to homeowners' associations.

In this phase the Romanian government attempted to introduce a comprehensive housing policy reform and sought international support for it. Despite strong efforts to implement parts of the new legislative framework, in particular a PPP housing scheme based on social housing models in Austria, the Netherlands, and some Nordic countries, hardly any reforms were ultimately carried out.

From 2008 to the present: The Economic Crisis and Return to Ownership Policies

After 2008, the housing market was hit hard by the effects of the financial crisis: the program of Rental Housing for Young People was reduced in size, the state premium payment for Bauspar banks was postponed for about one year and decreased from 7.4 million U.S. dollars in 2005 to 1.8 million U.S. dollars in 2009, the volume of housing construction decreased significantly, and borrowing for new construction virtually stopped.

As an anti-crisis measure, in early 2009 the Romanian government unveiled its First House program, designed to support mortgage lending and bolster the construction sector (Governmental Urgency Ordinance 60/2009 and Governmental Decision 717/2009). Despite the substantial number of subsidized loans granted since 2009 under this program (an estimated forty thousand), the results are disappointing. Almost all the loans have gone to the purchase of existing apartments and there has been almost

Table 13.2 Social Housing Programs in Romania

	2001	2002	2003	2004	2005	2006	2007	2008	2009	2012
Rental Housing for Young People (ANL program)	106	2,096	4,937	4,272	3,435	2,773	2,671	2,166	3,455	1,602
Social rental housing (Law 114/1996)	441	607	1,339	926	190	242	n.a.	n.a.		
Necessity housing (Law 114/1996)	n.a.	n.a.	n.a.	n.a.	n.a.	n.a.	n.a.	n.a.	1,225	578
Social rental housing for tenants evicted from restituted housing (Law 233/2008)	n.a.	n.a.	n.a.	n.a.	n.a.	n.a.	n.a.	n.a.	1,259	824
Privately-owned housing (G.O. 19/1994)	1,096	788	430	819	182	201	0	0	0	0
Privately-owned housing through mortgage loans granted by banks (ANL program)	295	512	142	313	107	94	113	335	597	364
Total Units	1,938	4,003	6,848	5,758	3,914	3,310	n.a.	n.a.	n.a.	n.a.
Total mill. LEI	161	359	433	472	270	258	n.a.	n.a.	n.a.	n.a.
Total mill. USD*	81	151	151	153	98	96	n.a.	n.a.	n.a.	n.a.

Source: Ministry of Regional Development and Tourism, National Housing Agency, exchange rate as of January 2012

no boost to new construction, which has benefited from less than 5 percent of total lending. Alongside this program, in 2009 the government agreed to a limited VAT exemption for new housing construction for apartments no larger than 120 square meters, using a land area of no more than 250 square meters and with total costs of no more than 117,100 U.S. dollars. The effects of this program are not yet apparent.

In 2009 the Romanian Parliament approved a document restating the guidelines of the public housing sector programs and their implementation priorities. This is today the only official (and very limited) document indicating the state's housing policy goals. The actual results of the social housing programs introduced between 2001 and 2010 are shown in Table 13.2.

INSTITUTIONAL SETTING

Major decisions affecting housing policy are set out in legislation and government ordinances. The institution responsible for the design, promotion, and implementation of housing policy and programs in Romania is the Ministry of Regional Development and Tourism. Yet, the Romanian government's competence in the area of the housing sector is largely dispersed among various institutions. This situation has not changed since the UNECE's criticism in 2001 (UNECE 2001, 52, 92), when the fragmentation of responsibilities was assessed as an impediment to lasting housing policy reform. There are now six ministries with partly overlapping responsibilities in housing. The funding of housing programs and technical and physical management of the housing stock are assigned to the Ministry of Regional Development and Tourism. The Ministry of Administration and the Interior oversees the provision of heating and hot and cold water subsidies to low-income families, and it formulates and implements regional development policies and ensures the coordination of state and local government interests. Issues related to energy use are decided by the Ministry of Economy, Trade, and Business Environment. The Ministry of Justice is responsible for the real estate register. The Ministry of Agriculture manages land matters, and the Ministry of Finance facilitates the financing of the sector through budget allocation.

The local authorities are primarily responsible for social housing administration, the management of public services, and social issues (Laws 215/2001 and 286/2006). Municipalities are allowed to outsource social housing services to private or publicly owned management companies.

A main player in Romanian social housing is still the ANL, which operates under the authority of the Ministry of Regional Development and Tourism. Its main objectives are the promotion of housing markets, the stimulation of new housing construction, and the rehabilitation of the existing housing stock. Since its establishment this institution has been regarded as a practical instrument for solving existing housing problems and an adequate channel through which the state may provide assistance to its citizens. ANL has a national network of territorial offices and collaborates with builders, financial institutions, local and central administration authorities, and foreign organizations. ANL programs focus on mortgage-financed, privately owned housing construction; the provision of rental housing for young people; and a pilot program for Roma families (there are three hundred housing units for the Roma; see Niţă 2009). There is also a new program that focuses on attracting young professionals to move to rural areas.

THE MAIN ISSUES OF ROMANIAN SOCIAL HOUSING

Target Groups and Housing Allocation

Given the substantial economic benefit of qualifying for a social dwelling, access to social housing is of high political significance at the local level. Local mayors are authorized to appoint a special interdepartmental committee to analyze applications for social housing, and it prepares the final approved selection of applicants made by the local council. The decision to grant social housing is made on the basis of approved and detailed allocation criteria. However, in practice, there are no statistics available for further analysis of the allocation process of social dwellings. Demand, however, far exceeds supply.

Rent Regulation

The rent level in social rental apartments is determined by a complicated formula, but should in no case exceed 10 percent of the household's disposable income. If, as frequently happens, the calculated rent is not enough to cover all the annuities, housing management and maintenance costs, and local taxes, the local authorities are obliged to cover the gap with an adequate allowance scheme. Such income-tested rents result in heavily subsidized apartments. There is little motivation for tenants to leave such dwellings. Hence, housing mobility in this sector is extremely low. The existing stock of social housing contributes very little to the supply of affordable rental housing for eligible households; most of it has to come from new construction. This makes this scheme rather costly for the state.

Leases in social housing are usually limited to five years, with an option to extend the lease if income eligibility is proven. In a survey conducted in 2002, it was shown that rent arrears are very common in the social housing stock, ranging from one-third of all dwellings in larger cities to one-quarter in smaller cities (Pascariu and Stanculescu 2003, 281). A tenant can only be evicted by an irrevocable court decision, but this rarely happens, as such practices are unpopular and mayors consequently try to avoid them. There are, however, cases of forced collective evictions of Roma people by some local authorities, sometimes accompanied by police brutality (Rughinis 2004; Niţă 2009, 5).

The Maintenance and Management of Social Housing

According to the Housing Act, tenants (in social housing) are required to properly maintain their apartment and facilities: the tenant has to repair or replace defective building elements and installations in private and shared use. Also, the tenant is responsible for paying all utilities, either directly to the provider or through the homeowners' association. In practice, like in many other

Central and Eastern European (CEE) countries, maintenance schemes are poorly implemented. Very few residential buildings have a repair fund, which is an important precondition for financing major repair work, such as thermal refurbishment. Some bigger municipalities have set up publicly owned special companies for this purpose (Pascariu and Stanculescu 2003, 278).

Social Housing Finance

Public housing is basically financed out of the very tight local budgets, in accordance with Act No. 189/1998 and within annually approved budgetary limits. The state assists in the construction of public housing through transfers from the national budget, and these are annually set aside in the budget of the Ministry for Regional Development and Tourism. Local authorities are responsible for preparing development plans and ensuring the provision of infrastructure to support development. Most programs rely on the municipality to provide building land and infrastructure free of charge. Some programs (e.g., Rental Housing for Young People) have funding from international financing institutions such as the CEB, the Council of Europe Development Bank, or Deutsche Bank AG.

CONCLUSION

Because there is no monitoring or documentation of the various and frequently changing social housing programs that exist among the local authorities, it is very difficult to evaluate social housing policy in terms of its equality of treatment and effectiveness at providing housing for poor and vulnerable households. However, some preliminary conclusions can be drawn from our observations.

In quantitative terms, between 1997 and 2007, the ANL proved to be an effective implementation unit for national and local housing policy. Social housing in new buildings constructed before the crisis was on the way to establishing itself well, with a share of total housing production close to the EU average (6 percent in 2010, but 9–12 percent in the years before). Some EU countries place particular emphasis on social housing construction, which can account for as much as 30 percent of total construction; others have no social housing construction at all. It is difficult to define an appropriate benchmark for a reasonable volume of social housing construction. Yet, in Romania, there is a clear lack of qualitatively high yet affordable housing owing to shortages in the existing housing stock, the small average floor space per capita, and the weakly developed commercial market in rental housing. Housing affordability is a major challenge for Romania, where the housing cost overburden rate ranks among the highest in the EU.

There is some continuity of housing policy. Although the Housing Act has been amended more than ten times since it was enacted in 1996, very few substantial changes to housing models and subsidy schemes have taken place so far. The reluctance to carry out a major housing reform may be explained in part by the fact that housing policy is not a priority for European integration, but it is also due to the frequent changes in the division and distribution of government responsibilities during the transition. Housing reform in many cases has the character of ad hoc decisions, made in reference to an immediate emergency but with no long-term strategy. There is no long-term housing policy in place. Consequently, there is no regular assessment of (or reliable data on) policy implementation.

Housing policy reform has not yet improved consumer choice of housing tenure. The ownership ideology is very strong in Romania, and housing policy programs have contributed to it. Attempts to make rental housing a secure and economically rational alternative have been insufficient. Rental housing is divided into extremely unequal market segments, with rents that are much too low in the small social housing stock and rents equal to international levels in the private market (UNECE 2001, 25). Rental housing is largely inaccessible owing to the small amount of available social housing units, unaffordability (high market rents), or legal insecurity (informal leases).

In general, there is an urgent need to increase housing production as a whole. Given the demand, Romania should set a target of construction of one hundred thousand housing units per year. This is 4.8 newly constructed units per one thousand inhabitants, which is close to the EU average. Action is required to adapt the housing supply to meet demand in terms of location and affordability. As a housing developer, for organizational and financial reasons, ANL is incapable of providing the whole volume of necessary affordable housing. The social housing programs in operation heavily rely on public funds, especially at the level of the local authorities, a problem that could be dealt with by making more use of private funds and players (Amann 2005, 2006; UNECE 2005, 60–67, Dübel et al. 2006).

In order for a more effective social housing construction to take place, there needs to be a thorough improvement in the legal framework that regulates housing (Amann and Mundt 2010). This relates particularly to legislation on rent regulation (beyond just contract law); consumer protection (e.g., pertaining to the purchase of housing); and the effectiveness of owners' associations, housing management, and maintenance (facing the challenge of thermal refurbishments). Some of these observations apply both to Romania and other CEE countries. For many of them, the transition has not ended yet, at least not in the field of housing policy.

REFERENCES

Amann, W. 2005. "How to Boost Rental Housing Construction in CEE-/SEE-Countries." *Housing Finance International* 12:24–31.

———. 2006. "Rental Housing for Middle Income Groups a Challenge for PPP-Models." Presented at the Proceedings of the World Bank Conference Housing Finance in Emerging Markets, March 15–17.

Amann, W. and Mundt, A. 2010. "Designing a New Rental Housing Law for Romania." *International Journal of Law in the Built Environment* 2 (2): 157–77.

Dawidson, K. 2004. "Conflicts of Interest in the Restitution and Privatisation of Housing since the Fall of Socialism: The Case of Central Timosoara City—A Problem of Democracy." *Euro-Asia Studies* 56 (1): 119–41.

———. 2005. "Geographic Impacts of the Political: Dealing with Nationalized Housing in Romania." *Political Geography* 24:545–67.

Dübel, H.-J., Brzeski, W.J., and Hamilton, E. 2006. *Rental Choice and Housing Policy Realignment in Transition, Post-Privatization Challenges in the Europe and Central Asia Region.* Washington, DC: World Bank.

IIBW. 2008. *Implementation of European Standards in Romanian Housing Legislation.* Final Report. Unpublished research study commissioned by the Romanian Ministry of Development, Public Works and Housing. With the collaboration of Wolfgang Amann, Ioan A. Bejan, Helmut Böhm, Nadeyda Komendantova, Mihai Mereuta, Alexis Mundt, Theo Österreicher, Ciprian Paun, Gerhard Schuster, Andreas Sommer, Arin O. Stanescu, Walter Tancsits. Vienna: IIBW.

Nae, M. and Turnock, D. 2011. "City Profile: The New Bucharest. Two Decades of Restructuring." *Cities 28(2): 206–219*

Niţă, D. L. 2009. *Romania. Raxen National Focal Point.* Thematic Study. Housing Conditions of Roma and Travellers. Center for Legal Resources. Study commissioned as comparative report on housing conditions of Roma and Travellers in EU Member States by the European Union Agency for Fundamental Rights. http://www.fra.europa.eu/fraWebsite/attachments/RAXEN-Roma%20Housing-Romania_en.pdf accessed March 20, 2011.

OTB. 2010. *Housing Statistics of the European Union.* The Hague: Ministry of the Interior and Kingdom Relations.

Pascariu, S. and Stanculescu, M. 2003. "Management Improvement and Quality Standard Challenges. Local Government and Housing in Romania." *Housing Policy: An End or a New Beginning?* Budapest: OSI/LGI.

PRC Bouwcentrum International. 2005. "Sustainable Refurbishment of High-Rise Residential Buildings and Restructuring of Surrounding Areas in Europe." *Report for European Housing Ministers, Conference Proceedings 14–15 March 2005 held in Prague.* Bodegraven, The Netherlands: PRC.

Rughinis, A. C. 2004. "Social Housing and Roma Residents in Romania." *Central European University Center for Policy Studies, CPS International Policy Fellowship Program 2003/2004.* http://pdc.ceu.hu/archive/00001919/01/rughinis.pdf accessed April 19, 2011.

Stephens, M. 2005. "A Critical Analysis of Housing Finance Reform in a 'Super' Home-Ownership State: The Case of Armenia." *Urban Studies* 42 (10): 1795–1815.

Tsenkova, S. 2009. *Housing Policy Reforms in Post-Socialist Europe. Lost in Transition.* Heidelberg: Physica-Verlag.

UNECE. 2001. *Country Profiles on the Housing Sector Romania.*Geneva:UN

———. 2006. *Guidelines on Social Housing.* Geneva: UN.

14 Russia

The Persistence of the Socialist Legacy?

Alexandr Puzanov

INTRODUCTION

This chapter sets out to describe the current situation in the social housing sector in Russia. Notwithstanding twenty years of market reforms, social and 'nonsocial' housing have yet to form to full distinct sectors, as will be shown in the following. There are some 'traces' of social housing in all segments of the housing stock. For example, although homeowners are legally responsible for all expenses related to the 'burden of ownership', in practice the state and the municipalities continue to finance capital repairs of multifamily buildings, irrespective of the tenure status of the housing units they contain. The Fund for the Promotion of Housing and Utility Sector Reform, set up in the Russian Federation in 2007,[1] cofinances regional and municipal budgetary expenditures for capital repairs. Currently, the fund requires 5 percent of the total cost of regional capital repairs be paid by the owners of housing units.

Under the existing legislation, owners are not required to insure their housing property. As a result, when people lose their housing to natural disasters, the government will usually finance the provision of housing for displaced people out of the state or municipal budget. As a result, there is still no big difference between the housing expenditures of people who own their housing and those who rent public housing. At present, owners pay a 'housing unit tax', which is very small, whereas renters pay a 'pure rent' component (see the following), which is also a small share of the total payment. Other expenditures on maintenance and utilities are currently almost the same for owners and renters.

In this chapter, we shall work with the definition of social housing as housing that is rented out on terms that differ from market conditions using a certain administrative procedure that regulates access to such housing.[2] Only two exceptions will be made to this general approach. Firstly, we shall also examine the housing allowances program as a pivotal component of social housing policy, but that is applied to all types of housing stock. Secondly, in the final section we describe the future of social housing policy, the key element of which is to expand the narrow perception of social housing.

The first section presents the historical background of social housing in Russia, its development and its current condition in the context of the transition from a centrally planned housing sector to one governed primarily by market relations. The second section is devoted to an analysis of the key structural elements of the social housing sector. Subsequent sections contain an expert evaluation of how well social housing works as a mechanism for improving the housing conditions of the poor and vulnerable groups of the population, the legal status of tenants of social housing, rent-setting policies of setting rent rates, and the problems of social housing finance. The final sections focus on an analysis of the main development opportunities, and the main challenges, for housing policy with regard to the social housing sector.

THE GENERAL CONTEXT: ROOTS OF SOCIAL HOUSING

At the beginning of the transition period Russia's housing stock was characterized by an overwhelming state presence. Nationally, 67 percent of the stock was state owned, managed by either the municipalities or state enterprises and by government agencies. In urban areas, 79 percent and in larger cities as much as 90 percent of housing was owned by the state. The importance of state ownership in Russia's housing sector dwarfed the corresponding role of the state in Eastern European countries at the start of the economic reform period (Kosareva and Struyk 1997, 1–5). And about 6 percent of the housing stock (and up to 10 percent in larger cities) was made up of housing cooperatives,[3] which received considerable state support, including access to cheap bank loans.

The key attributes of the system that developed and maintained the state dominance, which affected the development of the social housing system in the transition period, are:

- There is centralized distribution of all resources and strictly formalized planning of the volume and distribution of new housing construction.
- There is heavy subsidization of activities by state housing maintenance and management organizations; rent on state units covers only a fraction of total operating costs and none of the capital costs; rent controls result in the poor targeting of subsidies; in the early 1990s only a third of costs was covered by residents' payments and the sector was heavily subsidized (Puzanov 1997, 57–75) .
- Tenants enjoy extremely strong occupancy rights, which can be bequeathed to other residents registered at the same address; this special status has been conceptualized as termed 'quasi ownership' (Lux 2003).
- Distribution of housing through waiting lists maintained by municipal authorities and state enterprises was the predominant means of

acquiring housing; by 1990, 9,456,000 households were put on waiting lists (26 percent of all households), and 1,158,000 were given free housing (12 percent of those on the waiting list). At the same time only fifty thousand units were acquired through housing cooperatives and seventy-two thousand were built by individuals as private housing.
- Enterprises were important providers of state housing; a separate system for the production, allocation, and maintenance of housing existed parallel to the municipal housing system.

Two main processes were launched at the beginning of the economic transition: housing 'municipalization'—the transfer of the state-owned housing stock to municipalities under enterprise housing divestiture schemes[4]—and housing privatization, enabling tenants to acquire their unit (initially at little cost and since 1992 for free) simply by requesting transfer of ownership to them.

Several aspects of the decision on privatization offer significantly shaped development in the social housing sector. Firstly, tenants were able to decide themselves whether they wanted to privatize their flat, and this resulted in the current situation where almost every apartment building in Russia contains units in both private and public ownership. This is compounded by the use of the condominium model (Lujanen 2010) for apartment building management, which has considerably complicated management of the social housing sector (see the following). Secondly, the decision to launch the privatization process was not accompanied by a discussion of what part of the housing stock should remain in public ownership and be used as social housing, thus leaving open the possibility that all state and municipal housing stock could be privatized during the transition period.[5] Also the government decided that housing units that had been privatized but not involved in any subsequent transactions (about one-half of the privatized stock) could be deprivatized at any moment until 2013 and thus end up in the social rental housing stock. The amount deprivatization is currently rare at the moment, but the situation could change significantly if certain changes are made to real estate taxation, insurance, and so on. There are no restrictions for deprivatization in practice.

The highest rates of privatization occurred during the first three years: by the end of 1995, 12.5 million units or 36 percent of the housing stock eligible for privatization had been privatized. The privatization of state and municipal housing has occurred in waves, occasionally surging in response to rumors of a possible privatization deadline, which has been shifted several times. For example, in 2002 68 million square meters of housing was privatized, in 2003 42 million square meters, in 2004 again 69 million square meters, in 2005 89 million square meters, and so on. By the end of 2008, 26.4 million housing units (1,306 million square meters) or 70 percent of the housing stock eligible for privatization had been privatized.

No explicit concept or policy for developing social housing was formulated in Russia. One may conclude that social housing in modern Russia emerged out of the leftovers from nonprivatized state or municipal housing stock.

Current legislation extends the regime of free and 'conditionless' privatization until 2013. Therefore, up to 2013 the parameters of the social housing stock will depend, to a great extent, on the rate of the housing privatization (and deprivatization) process. This in turn will be influenced by various housing market incentives, the structure of state subsidies, the tax regime, and so on. Until 2013 municipalities will not have clear incentives for increasing the volume of housing construction for subsequent social rental. The current status quo also means that municipalities are unable to construct and maintain social rental housing as 'buildings', and instead social housing is represented by individual flats in mixed ownership property condominiums.

Access to waiting lists to acquire state or municipal housing was unrestricted for (the first) fifteen years of the market economy development: every household whose housing consumption was below a certain level could join a waiting list. Since the new Housing Code was enacted in 2005, only low-income households and several other categories[6] could be put on a waiting list for state or municipal housing.[7] However, the state was still obliged to provide housing to anyone whose name went on a waiting list before 2005, regardless of the person's income level or financial status (data from the State Committee for Statistics 2009).[8]

THE KEY CHARACTERISTICS OF SOCIAL HOUSING

Definitions and Structural Elements

When describing the current Russian social housing system it is important to distinguish social housing (as rental housing provided under nonmarket terms through an administrative procedure) in its narrow and broad senses. The 'narrow concept' of social housing is the one defined in Russian housing legislation. In Russian law *social housing* means housing provided under a social rental agreement. At present, it accounts for almost 85 percent of the total state and municipal housing stock (see Table 14.1). The remaining 15 percent is special purpose housing, such as boardinghouses (dormitories), and recently housing provided under 'for-profit rental' agreements or gratuitous use agreements. Obviously, special purpose housing performs a social function and can therefore be categorized as 'social housing' in the broad sense of the term and the same is true of housing provided under a gratuitous use agreement.

The situation with 'for-profit rentals' is even more complicated. Currently, Russian legislation does not recognize nonprofit housing rentals as a special type of agreement, so from the legal point of view all housing (including the

Table 14.1 Structure of Russia's Rental Stock (Public Housing and Housing Owned by Legal Entities)

	2006		2007		2008		2009	
Housing stock, total (mln m2)	3,003		3,058		3,116		3,177	
1. Public housing stock (mln m2)	605		575		549		492	
% of total housing stock	20%		19%		18%		16%	
Including:	mln. m2	% of public housing stock	mln. m2	% of public housing stock	mln. m2	% of public housing stock	mln. m2	% of public housing stock
1.1. Housing stock under social rental agreement	252.6	41.8%	242.8	42.2%	233.7	42.6%	224.7	45.6%
1.2. Special purpose housing stock	48.0	7.9%	50.2	8.7%	50.4	9.2%	48.0	9.8%
Including:								
Tied accommodation	1.4	0.2%	1.8	0.3%	2.5	0.5%	2.8	0.6%
Dormitories and other special purpose housing stock	46.7	7.7%	48.4	8.4%	47.9	8.7%	45.3	9.2%
1.3. Housing, provided under 'commercial' (non-subsidized) agreements	6.7	1.1%	6.4	1.1%	9.6	1.8%	6.4	1.3%
1.4. Other public housing stock (unclassified)	297.3	49.2%	275.4	47.9%	254.8	46.5%	213.2	43.3%
2. Rental housing owned by legal entities	95		94		100		102	
% of total housing stock	3.2%		3.1%		3.2%		3.2%	

Note: Calculated using data from the Federal Statistical Survey, Form 1-Housing.

portion of state and municipal housing that is neither social—in the narrow sense—nor special) is provided under commercial (or 'for profit') agreements. However, one could argue that all this housing is allocated under nonmarket principles and for rents below the market level.

So, in the broad sense, social housing comprises almost all public (state and municipal) housing stock and most of the housing stock rented out by private entities.[9] For the purposes of this article, we shall refer to social housing in the narrow sense (as defined in Russian legislation) as 'housing provided under a social rental agreement' or 'social rental housing'.

Table 14.1 illustrates the structure of and recent dynamics in the housing stock in Russia.

Table 14.1 shows the continuous decrease in the size of the public housing sector, including housing provided under social rental agreements. The large amount of public housing with an 'unclassified' type of use reflects the fact that the inventory of public housing covered under the current legal framework is far from exhaustive. Although one would expect the distribution of 'unclassified' types of housing to be similar to that of the already classified housing, we estimate the amount of social rental housing in 2009 at 418 million square meters or 85 percent of the total public housing stock. The total social housing may be estimated at 594 million square meters or 19.2 percent of the total housing stock.[10]

Problems of Housing Stock Management

Currently nearly all social rental housing consists of flats in condominium buildings. The situation is more or less the same in special purpose housing and rental housing owned by legal entities. This causes numerous problems resulting from the municipality's conflicting interests, as the municipality may at the same time be (a) the co-owner of the common property in the condominium building, (b) the owner or quasi owner of the housing management and utility companies, and (c) a public entity (regulation, budget support allocation).

Housing legislation contains some incentives for 'consolidating' the existing municipal stock in the future: if the owners of the units in a condominium decide to increase maintenance or repair fees the decision does not apply to housing with social rental agreements, then the municipality either has to pay the difference for these units out of its own funds or it must sell the unit and provide the tenants with a social rental housing unit in a different building with lower fees.

Targeting

The targeting of social rental housing has largely been determined by the fact that it emerged out of the leftover housing from the nonprivatized state or municipal stock. The factors that drove housing privatization in Russia

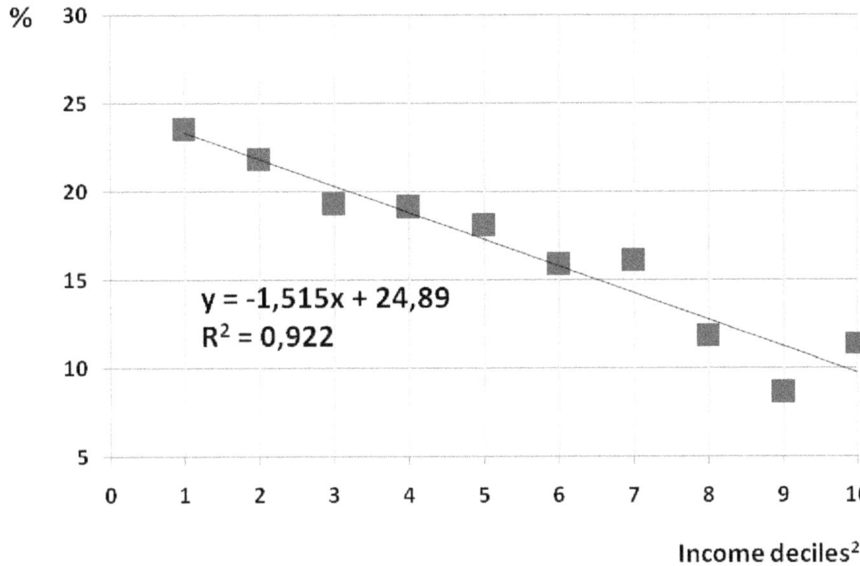

Figure 14.1 Share of tenants in public housing by income deciles, 2007.

were examined by Daniel and Struyk (1994), who found that certain low-income categories (lone pensioners) had a higher incentive to privatize. As a result, in the mid-1990s the average income of renters was 1.06 times higher than that of owners.[11] Recently the situation has changed and the concentration of low-income households in public housing is much higher, but a considerable portion of higher-income households nonetheless remain in public housing (Figure 14.1).

So the targeting of social housing is moderate at best. There are also no big differences in housing consumption between the 'social' and 'private' segments of the housing stock.

The average crowding rate in the state and municipal housing stock is 22.1 square meters per person compared to the national average of 22.5 square meter s(data for 2009). In the housing stock provided under social rental agreements, the occupancy rate is higher, and it matches the national average.

THE DEMAND FOR SOCIAL HOUSING AND THE DYNAMICS OF WAITING LIST ADMISSION AND ALLOCATION

A general idea of the real demand for social rental housing may be provided by the national household survey of 2003 (Kosareva et al. 2004).[12] Of those not satisfied with their housing conditions (61 percent of households), one-fifth of respondents said that they saw no alternative to waiting for social housing after being put on a waiting list. Thus, almost three million households currently are currently relying on social housing allocation instruments.

As described in the preceding, until 2005 any citizen with less housing space than he or she was entitled to had a 'no-cost' opportunity to apply for social housing. Obviously, the status of an applicant did not automatically grant him or her a real chance of getting social rental housing: annually only 4–5 percent of households on a waiting list improved their housing conditions. Therefore, there are many people who do not expect to obtain social housing by waiting on a list, evidence of which is proved by the fact that between 1995 and 2005 the waiting lists for social housing considerably 'shrank', mainly due to natural changes in the size of some applicants' households so that they were no longer eligible for assistance with housing allocation. Moreover, some households on the waiting list managed to improve their housing conditions without state or municipal assistance. Finally, the estimated total number of households that have to rely on social housing allocation instruments (three million households) exceeds the number of households currently on a waiting list (2.8 million households), and many of the latter may have other means of improving their housing conditions but prefer instead to take the no-cost opportunity to be on the waiting list.

The owners of the housing stock have full authority to set the rules for 'intake' to their waiting list, so the system is decentralized. Since 2005, public authorities have been able to regulate admission to waiting lists by setting certain 'low-income' criteria for household eligibility.[13] As a result, in 2009 the number of new admissions and the number applicants that

Table 14.2 Waiting List Dynamics

	1995	2000	2001	2006	2008	2009
Number of households on the waiting list (as of the end of the year), million households	7.0	5.42	4.86	3.12	2.86	2.83
Number of households that got housing and improved their housing conditions (per year), million households	0.65	0.25	0.24	0.14	0.14	0.15
Households that got housing and improved their housing conditions as a proportion of the total number of households on the waiting list (%)	8.4%	4.6%	4.9%	4.5%	5.0%	5.2%
Households on the waiting list as a proportion of the total number of households (%)	15	11	10	6	6	6

Source: Fankhauser and Tepic (2005).

dropped off the waiting lists were almost equal—263,000 households. Of those who dropped off the waiting list, only 56 percent received housing assistance from the public authorities, whereas others quit for various reasons described in the preceding.

A few categories (orphans graduating from state institutions, people who had lost their previous social rental housing units, etc.) had priority access to social rental housing without having to join a waiting list.

Nationally, only 31 percent of those who joined a waiting list in 2009 belonged to a 'low-income' category. This means that the assumption in the Housing Code that the waiting list system would be used primarily to provide housing to low-income citizens is not supported by current practices. The structure of housing allocation (Table 14.3) explains this phenomenon. Up to

Table 14.3 Structure of Publicly Supported Housing Allocation, 2009

	In total	Households that got housing in newly constructed buildings: In total	Households that got housing in newly constructed buildings: As % of households that got housing and improved their housing conditions
	Thousands	Thousands	Percentage
1. Households that got housing and improved their housing conditions	146	51.7	35.4
Of which			
1.1. From "Off" the waiting list (orphans and other special categories)	27	8.0	29.6
1.1.1. Under social rental agreement	20.7	7.3	35.3
1.2. From the waiting list	119	43.7	36.7
1.2.1. Under housing ownership support schemes	67.8	23.4	34.5
1.2.1.1. With federal subventions	35.4	6.2	17.5
1.2.1.2. Through subsidized mortgages	10.6	6.7	63.2
1.2.1.3. Via other schemes	21.8	10.5	
1.2.2. Under social rental agreements	46.9	16.5	35.2
1.2.3. Under other schemes	4.3	3.8	88.3

Note: Calculated using data from the Federal Statistical Survey, Form 4-Housing.

60 percent of households on a waiting list acquire housing in ownership under various schemes that offer substantial deductions compared to market rates. There are several categories of households that are entitled to federal and/or regional subsidies (the most common one is 'young families') or subventions (war veterans). Therefore, one can assume that the municipalities admit to the waiting lists households that are able to 'attract' federal subventions or subsidies or have the funds to cover at least part of the housing price when purchasing housing. In the latter case housing is offered to them either at special prices or under heavily subsidized mortgage schemes—so-called social mortgages. Both schemes are nontransparent and potentially prone to corruption. There are, of course, also households that joined a waiting list before 2005 (before the income criterion was set), and they are offered a trade-off: they can either wait for an indefinite period for free-of-charge social rental housing or purchase housing at a below-market price. The local authorities thus still seem to 'favor' households that are able to cofinance their housing purchase.

Table 14.3 shows that only 35 percent of households on the waiting lists obtained social rental housing in a newly constructed building. Others improved their housing conditions through housing chain mechanisms or when public flats were vacated and were available for other reasons. In practice, only Moscow and several other jurisdictions continue to finance public housing construction from their budgets.

THE LEGAL STATUS OF TENANTS IN SOCIAL RENTAL HOUSING

Eligibility

In 2005–2007, most of the constituent entities of the Russian Federation approved regulatory legal documents defining the criteria for categorizing citizens as 'low income' and the procedure for registering citizens for housing and evaluating their financial status. The authority sets exact income limits (adjusted to the value of the property owned by a household) and the threshold of housing space per person for eligibility to join the waiting list lie with the owner of the housing stock. If the state or regional authority does not impose any special requirements for eligible categories defined in federal or regional laws or presidential decrees, the rules established by the municipality in which the housing unit is provided are the rules that apply. Thus, the municipalities have some opportunity to regulate the number of 'low-income' people on their waiting lists. However, households that do not belong to the low-income category continue to be eligible (see the following).

The Social Rental Agreement

Tenants with a social rental agreement have a pretty wide range of rights, which transforms their status to 'quasi ownership'. First of all, the social rental agreement is signed for an indefinite term. Second, since Soviet times, a tenant has been able to use the mechanism of a “replacement of the tenant” under an agreement to engage in ‘tenant exchange’ practices, where two tenants with social agreements exchange flats or one subleases to another, and so on. Consequently, tenants essentially used to possess surrogate tools enabling them to effectively dispose of the housing that they occupied—by passing it on to heirs, renting it out, and so on.

The new Housing Code imposed only minor restrictions on these powers. Combined with the absence of conditions that would allow owners of housing to fully exercise their rights (i.e., make decisions on how to manage their housing, e.g., when they make a decision on multifamily building capital repairs) and meet their obligations (in practice owners cover only a negligible share of the capital repairs in multifamily buildings), this makes the legal status of participants in the residential real estate market vague, and that undermines the efficient functioning of the market. Thus, the differences between social and nonsocial housing segments are still not very clear.

RENT IN THE SOCIAL RENTAL SECTOR

Public housing rent was one of a few household expenditures that were not subjected to the price liberalization introduced in January 1992. As a result, by the end of that year households were covering only 2–4 percent of housing maintenance costs. In December 1992, a rent reform program was developed as part of the housing reform framework law passed by the national legislature. The law declared that the full costs of maintenance and repair of housing and utility services must be covered by the residents who occupy residential premises in state and municipal housing under social rental agreements. The transition to this new system of housing and utility payments required the simultaneous introduction of housing allowances to all eligible families.

Rent in public housing is set annually by a municipal regulatory act and applies to both state and municipal stock in a particular jurisdiction. Rent consists of two components: (a) the pure rent, payment for renovations, and (b) a fee for maintenance and current repair services. The amount of both components is determined based on the number of square meters of the flat. The half-dozen utility charges that exist are calculated and paid separately.

The municipalities usually individually determine the amount of ‘pure rent’ and the fee for maintenance and repair services by type of buildings depending on the building’s physical condition, amenities and location. As a result, an enormous gap (by an order of magnitude) persists between rents paid by tenants of social rental housing and market-level rents.

There are no legal limits on the amount of the pure rent, except for the legal provision that tenants that have ‘low-income’ status do not pay the pure rent component. In practice the pure rent is symbolic and covers only a small fraction of renovation costs. It is usually a much smaller amount than the second component. The fee for maintenance and current repair services should not exceed the actual cost of such services. Municipalities could set maintenance fees at a lower level and subsidize the difference from their budgets. Currently, statistics report rates averaging 95 percent of expenditures. Expenditures on capital repairs are not included in the calculation of fees. There are caps on annual rent and utility tariff increases. The Federal Tariff Service sets individual caps for the regions, whereas regional regulatory bodies set them for the municipalities. But the cap applies to the whole housing and utility bill, and there is always a trade-off between increases in maintenance rates and tariffs. As a rule, utilities account for 66–85 percent of the total bill.

In 1993 housing allowances were introduced to help low-income households pay their housing and utility fees. This was particularly important during the period of transition, because service providers had difficulties in collecting the fees and covering the expenditures on housing and utility services. Both tenants in public housing and owners of housing units were eligible for the housing allowance. However, the allowance does not cover pure rent. Prior to the recently adopted legislative changes, there was no uniform housing allowance scheme in Russia. The current housing allowance formula was introduced by the new Housing Code in 2004:

$$S = MSR—a^*t^*Y,$$

where

a = 1, if per capita income of the recipient household is not less than the officially set subsistence level;
a = PCI/SL, if per capita income of the recipient household (PCI) is less than the officially set subsistence level (SL).

Since the new Housing Code was adopted in 2004 the key parameters of the housing allowance program are set by the regions, which are also responsible for financing the allowance payments through grants to the municipalities. The municipalities can, however, change the parameters to make the program more generous. Under the new Housing Code tenants in the private rental sector are also eligible for the housing allowance, but the formula used to determine the amount of the allowance is based on rates and tariffs in the municipal sector, which are several times lower than in the private rental sector.

Housing allowances were most important during the period of transition to the point where the public/people were financially able to afford to pay their own housing and utility services (1993–2005). In 2003, 15.2 percent of all households were receiving the housing allowance. Since then the program has gradually been downsized, and by 2009 the figure had fallen to 8.3 percent. However, housing allowances in Russia still considerably differ from similar programs in Western European countries: (a) they do very little to improve the affordability of private rental housing, and (b) Russian housing allowances make it easier to pay only current costs related to the delivery of housing and utility services, but, for example no outstanding payments or arrears can be covered.

FINANCING SOCIAL HOUSING

Financing social rental housing construction and capital repairs is the legal responsibility of the municipalities from their municipal budgets (or state authorities from corresponding state budgets, if the state decides to build such housing, but the obligation to provide social rental housing to those on the waiting list lies with the municipalities). In practice, they more often use an alternative option and acquire housing units for use as social housing by entering into an 'investment contract' with a private developer (this usually involves some kind of reciprocal agreement where the municipality provides the developer with land and access to infrastructure under nonmarket terms in exchange of housing units). However, the physical parameters of these housing units make them often unsuitable for social housing purposes.

The obligation to provide housing to households on the local waiting list clearly exceeds the budgetary resources of the municipalities. Providing social rental housing to the 2.8 million households in the country that are currently on a local waiting list would require a total of 140 billion U.S. dollars (assuming that the average unit size is 50 square meters, and the cost of one square meter is approximately 1,000 U.S. dollars[14]). This is equal to 171 percent of the total consolidated budget of all the municipalities in 2009. In fact, in 2009 the municipalities spent less than 10 billion U.S. dollars on the development of new social rental units (this estimate includes hidden budgetary subsidies provided under investment contracts with private developers).

Until 1999, housing allowances were funded from local government resources, although the regions provided fungible grants to municipalities that could be used for this purpose. In fact, an increase in fees for housing and utility services nearly always generated more revenue than necessary for the payment of housing allowance benefits, providing extra revenue to the city budget. Consequently, the 1999 legislation recognized a federal responsibility and led to the creation of federal grants to partially compensate for local allowance payments. The grant amount is based on program parameters for calculating household subsidies established by the federal government. Communities in which the established cost recovery rates and household contribution rates (*t*) meet or exceed the federal parameters get their full grant allocations, whereas others receive less. In 2009, federal subsidies for regional housing allowance programs amounted to 3.9 billion U.S. dollars. Total (state) budget expenditures on housing allowances reached 1.9 billion U.S. dollars in 2009, and expenditures for further benefits to selected categories of households equaled an additional 5 billion U.S. dollars (data for 2008).

Total socially targeted budgetary expenditures on housing in 2009 can thus be estimated to be in the range of 7–8 billion U.S. dollars. This amount consists of expenditures on the provision of new social rental housing units, housing allowances, and some budgetary expenditures on covering some further privileged subsidies. The latter component relates to the system of granting privileges to certain categories of the population, not all of whom could be considered vulnerable, which was inherited from the Soviet period (usually in the form of a 50 percent discount to housing and utility bills). One might also consider adding to this estimate the approximately 0.8 billion U.S. dollars of budgetary subsidies to support housing acquisition for certain categories of population (e.g., young families, military personnel, civil servants). This policy measure is oriented more towards the promotion of homeownership. However, recently incentives were created to stimulate affordable (rental) housing provision to meet this budget-supported demand.

If we compare this with socially nontargeted budgetary expenditures in the housing and utility sectors (about 20 billion U.S. dollars in 2009) we can conclude that the efficiency of budgetary expenditures is rather low.

THE SOCIAL HOUSING STRATEGY

So far, housing policy in Russia has been based on the concept of a maintaining a moderate volume of social rental housing used to supply housing only to the neediest households. The expectation is that after the transition period most households would be able to satisfy their housing needs with the help of market tools. However, it has become obvious that this view needs to be revised. Firstly, only a minority of households are able to make real use of the advantages offered by the housing market to improve their housing conditions. Large parts of the population have no prospects for improving their housing conditions with the help of state subsidies or in the social housing sector.

In 2010 only about 20 percent of households could afford to buy standard housing without state assistance. It is expected that by 2020, assuming that economic growth and the growth of real household income continue, as much as 50 percent of the total population will be able to purchase housing using their own means and credit resources and without any other assistance. However, even with this optimistic forecast (for future homeownership) it is obvious that the current volume of social rental housing is far from sufficient, and development of more social housing is limited by budget constraints and a lack of motivation of the major actors.

Secondly, the existing social rental housing, which accounts for less than 20 percent of the housing stock and has been shrinking every year as a result of the ongoing privatization, is not used efficiently enough from the point of view of meeting the housing needs of the poorest households. The average waiting period for such housing is more than twenty years, which clearly demonstrates that the institute of social rental housing in its current form is not serving its purpose. At the same time, the housing rights of those who do obtain social rental housing are excessively broad in some cases and resemble quasi ownership.

Thirdly, many households that became owners through privatization discovered that they are unable to afford the full financial burden of homeownership. This has especially created problems for the rehabilitation of apartment buildings.

By the end of the first decade of the twenty-first century, all of the aforementioned issues began to be seen as political issues. Voices began calling for a more differentiated approach to the assessment of the housing needs of different population groups and for a shift towards a broader concept of social housing. At present a revision of the current social housing policy is being discussed by experts and policymakers.

State and Municipal Social Rental Housing Stock

The state and municipal social rental housing stock should be developed to the extent where it is able to provide housing supply to low-income households and other citizens who are on the 'waiting list' to improve their housing conditions. Obviously, in the foreseeable future, the budget capacity of the municipalities will not allow them to considerably increase the volume of construction of new social rental housing. Nevertheless, it is important to create incentives for increasing budget spending in this area (currently no such incentives exist). There should also be a continued search for ways in which to encourage households that are on a waiting list but are not in the category of low-income households to use alternative means to improve their housing conditions. This would help to reduce the volume of public obligations with regard to social rental housing allocation. This would help to cut the waiting period for social housing from the current level of more than twenty years to just four to five years. Only once the waiting period is reduced to a reasonable length of time will we be able to talk about the effectiveness of the institute of social rental housing in Russia.

Rental of State and Municipal Housing, Nonprofit Rental

There is a clear need for rental housing that can be offered at below-market rates but is not as heavily subsidized as social rental housing. The demand for such housing comes from moderate-income households, which are unable to purchase or rent housing at free market prices but at the same time could not be classified as 'low-income' households. In some cities (e.g., in Moscow and Chuvash Republic) attempts have already been made to create a nonprofit (unsubsidized) socially oriented rental sector, which will target a wider circle of citizens (e.g., young families, public sector employees). These attempts are still of an experimental nature (6 apartment buildings in Moscow by the end of 2010). As it was described earlier, such housing is legally distinguished as 'for-profit' or 'commercial use' housing. Special regulations are thus needed to give a real start to nonprofit housing development. At least two things need to be legally addressed: (a) creating the special legal status of a nonprofit housing developer, owner, and manager, and (b) creating the special status of a long-term nonprofit rental agreement. This kind of nonprofit/unsubsidized rental housing should not be aimed at making a profit. However, unlike social rental housing, it must ensure that the owner is able to recover not only the maintenance expenses of the housing, but also capital expenditures on construction.

Today, civic legislation deems the term of a rental contract (other than social rentals) to be one of its material provisions and that it should not exceed five years. In spite of regulatory norms on the preemptive right to sign an agreement for a new term, this legal framework is fraught with serious risks for tenants of nonprofit housing.

The practices of similar nonprofit housing organizations in Europe may be fully applied in Russia. However, we should take into account the fact that European nonprofit housing associations have a long history and in their work they are able to rely on public institutions well established in the past two centuries. Because Russia lacks all this, we can assume that the process of creating such organizations will be very painful and prolonged.

Enterprises are now aware of the growing role of housing as a means of attracting and keeping skilled personnel in their employ. Nevertheless, so far their actions have not been supportive in terms of creating incentives for the development of noncommercial rental housing. Some enterprises in Russia do currently provide housing to their employees, including those who would otherwise be eligible to apply for social rental housing, on terms similar to those of social rental or special purpose housing rental. In the light of this fact, the practice of signing trilateral agreements between enterprises and local government bodies/entities of the Russian Federation should be encouraged. In the foreseeable future such enterprises could become the founders of nonprofit housing organizations.

Expanding the Housing Allowances Program

As discussed in the preceding, housing allowances granted to citizens to cover housing and utility payments are calculated according to the level of such payments in the sector of social rental housing. When a nonprofit housing rental sector develops, there may be a problem with the affordability of such housing for citizens with moderate income. In addition, it is expected that an increasing number of citizens will try to address their housing problems by renting housing at free market prices. To maintain and enhance the sustainability of this foreseeable process, it is recommended that a new housing allowance model be introduced that reflects the expansion of rental housing into the market and nonprofit sectors.

Housing Construction Cooperatives

We expect that housing cooperatives that have some characteristics of social housing providers will enjoy considerable state support in the nearest future. Because the main goal of such associations is to provide housing to citizens/members of the cooperative rather than to make profits, there are motivations for reducing housing costs by excluding the developer's monopolistic profit aim and guaranteeing a demand for such housing. Currently consideration is being given to how to amend the legislation currently in effect in order to restore the legal framework of 'full-fledged' cooperatives (we use the word *restore* because a similar institution function in the 1960s–1980s in the form of Soviet era housing construction cooperatives).[15] These 'full-fledged' cooperatives will be less attractive to both speculators and to investors. Such would be the necessary prerequisites for state support for housing cooperatives. One suggested approach to creating cooperative housing is that a 'full-fledged' cooperative would be set up by people in a local waiting list for housing who are not 'low-income' households, and they would obtain for free a plot of land for the construction of housing and would receive subsidies and other forms of organization support from the public authorities.

CONCLUSION

After twenty years of economic transition social housing in Russia is still in a transitory phase. Neither the internal structure of social housing nor the difference between the social and market segments of the housing stock is well defined. A state policy has been formulated only for state and municipal housing provided under social rental agreements, but even in that area adequate instruments for policy implementation are lacking. Recently, the need for a comprehensive concept of social housing development has emerged as an issue of housing policy debate. However, visible changes can only be expected after the housing privatization regime expires in 2013 and once legislation to regulate nonprofit and cooperative housing is finally adopted.

NOTES

1. Federal Act No.185-FZ on the Fund for the Promotion of Housing and Utility Sector Reform, dated July 21, 2007.
2. It will be shown in the next section that this interpretation of social housing in Russia in turn comprises both a narrow and a wider definition.
3. Meanwhile, access to cooperatives was regulated by the state authorities. In practice, this opportunity was available only to residents of large cities. The right to use a housing unit in a cooperative was granted only on the basis of membership in the cooperative. Soviet era cooperatives were not rental cooperatives, which made them different from cooperatives in a number of other countries.
4. The privatization legislation required that state housing stock possessed by state enterprises should be excluded from 'privatization en masse' and transferred to a municipality where an enterprise is located.
5. In some post-Soviet republics, 'voluntary-compulsory' privatization ultimately resulted in the near disappearance of all state and municipal housing.
6. Such categories could be determined by federal or regional laws and decrees of the RF president.
7. Waiting list procedures are further discussed in the section "The Demand for Social Housing and the Dynamics of Waiting List Admission and Allocation".
8. We estimate that out of the 2.8 million households currently on a waiting list about two million were put on it before 2005. Nearly 48 percent households have been on a waiting list for more than ten years.
9. For-profit private rental as a commercial enterprise under current conditions is not economically viable in Russia.
10. Approximately twelve million housing units or more than 20 percent of all housing units. Unfortunately, Russian statistics do not provide a breakdown of housing units by tenure.
11. Calculated using data from the Russian Longitudinal Monitoring Survey (RLMS) (1994).
12. The project was implemented by the workgroup on the development of an affordable housing market set by the Center for Strategic Research. Vneshtorgbank (VTB) was the customer under the project, and the Institute for Urban Economics (IUE) was the main contractor working in partnership with the Research Centre of the Russian Marketing Association (RMA Research Centre), the Centre for Information and Economic Research in the Construction Industry, the Development Centre of the Economic Research Foundation, the Agency for Housing Mortgage Lending (AHML), and the AN SAVA Joint-Stock Company.
13. Public authorities (mostly municipalities) can also set the 'intake norms' for housing provision.
14. Based on official estimates of the RF Ministry for Regional Development for the second half of the year 2010.
15. According to current Russian legislation, once a member of a housing cooperative repays his or her stake in the cooperative, the member automatically becomes the owner of the housing premises he or she occupies. This makes housing cooperatives an interim (rather than a permanent) organizational form, because after the repayment of the first installment by their members, the operations of such cooperatives should be regulated by the laws on the associations of owners.

REFERENCES

Daniel, J. and Struyk, R. 1994. "Housing Privatization in Moscow: Who Privatizes and Why?" *International Journal of Urban and Regional Research* 18 (3): 510–25.

Kosareva, N., Rogozhina, N., Tumanov, A., and Yakoubov, M. 2004. *Evaluation of the Scale and Dynamics of Changes in Effective Housing Demand and Housing Construction in Russia.* Report. Moscow: The Institute for Urban Economics.

Kosareva, N. and Struyk. R. 1997. "Chapter 1: Reforming Russia." *Restructuring Russia's Housing Sector, 1991–1997.* Washington, DC: Urban Institute Press.

Puzanov, A. 1997. "Chapter 5: Rent Reform and Housing Allowances." *Restructuring Russia's Housing Sector, 1991–1997.* Washington, DC: Urban Institute Press.

Lujanen, M. 2010. "Legal Challenges in Ensuring Regular Maintenance and Repairs of Owner Occupied Apartment Blocks." *International Journal of Law in the Built Environment* 2 (2): 179–86.

Lux, M. ed. 2003. *Housing Policy: An End or a New Beginning.* Budapest: OSI/LGI.

"Russia Longitudinal Monitoring survey, RLMS-HSE", conducted by HSE and ZAO "Demoscope" together with Carolina Population Center, University of North Carolina at Chapel Hill and the Institute of Sociology RAS. Report 1994. (RLMS-HSE sites: http://www.cpc.unc.edu/projects/rlms-hse, http://www.hse.ru/org/hse/rlms)

15 Serbia

A Patchwork of Local Options

Mina Petrović

INTRODUCTION

Historically speaking, Serbia has never developed a full-fledged social housing policy, and the housing policy challenges of the interwar period were very similar to those that exist today. Some parallel issues are (a) the need to develop a complex strategic approach to housing at both the national and local levels as a precondition for economically efficient and socially effective social housing programs; (b) tackling the effects of the lack of coordination of housing construction for the poor; and (c) the 'slumification' and ghettoization of housing for the poor, in part due to informal construction strategies (Vukasnović-Macura 2011).

Since the interwar period, of course, the social context has significantly changed. But because of the specific distribution of power in Serbia a strategic approach to social housing is still lacking (Kemeny 1992; Harloe 1995). Therefore, even though it is more common to view post-socialist development as a complete break with the socialist past (Scanlon 2008), we think it is warranted to discuss the role and type of social housing from a path dependency perspective, combining path-shaping and path-breaking factors (Reinprecht et al. 2008).

This chapter opens with a discussion of the socialist legacy and the current ambivalent conditions. In the subsequent analysis, the context and dominant approach to social housing in post-socialist Serbia are described. The chapter is divided into two sections: the first reviews factors that (might) generate demand for social housing, and the second discusses the legislative and financial framework and concrete programs of subsidized housing provision in Serbia. The conclusion reflects on effectiveness and efficiency issues.

THE DEFICIENT APPROACH TO SOCIAL HOUSING: SOCIALIST LEGACY AND POST-SOCIALIST AMBIVALENCE

Under socialism, subsidies generally targeted public housing production and the state (through socially owned enterprises) was responsible for the distribution of flats. The low-income policy meant rents were also low, set at levels that did not cover the investment and maintenance costs. Other types of housing provision were strictly controlled through land policy, the provision of construction material, bank loans, and so on. Private property was tolerated, but homeowners' rights were limited to personal consumption. Tenants' rights were very similar to homeowners' rights, such as the right to transfer or inherit homes (see Petrović 2001).

All new housing policies were supposed to be designed in conformity with the socialist housing policy model. In reality, however, this did not happen: the predominance of privately owned flats (77 percent), even in urban settlements (61 percent), with the exception of Belgrade (46 percent), clearly demonstrates how socialist housing policy failed. The largest share of socially owned flats were in major administrative and political centers in the country, housing the elites, professionals, and highly qualified workers, whereas in small towns, even important industrial ones, the share was much smaller.

Economic inefficiency resulted in a decrease in social housing production (Hegedüs and Tosics 1996; Petrović 2001, 219). Social housing was allocated to higher-status social groups, so socially owned flats had a significant role in reproducing the polarized political power structure and income distribution (Mrkšić 1987), but housing allocation was open to various groups, the priority of which changed from time to time. This continuous change prevented selected groups from getting access to social housing in large numbers, and other groups were left out of the allocation procedures. In these circumstances, the right to housing was never defined as a social right.

Social policy in general was not perceived as a separate policy arena. It was based on four pillars: full employment, price control, the universal availability of goods, and full employment as an important distributive channel of social goods, including housing (Dixon and Kim 1992, 4). However, the issues of poverty, poor housing, and homelessness were ignored, and poor people were left to find their own solutions to problems that did not fit into the ideological vision of socialist society (Rus 1991).

Lower-income social groups were forced to develop 'exit' housing strategies (Hegedüs and Tosics 1996, 19–22). As a result, self-built housing, often constructed illegally, mainly owing to restrictive urban planning,[1] emerged as the 'unofficial social housing policy'; it was tolerated as an inevitable side effect of the official housing system (Petrović 2001, 2004). The only reform that tried to incorporate social issues into housing policy was introduced in 1974, with the foundation of the so-called solidarity flats that were created for workers employed by less successful enterprises. Although the program was coordinated by the municipalities, this did not mean that it was decentralized (Petrović 2001, 2004).

In the post-socialist period, Serbian politicians had to accept the new logic of state interventions in a market environment. New policy instruments that had never existed under socialism, or even before that time, had to be developed for the first time, including the very institution of social housing. Still, the process took long: except for the privatization process in the early 1990s, housing was not a policy issue until the beginning of the 2000s. The privatization of housing on a mass scale played the role of a shock absorber (Struyk 1996), as it was a tool for the increasingly impoverished middle class. Throughout the period of blocked transformation (Lazić 2000), the political elite did nothing to curtail the spread of illegal construction, which ceased to be just a phenomenon observed among lower-income groups and turned into a widespread strategy in response to the unaffordability of housing and the increasing pressure on the housing market, exacerbated by the increased demand caused by an influx of refugees from the Balkan conflicts.

Serbia entered the first phase of the institutional transition towards a market society only after 2000, and the transition process has again been slowed by the global economic crisis since 2008.[2] Housing policy slowly made its way onto the political agenda, but it has constantly had to compete over limited budget resources with the priorities of economic growth and social protection, and there is also the challenge of defining a policy's target groups. Consequently, there are almost no sound laws governing the sphere of social housing, and this fuels the inertia of political voluntarism that emerged under socialism and constantly reinforces the 'weak state' syndrome (Woolcock 1998) at every level of government. Moreover, with no legislative framework to define the social aims and rights of housing, poor and marginalized people remain powerless actors who have no way of influencing the formulation of social housing policy from the bottom up. They mostly depend on illegal construction and micro-networks driven by force of necessity, and although this provides for survival strategies, it impedes efficient social integration. This is all the more complicated given that many of these households live in substandard housing served by poor social infrastructure.

Housing privatization made Serbia a nation of homeowners. Public rental housing was always perceived more as a form of homeownership than rental tenure under socialism and was viewed to be as 'safe' and transferable as ownership. New social housing in the public sector that has no right-to-buy option is rather unpopular.

There is now a move away from the social housing concept based on solidarity (and aimed at key workers) towards a concept based on efficiency, which should be achieved by providing 'very social' housing for the most excluded and marginalized members of the population (Reinprecht et al. 2008). This makes defining social housing a complex task, because both concepts represent a departure from Serbia's socialist legacy and inherited institutional capacities, not only because the public rental sector had shrunk, but also because a new social housing definition presupposes a shift in the policy approach: from assistance to integration.

THE DEMOGRAPHIC, HOUSING AND SOCIOECONOMIC CONTEXTS: SUPPRESSED DEMAND

The size of the population in Serbia has been decreasing since 1991, despite enormous immigration flows of refugees and internally displaced people (IDPs).[3] The population is significantly aging, which usually increases the demand for social housing in modern individualized societies. In Serbia, there has been only a modest increase in the number of households between 1991 and 2002, which is basically related to the slow emergence of varieties of household types and to sluggish individualization due to, among other things, limited income and housing affordability (Petrović 2009). Between 1991 and 2002 refugee households (130,730 in 2002) came to make up the majority of newly formed households in the country (82 percent), and this put substantial pressure on the housing market and increased the number of people in need of social housing, which, together with various support services, should have served as a means of helping the integration of refugees.[4]

According to the last available census data (2002), 83 percent of households are homeowners, only 2 percent rent publicly owned flats, around 4

Table 15.1 Ownership Structure of the Housing Stock, in Thousands

	1991			2002		
	Total	Private	Public	Total	Private	Public
Total stock	2,713			2,956		
Total number of dwellings for permanent living	2,546	1,955	592.0	2,744	2,686	58.0
Occupied units	2,446	1,864	581.0	2,409	2,359	50.0
Unoccupied units—temporary				277.0	271.0	6.0
Unoccupied unites—left				58.0	56.0	2.0
	out of which					
	1991			2001		
	Total	Individual ownership	Other	Total	Individual ownership	Other
Homeownership	1,565	1,565	0	1,965	1,965	0
Tenants—public	558.0	24.0	534.0	62.0	17.0	35.0
Tenants—private	72.0	64.0	8.0	106.0	98.0	8.0
Relatives	72.0	64.0	8.0	145.0	140.0	5.0
Other	178.0	147.0	2.0	130.0	128.0	2.0

Source: Republican Statistical Office: Census 2002.

percent rent privately owned flats, and nearly 6 percent of households share flats with their relatives.

Overcrowding is a serious component of the housing problems in Serbia. Households that reside with relatives represent a latent demand for housing in general, and for rental housing in particular. Over 15 percent of the housing stock (380,000 flats) is overcrowded;[5] almost 333,000 flats are not built of solid material (25 percent of them have no other utilities but electricity or no communal facilities); around 360,000 flats are without sewage facilities; 124,000 flats are occupied by more than one household; and almost eighteen thousand households live in spaces not suitable for housing. All these are robust indicators of a considerable housing shortage.

The social housing sector decreased from 22.8 percent in 1991 to 2 percent of the housing stock in 2002, from almost six hundred thousand to fifty-eight thousand units, of which fifty thousand have permanent tenants (Table 15.1). In 1991, almost all tenants with protected rents lived in publicly owned flats (96 percent).[6] In 2002, the share of tenants with protected rents who lived in privately owned flats rose to 43 percent, although their absolute number decreased radically.

Today, almost 50 percent of the public rental housing that has not been privatized is composed of flats that were nationalized during the socialist period and are now occupied by protected sitting tenants who have no right to buy and are renting at fixed rent levels.[7] Also, an estimated 20–30 percent of flats not privately owned are in the process of privatization, because a considerable segment of housing produced by state enterprises during the 1990s was put up for privatization. In that sense, the share of the *de facto* public rental sector is less than 0.5 percent, but given that most tenants possess a right to occupy the flat permanently without any eligibility testing, these dwellings almost never become available to new households.

In the past two decades Serbia has faced a paradoxical development in the housing sector, as the number of households has increased without a corresponding increase in the number of occupied flats. This has to do with the continuous decline in new housing production (related to completed legal flats) that occurred in the 1990s, but also with the significant increase in the number (335,000) of flats left vacant, according to the 2002 Census data. This could be linked with the effects of emigration and/or the shortage of finance available for completing legal or illegal construction. By the mid-1990s, new legal housing production dropped to 28–30 percent of its 1990 level.[8] It subsequently fluctuated, and by 2006–2008 it reached the replacement level of the housing stock in the 2006–2008 period. It is worth noting that in 1990 new housing production financed by the public sector made up 30 percent of all new annual construction; it then decreased, but it still accounted for a considerable amount of new legal construction. However, the largest share of most new public housing construction was ultimately privatized.

Between 2004 and 2008, Serbia's GDP grew significantly and average household income rose, but so did the unemployment rate until 2007. The gray economy remained significant and income inequalities increased. The average price to income ratio has been constantly high, exceeding fifteen for newly built flats and eleven in the secondary housing market. Rents are typically high in the private rental market because of the limited supply of rental housing, especially in large cities, and because of insolvent demand, above all in cities affected by high immigration of refugees and IDPs.[9] The rent to income ratio is above 0.45 in big cities.[10]

Housing expenditures exceed 50 percent of household income for 6.6 percent of households in Serbia, and this is the case of every third household in the bottom two income deciles (RSO 2010). The 2007 Household Budget Survey data indicate that 17 percent of households had difficulty paying their utility bills and were behind in their payments (RSO 2007).

Despite a decrease in poverty between 2003 and 2008, it is still widespread. There seems to be no connection between household income and the type of housing people live in, so the risk of poverty is also unrelated to tenure status.

Most poor people own their housing. The quality of the housing, however, is lower than the average, and renting is rarely an option for the poor, as both sectors (public and private) are beyond their means. Poor housing conditions coincide with other dimensions of material deprivation. Data on social exclusion (Government of Serbia 2009) confirm that 80 percent of households with insufficient levels of income lived in very bad housing conditions, compared to 10 percent of all households.[11] In large and expanding cities there are vast illegal and unhygienic settlements that house the poorest strata of society. For instance, within the greater Belgrade area there are twenty-nine slums and sixty-four settlements that are home to approximately twenty-five thousand people that do not meet even the minimum hygienic standards (Institute of Urban Planning 2003). In the case of the Roma population in Serbia, out of 593 registered Roma settlements (with roughly 250,000 inhabitants), 43.5 percent are slums that do not have basic hygienic facilities (Jakšić and Babić 2005, 32).

There is no official estimate of the demand for social (rental) housing. One reason for this is that there is no official definition of who should be the target of social housing. Begović et al. (2010) claim that there are ten thousand refugee households without housing (sixty-five hundred of whom are still living in collective centers), and they estimate that for one-quarter of this group the best policy option would be to buy for them housing in rural areas. Another three thousand households should be provided with support to self-help strategies, that is, help with the purchase of construction materials. Some five thousand households would need social housing, which would have to be built for them.[12] In addition to these groups, the population currently receiving social assistance (in the form of material support for families—MSF and the child allowance, which means almost

280,000 households) could be one target group.[13] If we assume that their housing conditions are among the poorest, at least 50 percent of this population group will need some kind of support. And if we apply the analogy of how to cover the housing needs of refugees to this population, at least another seventy thousand poor households will need social rental housing, most of them in bigger cities.

THE PATCHWORK PROVISION OF SOCIAL HOUSING

In Serbia, the links between different social housing programs are only loose and random, responsibility for the sector is scattered between different players and institutions, and there is a lack of capacity and resources. The basic problems stem from the lack of necessary legislation, laws that are outdated or poorly coordinated, a shortage in the number of available dwellings, the absence of any normative standards for social housing, and problems of public acceptance of social housing in designated neighborhoods.

The Legislative Framework

The latest Housing Act was adopted in 1992. It stipulates that the state should create the necessary conditions for the construction of housing and for solving the housing needs of socially vulnerable persons, whereas local government is responsible for the social safety-net function of housing. The Planning and Construction Act (2003) assigns the municipalities with the responsibility for identifying public land that can be used for social housing programs, but the issue of municipal ownership of land (and even affordable rental flats) has not yet been resolved. The Act on Means in State Property (1995) stipulated that the state is the owner of all goods of public interest until the new Law on Public Property, adopted in 2011, which has recognized the municipal property over the land and social housing. However, its implementation goes rather slow and no effects have been visible yet.

The right to buy socially owned flats was introduced by the Housing Act in 1990, the idea being to establish a fund for new social housing construction (as the previous system was not meant to have a safety-net function, but the necessary bylaws were never adopted). Inflation and the decentralized system of privatization (the owners of privatized property were enterprises and public institutions, not the central state) diminished the financial benefits of the mass privatization in the first half of the 1990s, when almost 90 percent of social flats were privatized. The right-to-buy option was initially schedule to expire at the end of 1995, but later this limit was canceled.

The only mechanism related to the provision of new social housing established the Solidarity Housing Funds (SHFs), which lasted up until the middle of 2004. SHFs functioned mainly as a mechanism for delivering highly subsidized owner-occupied housing to middle-income groups.[14] It is estimated that fifteen thousand to eighteen thousand housing units were built using SHFs in Serbia between 1991 and 2004. Although the public institutions were the builders of this new housing, the number of units built did not contribute in any way (much) to the supply of social housing (Damjanović and Gligorijević 2009).

Rent setting and permanent tenancy rights are part of the socialist legacy: rents are administratively set well below real costs, and although deregulation has been planned it has never been implemented, nor has the plan to set the rent on new leases at cost level (based on 3 percent of the annual replacement value of the flat). As the issue of nationalized flats has not yet been resolved, no real policy changes could be introduced that would change, for instance, the rent allowance system, the management of rent arrears,[15] or evictions in both the public and private sectors. The private rental sector, although recognized, is entirely unregulated (there is no rent monitoring, supervision of contracts, tax regulations, etc.). A few attempts to stimulate renting in the private sector through tax incentives (VAT exemptions on rent) failed at the first step when it came to reporting the rent revenue and registering at the tax office (see Damjanović and Gligorijević 2009). The sector continues to operate as a black market.

The Act on Social Protection does not deal explicitly with social housing (or housing allowance programs). It mentions only the responsibility of local government to provide shelter for the homeless, and this is done just in Belgrade, Novi Sad, and Niš (with a total capacity of only five hundred beds). On the other hand, the Act on Local Self-Government (2002, 2006) stipulates that it is the responsibility of municipalities to give social assistance to households living below the poverty line, not to help them obtain access to housing but just to mitigate the negative social effects that price liberalization has on the housing-related expenditures of low-income households. In Belgrade, for example, almost sixty-eight thousand households are eligible for a discount of between 10 percent and 50 percent of total utility costs (without electricity); eligible groups include low-income households, people disabled by the war, MSF recipients, households with disabled or seriously ill members, and foster families.

SOCIAL HOUSING PROGRAMS FOR REFUGEES AND IDPS

In 2002, the government of Serbia adopted the National Strategy for Resolving the Issue of Refugees and IDPs, which stipulated the closure of the collective centers serving as temporary housing for refugees.[16] However, the implementation of this strategy ran up against a number of problems connected with the inadequacy of (the state's) legislative and financial framework.[17] Around four thousand rental flats were built through different programs financed mostly by international donations and partly out of the state budget (with *ad hoc* dedicated resources), but this was not enough to be able to close the collective centers. Besides refugees, who represented 80 percent of the beneficiaries of this program, the low-income local population was also included, the idea being to facilitate the social integration of refugees.

The flats are modest in size (ranging from 22 square meters for one person to 55 square meters for a larger family) and rented on a permanent basis for a symbolic social (or zero) rent. Initially, the rents were based on the household's income, and the flat's operating costs were costs shared by the municipality, the Ministry of Social Welfare, and UNHCR, but the administration of the programs was weak and no real monitoring or enforcement system was set up. Even the selection schemes were somewhat arbitrary (Economic Commission for Europe [ECE] 2006). Besides social rental housing, around two to three thousand households were provided with subsidies in kind (land and construction material) or with small grants (for building, renovating, or finishing the construction of houses).

A similar rental housing initiative was the Settlement and Integration of Refugees Program (SIRP), which aimed not only to provide housing, but also to initiate a more sustainable institutional framework for social housing, at least at the local level. It was implemented in seven municipalities, where the local SHFs were transformed into Municipal Housing Agencies[18] that developed local housing strategies (until the beginning of 2012, when the National Strategy on Social Housing was adopted, [19] these were the only strategic documents on housing in Serbia). The program created a small experiment of 'cost-based' rental housing and produced 530 flats (Program for Urban Development [PUR] 2009, 37). Since May 2008, the flats have been rented for a limited time period (three years) to refugees (80 percent) and domicile lower-income households (20 percent). Eligible households were those able to pay nonprofit cost rent. The program planned to set the rent at 135 U.S. dollars per household, thus effectively excluding low-income households from eligibility, but additional donations to the program made it possible to reduce the rent and make these homes affordable for very low-income households. The program regulations required the rent to be equal to 2 percent of the annual construction costs, which resulted in rents at 1.7–2.1 U.S. dollars per square meter (40–60 percent below market rents but still higher than existing social rents[20]). To date, the Municipal Housing Agencies have been managing these flats and their maintenance (the costs are covered by the rent). This small project is still unique in Serbia (Ramirez et al. 2008).

THE SOCIAL HOUSING ACT

The SIRP program successfully contributed to the formulation and adoption of the Social Housing Act (SHA) in August 2009, fueled by the European integration process and the need to create a basis for future absorption of European Structural Funds. There are a number of ambivalences in the SHA. The definition of social housing does not specify targeting and allocation, management, and social purpose, it only states that "social housing is housing with adequate standards provided with the assistance of the state for households that are not in a position to provide a dwelling under market conditions for social, economic or other reasons" (Law on Social Housing 2009, Article 2), which basically encompasses the average-income (middle-class) population with affordability problems.[21] Moreover, the definition leaves undetermined what the adequate standards are that the state should support in the case of both social rental and affordable nonprofit dwellings.[22] This broad definition—which is clearly not in conformity with EC regulations on social housing as a service of general economic interest—represents a continuation of the socialist tradition, which used to target key workers in the public sector and provide them with housing under the Solidarity Housing Fund.[23]

Implementation of the SHA has been slow. The National Housing Fund that was supposed to be set up to support housing construction through several funding instruments and institutions is not yet operational, and the local Municipal Housing Agencies that should be responsible for strategy development have not been formed.[24] Although it seems that the act aims to strengthen the role of the municipalities, it does not specify whether they can set the rents;[25] choose different types of rental contracts (social, cost, or market rent); decide on allocation procedures; determine the conditions of sale of affordable nonprofit dwellings; and so on. Nonprofit organizations are also assigned an important role in the SHA, but there is no legislation that properly defines the profile of a nonprofit (or with limited profit) housing association.[26] In practice, there has been no involvement of the private sector in providing and managing social housing and no public–private partnership (PPP) arrangements, so the Municipal Housing Agencies remain the sole actors in social housing provision at the local level.[27]

SOCIAL HOUSING PROGRAMS: THE CASE OF BELGRADE

In 2003, the Belgrade city government initiated a program to build eleven hundred nonprofit housing units each year; however, without a steady budget line, housing production was much lower than planned.[28] Consequently, around three thousand flats had been built by the end of 2009. All the housing constructed under this program could be privatized at about 30 percent below their market price and with very favorable buying terms (20 percent down payment, twenty-year repayment period with an interest rate of just 0.5 percent). Eligible households are primarily those employed in the public sector,[29] but also young married couples, people disabled in the war, families with disabled children, self-employed artists, and distinguished sportsmen, whose income is at least 200 percent of the monthly repayment installment, with no upper income limit. The allocation process is based on a controversial set of criteria: no housing quality indicators are used, whereas education and years of employment are given more weight than health status or family size.

In 2010, 180 flats were built and 2,333 applicants competed for them.[30] Only 15 percent of the flats built under the program target households in extreme social need;[31] education and employment status are favored over social deprivation. In addition, there is obvious confusion over the purpose of public rental housing, as, according to the 1992 Housing Act, it should be used for resettling tenants from restituted flats. The scheme does not support social mixing either, as households from nationalized flats are mainly allocated flats that are meant to be sold.

Between 2003 and 2009, 320 'very social rental' units were built in the periphery of Belgrade;[32] they are modest-size flats rented for five years at a rent level defined in the Housing Act. Eligibility is checked every second year. There are no monitoring mechanisms in place, except for following up on arrears, based on which eviction procedures can be launched. The flats cannot be privatized. Interestingly, the city government has not appointed an institution to assume responsibility for managing these flats. As a result, the housing stock is poorly maintained and is rapidly dilapidating.[33] By concentrating poor families in peripheral locations, a kind of ghettoization has occurred, particularly owing to the inclusion of the Roma among the eligible households in this program.[34]

In 2003, the city of Belgrade began building five thousand housing units for resettling people, mostly the Roma, from slums and illegal settlements. The initiative was blocked by huge protests from the local population in the neighborhoods where the housing was to be built. Therefore, the city government has been using container accommodation as a temporary housing solution for people awaiting resettlement since 2009 (see Chapter 6, this volume).

PROVIDING AND SUBSIDIZING HOUSING LOANS

The housing affordability problems of middle- and upper-middle-income households are the focus of the process to reestablish the housing finance system. There are various housing finance programs in place, of which the state (mortgage) guarantee program and the housing loan subsidy program are the most important ones.

Since 2004 the National Corporation for Ensuring Housing Loans (NCEHK) guarantees mortgage credits up to 75 percent of the real estate's value, thus decreasing the bank risk and interest.[35] By April 2010 around forty thousand loans had been provided. The housing loan subsidy program has become the biggest budget subsidy since its introduction in 2006. The state pays 20 percent of the loan's down payment, and the holder covers 5 percent and repays the rest of the down payment in five years with only 0.1 percent interest. The eligibility conditions are redefined every year. In 2009, the scheme favored young, first-time buyers. The maximum loan was set at 50,000 U.S. dollars for flats below 50 square meters. By the end of 2009 roughly six thousand loans had been subsidized. In 2010 the scheme targeted newly built flats or even flats under construction in order to stimulate the construction industry, and loans were linked exclusively to housing projects initiated by the Government Act on Subsidized Housing Provision Loans, which was adopted in January 2010 and should result in the construction of ten thousand flats in various larger cities.[36] The first housing project is planned for realization in Belgrade's second zone by converting military land into a residential complex of five thousand new housing units. It is not clear if 5–8 percent of the housing in this project will be earmarked as social rental housing, which would be in conformity with requirements set out in the Master Plan of Belgrade, which stipulates that a certain quota of social rental flats be set aside in housing projects with more than 250 flats (except in the first zone).

INDIRECT SUBSIDIES

There are also indirect subsidies to improve housing affordability. Since 2008 a tax exemption has been granted to first-time house buyers. The annual property tax, which increases housing expenses (and is a heavy burden) for many poor homeowners, will not be based on real estate market value until 2012, when the cadastre system is set up.

Widespread tolerance of illegal construction is another indirect subsidy.[37] Moreover, the intention of the central and local authorities in reducing the administrative costs (attached to building housing) was to encourage legal construction. For example, Belgrade (with the highest concentration of illegal housing) has been offering a discount of 60 percent on administrative costs and extending the payment period to 240 months. Still, the results remain poor.[38]

CONCLUSION

Serbia has so far failed to develop social housing institutions based on strategic state interventions. In general, housing is not on the policy agenda, or is it subordinated to short-term political decisions. At the same time, there is a pressing need for housing: the stock of (public) rental housing is too small and affordability issues remain unaddressed. In addition, whereas some housing stock is overcrowded (mainly occupied by homeowners), other flats are left vacant, indicating ineffective use of the housing stock in general. In the future, labor market flexibility will probably have to be encouraged by the rental sector, which is still not functioning properly.

It is difficult to evaluate the effectiveness of existing social housing programs. There are no real guidelines in the current policy context. Nevertheless, social justice, social norms, and values related to redistributive goals in housing exist and are a long-term tradition in Serbia. All measures but those creating financial mechanisms have been influenced by the inherited socialist logic. Affordable nonprofit housing is more subsidized than 'very social' rental housing, thus the vertical effectiveness of housing subsidies is poor (i.e., subsidies assist higher-income groups more than lower-income groups). Social housing programs aimed at the poor are still in embryonic stage and reduced to marginal local initiatives that have limited resources. Consequently, existing subsidies have little horizontal effectiveness, as they are inaccessible to many households in need within the targeted population. Besides that, the effectiveness of the subsidies used is reduced by the fact that target groups and eligibility criteria for social housing programs are inconsistently defined. This means that despite comparably large budget investments in various schemes, the neediest received only a fraction of the subsidies (primarily via social housing construction by international donations).[39]

The public rental sector inherited from the socialist period has almost disappeared; newly built housing is small in scale, residual, and segregated; and there is no regulation of the private rental sector. Creating a new social rental sector is very expensive, particularly when starting from scratch. Nevertheless, without connecting schemes with sufficient rent allowance programs extended to the private rental sector, or obtaining flats in public property at the second-hand market, public resources will be easily wasted. It is also true that, in Serbia, without the existence of permanent social housing, social housing policy remains vulnerable to political decisions. Thus, the Serbian politicians must come to see social (rental) housing as an important public policy for achieving social integration.

NOTES

1. Self-built construction was helped by income from Serbian guest workers abroad in the 1960s and by the shift in the primarily responsibility of (state) enterprises from providing flats to granting housing loans for employees to pursue their own private housing strategies in the 1980s.
2. Between 2001 and 2007 Serbia's GDP grew but did not manage to return to the level it was at in 1989, before the economic crisis.
3. Serbia has experienced large waves of emigration of young people since 1991, so refugee immigration has just mitigated the negative effects of negative natural growth. Almost one hundred thousand people have emigrated.
4. A survey on the living standard of IDPs from 2008 showed that 56 percent had their own flats in Serbia (compared to 90 percent of the domestic

population) and 10 percent lived in spaces unsuitable for housing (compared to 0.5 percent of the domestic population); 4,852 IDPs lived in collective centers and another 1,765 in hidden collective centers not covered by steady state support (Cvejić and Babović 2007).

5. Although there are no universally defined standards for minimum floor space per person from which to measure overcrowding, housing conditions with less than 10 square meters per person are taken as the critical threshold, below which family relations and group cohesion are jeopardized (De Lauwe 1960).
6. The rents are set according to the inherited socialist logic, not according to investment or maintenance costs.
7. According to the 1992 Housing Act, which is still in effect, owners of flats may not use or dispose of their flats until new housing is found for the sitting tenants. Local authorities are responsible for obtaining the flats, but do not have adequate resources, so the issue of nationalized flats and restitution is still unresolved in Serbia.
8. Taking into account that the estimated number of dwellings built without a permit equaled those erected with a permit in the mid-1990s, the total housing production was about 50 percent of its level in 1990.
9. Private rental supply mainly consists of letting or subletting housing by landlords who are typically income-poor owners, frequently unemployed or retired, and renting out their own units or individual rooms in it. Small rentals are generally *ad hoc*, often created when a household has some extra space, and such households tend to enter and exit the rental market according to the need for additional income, which makes the supply of private renting unstable (Petrović 2006).
10. The calculation is based on the assumption that the gray economy increases average household income by 30 percent, and the ratio of median private rental rent to household income is taken as the average for the population in general. Other data show varying ratios: according to the latest Household Consumption Survey, the ratio was 0.29, which is still rather unaffordable (representative sample for Serbian urban households).
11. Data based on the Household Consumption Survey do not include the Roma and other people living in illegal settlements, people who are homeless, and people living in collective centers.
12. The collective centers are state-owned hotels or similar buildings, usually very old, dilapidated, and located far from cities, that are used as temporary collective housing for refugees. The refugees do not pay rent or utility costs, but the living conditions in the centers are very poor, as are the chances for social integration.
13. There is no need to test their material situation because the material census reduces the potential beneficiaries of MSF and child allowance to those without real estate except the housing in which they live (no bigger than what is adequate for the household's needs, but it can be smaller), 0.5 acres of land, and movable property the value of which is not greater than six times the value of financial support they receive monthly. The disadvantage of directing state social housing support to beneficiaries of other programs is the increasing attractiveness of financial support and the redistribution of resources to one specific target group; on the other hand, it reduces the administration costs and offers relatively good economic efficiency and effectiveness, although with the threat of corruption (Begovic et al. 2010).
14. Only employed persons could apply for flats, which meant that a large proportion of the economically most vulnerable, unemployed population was excluded. The central government and local authorities maintained the

obligation to provide public housing (with right to buy) to their employees, whereas only a small share of flats (5–10 percent) was aimed at other target groups, defined according to different criteria: poor income or housing conditions, but also the need to resettle tenants from restituted flats or to support young scientists and artists, and so on.

15. Theoretically, a tenant might be able to stay for as long as seven months without paying, as landlords first have to give notice ninety days in advance, and if it falls in the period of December–February it must be extended one month more, plus the tenant can only be evicted after failing to pay for three consecutive months or for four months within a year. Evictions are very rare.
16. The idea was to develop both public rental units (for the most vulnerable refugee households) and owner-occupied units (aimed at more solvent households). The strategy of poverty reduction (2003) also highlighted the need for subsidies, not only for new construction of public rental housing, but also for the reconstruction of illegal settlements and self-built housing.
17. In 2001 the national government established an interministerial body for the strategic preparation and implementation of the Law on the Fund for Social and Affordable Construction, which was ultimately never adopted. Also, legislation required to regulate the right of refugees to use, buy, and/or acquire ownership of housing financed by donations or budget sources has never been adopted (although it was before Parliament in 2007).
18. This idea was based on the assumption that existing institutions could be adapted to the new environment by restructuring them and giving them new tasks. Nevertheless, municipal housing agencies within this project are responsible only for managing the flats, and they can make no decisions regarding allocation criteria, rent levels, and so on.
19. The Strategy is adopted in accordance to the Social Housing Act (2009, see further in the text), although general Strategy on Housing has not been adopted, yet.
20. The ministry responsible for housing defines the rent annually in a nontransparent manner, taking into account net incomes and different cost parameters. The rent is about 0.5 U.S. dollars per square meter.
21. In order to enforce the SHA, an NGO, Program for Urban Reconstruction, founded by experts previously engaged at SIRP, developed a project proposal for the Serbian government to apply for credit funds from the Council of Europe Development Bank (approximately 26 million U.S. dollars). The project aims to build seventeen hundred flats in different municipalities in Serbia, five hundred in the social rental sector, and twelve hundred for selling as affordable nonprofit housing (67 percent of the costs covered by a loan and 33 percent provided by the municipalities in kind). The idea is to use individual repayments (which should cover the full costs, i.e., including the costs to municipalities for providing serviced land) as investment in new social housing construction, which would allow an additional one thousand rental flats to be built over a twenty-five-year period. Again, this is a rather small-scale project used to illustrate the logic of economic sustainability, but the option has not yet been discussed by the government (Mojović 2011).
22. The eligibility criteria are: current housing conditions, income, health, disability, household size, and material situation. These should be combined with additional criteria: lone-parent households, young, aged (sixty-five plus), refugee status, Roma. It is not clear which criteria should be given priority or how the proxy criteria should be evaluated (as will be illustrated in the case of Belgrade).
23. The ECE country profile recommends that Serbia should focus on the poorest and most vulnerable households living in substandard and/or unsafe housing

conditions (ECE 2006, 83). The EC claims that government funds should only be used to subsidize housing for the poor (Ghekiere 2008).

24. The act recognizes the following sources: state budget allocations, donations, loans from domestic and foreign sources, revenues from the fund investments, repayments from loans issued by the fund, and revenue from the sale of state-owned dwellings.
25. This will collide with the existing Housing Act with regard to rent setting in the public rental sector and right-to-buy conditions. Nevertheless, as will be illustrated in the case of Belgrade, the terms for the sale of affordable nonprofit housing are set by the city government.
26. There is no law regulating specific saving schemes or contracts of housing cooperatives. Serbia has no experience with cooperative rental housing; cooperatives only exist during the construction stage and are designed to help people with substantial resources obtain owner-occupied tenure. After the introduction of VAT they no longer enjoy fiscal advantages and are unlikely to contribute to new affordable housing construction (ECE 2006).
27. Therefore, local governments are not in the practice of selling their housing stock (with sitting tenants) to private developers, who would then evict the tenants.
28. The Belgrade government has just recently established the Agency for Housing Investments.
29. The socialist legacy is challenged by suggestions to make those employed in the private sector as eligible, too, because they also contribute to the city budget.
30. As applicants mostly come from the private rental sector or from a shared household, social filtration process is not associated to the program.
31. Particular attention is given to lone parents and to families with a disabled child, a foster child, or a household member with 80–100 percent disability.
32. The poor transparency of the allocation procedure gave rise to protests and the last competition in July 2010 had to be repeated.
33. The Belgrade housing stock is formally managed by the Public Communal Enterprise 'Infostan'. Generally, the social housing stock is very poorly managed because the rents are low (and do not cover maintenance costs) and there are no institutions in charge. Most of the flats inherited from socialism are dispersed among condominium buildings (with a majority of privatized/privately owned flats, which, depending on the tenants' income and willingness to cooperate, also face maintenance problems, as the Act on Condominium Maintenance is insufficiently enforced). The situation is almost the same in new social housing, more concentrated in the same buildings but without positive effects on maintenance.
34. There are no data on the proportion of the Roma among the households included in the program. Bearing in mind the poor transparency of the allocation procedure and the low cultural and social capital of the Roma population, especially individual families, it is likely that they are underrepresented. In addition, the Roma sometimes have problems producing identification documents required to obtain social support.
35. If the corporation provides the loan, the highest interest rate might be 8.95 percent (if there is a down payment) or 7.45 percent (the deposit model). With the introduction of the Mortgage Act and completion of the cadastre, the state has almost set up all the necessary framework for providing accessible and functional housing loans.
36. A mortgage can be granted to a flat under construction if it is 80 percent finished. This is not necessary if the investor is credited by the same bank. Eligibility criteria have also changed, as instead of maximizing the flat size and

the amount of the loan, the holder's income has been capped at 120,000 RSD (about 1,550 U.S. dollars), which might have a regressive income effect.

37. According to estimates, almost 20 percent of the housing stock (five hundred thousand flats) has been built illegally, nearly half since 1990 (Petrović 2004; ECE 2006).
38. Bearing that in mind, the government has made a new proposal that would allow households that have no other flat to live in and have built housing no larger than 25 square meters per household member to be exempted from paying the legalization costs.
39. Between 800 million and 1 billion U.S. dollars have been invested in housing within the Solidarity Housing Fund program. Other programs also partly supported by the state budget have invested 155–195 million U.S. dollars, mostly after 2003. Belgrade has invested almost the same amount of money as the state in housing. State expenditures on the provision or subsidization of housing loans amount to around 94 million U.S. dollars (PUR 2009). Some estimates take into account the 7.8 billion U.S. dollars that were forfeited by the state through privatization (Damjanović and Gligorijević 2009).

REFERENCES

Begović, B., Matković, G., Mijatović, B. and Paunović, M. 2010. *Social Housing in Serbia (Socijalno stanovanje u Srbiji).* Belgrade: Sluzbeni glasnik.

Cvejić, S. and Babović, M. 2007. *Social and Economic Position of IDPs in Serbia.* LSMS draft report.

Damjanović, D., Gligorijević, Z., eds. 2009. *Social Housing (Socijalno stanovanje).* Belgrade: Palgo.

De Lauwe, Ch. 1960. *Famille et habitation (Family and Home).* Paris: CNRS.

Dixon, K. and Kim, H. S. 1992. "Social Welfare under Socialism." In: Dixon, J. and Macarou, D. eds. *Social Welfare in Socialist Countries.* New York-London: Routledge.

Economic Commission for Europe. 2006. *Serbia and Montenegro, Country Profiles on the Housing Sector.* Geneva: Economic Commission for Europe, United Nations.

Ghekiere, L. 2008. "Social Housing as a Service of General Interest." In: Scanlon, K. and Whitehead, Ch. eds *Social Housing in Europe II.* London: London School of Economics.

Government of Serbia. 2009. *Monitoring of Social Inclusion in Serbia (Pracenje socijalne ukljucenosti u Srbiji).* Belgrade: Republican Government Social Inclusion and Poverty Reduction Unit, RZS.

Harloe, M. 1995. *The People's Home: Social Rented Housing in Europe and America.* Oxford: Blackwell Publishers.

Hegedüs, J. and Tosics, I. 1996. "The Disintegration of East European Housing Model." *Housing Privatization in Eastern Europe.* London: Greenwood Press.

Institute of Urban Planning. 2003. *Belgrade Master Plan 2021.* Belgrade: Institute of Urban Planning.

Jakšić, B. and Bačić, G. 2005. *Umetnost Prezivljavanja—Gde i kako zive Romi u Srbiji (The Art of Survival—Where and How Roma in Serbia).* Belgrade: Institut za filozofiju i drustvenu teoriju.

Kemeny, J. 1992. *Housing and Social Theory.* New York—London: Routledge.

Law on Social Housing. 2009. Belgrade: Sluzbeni glasnik.

Lazić, M. 2000. *Racji hod.* Belgrade: Filip Visnjic.

Mojović, Dj. 2011. *Projekat izgradnje stanova za socijalno stanovanje kreditnim sredstvima Banke za razvoj Saveta Evrope, Nacionalna konferencija: Novi okvir socijalne stambene politike (Project for Construction of Flats for Social Housing Loan Funds, Development Bank of the Council of Europe, National Conference: The New Framework of Social Housing Policy).* Belgrade:Program za urbani razvoj

Mrkšić, D. 1987. *Srednji slojevi u Jugoslaviji (The Middle Class in Yugoslavia).* Belgrade: IICSSOS.

Petrović, M. 2001. "Post-Socialist Housing Policy in Yugoslavia." *European Journal of Housing Policy* 1 (2): 211–32.

———. 2004. *Housing Policy: Challenges and Possibilities (Stambena politika: Izazovi i mogucnosti).* Belgrade: ISI FF.

———. 2006. *Affordable Rental Housing, National Housing Conference: Towards a New National Housing Policy for Serbia.* Belgrade: UN Habitat, Government of Serbia.

———. 2009. "Domacinstva u Srbiji prema porodicnom sastavu: Izmedju (pre) modernosti I (post)modernosti." *Porodice u Srbiji danas (Households in Serbia According to Family Composition: Between the Premodernity and Postmodernity).* Belgrade: ISI FF.

Program for Urban Development. 2009. *Local Housing Policy (Lokalna stambena politika).* Belgrade: Program for Urban Development.

Ramirez, L., Mojović, Dj., Galassi, B., Čolić, R. and Vukasanović-Macura, Zl. 2008. *Knjiga o SIRP-u, Program stanovanja i trajne integracije izbeglica u Srbiji 2005–2008 (Book of the SIRP, The Settlement and Integration of Refugees Program in Serbia 2005–2008).* Belgrade: UN Habitat.

Reinprecht, Ch., Levy-Vroelant, C., and Wassenberg, F. 2008. "Learning from Histories: Changes and Path Dependency in the Social Housing Sector in Austria, France and Netherlands (1889–2008)." In: Scanlon, K. and Whitehead, Ch. eds. *Social Housing in Europe II.* London: London School of Economics.

RSO. 2007. *Household Consumption Survey.* Belgrade: Republican Statistical Office.

———. 2010. *Household Consumption Survey.* Belgrade: Republican Statistical Office.

Rus, V. 1991. "Social Policy between Negative and Positive Equality: The Yugoslavian Case." *Social Policy in Changing Europe.* Boulder, CO: Westview.

Scanlon, K. 2008. "Introduction." In: Scanlon, K. and Whitehead, Ch. eds. *Social Housing in Europe II.* London: London School of Economics.

Struyk, R. 1996. *Economic Restructuring of the Soviet Bloc: The Case of Housing.* Washington, DC: Urban Institute Press.

Vukasnović-Macura, Z. 2011. *Uslovi i oblici stanovanja siromasnih zitelja, Beograda izmedju dva svetska rata (1919–1941) (Forms of Housing Conditions and Poor Residents, Belgrade between the Two World Wars [1919–1941]).* Belgrade: Zaduzbina Andrejevic.

Woolcock, M. 1998. "Social Capital and Economic Development: Towards a Theoretical Synthesis and Policy Framework." *Theory and Society* 27 (2): 154–89.

16 Slovakia
On the Way to the Stable Social Housing Concept

Marek Hojsík

INTRODUCTION

Despite a long tradition of housing funded from public sources, the concept of social housing was formally missing from Slovak law. The Slovak Parliament adopted the Act on Social Housing only in 2010 (Act No. 443/2010 Coll. on Grants for Development of Housing and on Social Housing). Under the term *social housing*, the law grouped the principles, tools, and practices developed by the Slovak government during the transition since 1989. The housing situation in Slovakia differs from the other part of former Czechoslovakia and was shaped by settlement history in Slovakia and a distinct pattern of modernization after World War II.

Since the time of the Austro-Hungarian monarchy the territory of present-day Slovakia was unlike the Czech lands (Bohemia), prevailingly rural in character, owing to the historical system of land inheritance: property was divided among all descendants, in contrast to primogenital heritage in Bohemia. Strong urbanization only began to occur under the communist regime's modernization policy, which included the massive state-driven, centrally planned construction of new dwellings. For this reason, the current housing situation is not burdened by restitution issues to the same extent as many other Central and Eastern European (CEE) countries. Instead Slovakia has to deal with the consequences of the poor quality of construction and ineffective housing management under the communist rule, which will be discussed in the first section of this chapter.

The second and third sections of this chapter focus on the efforts of the new regime to set up measures to correct the distortions of the communist housing policy and at the same time tackle challenges related to the wider processes of the economic, political, and social transformation. This included the transformation of the centrally controlled and planned economy, decentralization of public decision making, and privatization of state-owned properties, including the housing stock. The mass transfer of dwellings to the ownership of tenants has caused the current shortage in available rental housing.

After a decline in construction following the collapse of communism, the Slovak authorities tried to restore housing development. In this context, social housing was not only a tool of welfare policy, but also a mean of stimulating the construction of housing and specifically of rental housing. This approach to social housing, described in the fourth and fifth sections of this chapter, can have a negative impact on its effectiveness from the point of view of the welfare economy, because it is not necessarily allocated to the neediest housing seekers.

THE HOUSING POLICY OF THE COMMUNIST REGIME

After the communist coup d'état in 1948 the construction of new housing became a high priority. The immediate reason was the need to replace the dwellings destroyed during the Second World War. But in line with the new state ideology, housing was also viewed as part of the country's welfare policy, and the right to housing was guaranteed by the paternalistic government. Most private land in the country and residential buildings in the towns were nationalized as a step towards the goal of the complete abolishment of private ownership. However, the private property of family houses survived in rural areas.

The right to housing, one of the social rights, was accommodated according to citizens' housing needs. However, in reality state-owned flats were allocated through the administrative decisions of the committees,[1] which considered not just applicants' needs, but also their political merits and the real or assumed public benefit of certain individuals (e.g., teacher, doctors, artists, or other professions). The allocation of a flat established a right of use, which was inheritable and could be transferred to other persons. This nontransparent system promoted nepotism, clientelism, and even corruption in the distribution of housing. It created a black market in flats and led to ineffectiveness in housing management. The administrative distribution of housing served as a means of reinforcing political, social, and professional loyalties; in the field of economic policy, it was used as a tool for the sectorial and regional distribution of the labor force (Šmídová 1993, 575).

Due to the prevailingly rural character of the Slovak part of Czechoslovakia, privately built family houses in the countryside remained a significant part of housing construction.[2] However, the state was the most important investor and developer of housing; construction was closely linked to the wider centrally planned economic and social policy. State ambitions in the housing policy field were hindered by a lack of construction materials, especially bricks (Ivanička et al. 2003, 38).

Construction of new housing was part of a larger program of modernization of rural Slovakia, which included developing the economy, advancing heavy industry, and promoting urbanization. The migration of the rural population into the towns required the mass production of new housing. Those factors led to the adoption of a program to industrialize housing construction in 1955, which was accompanied by the introduction of new technologies, including the prefab technology (the dominant construction system in Slovakia at that time),[3] and the erection of large urban neighborhoods composed of multifloor buildings. After 1959 new forms of housing development were introduced, in particular the practice of large companies building housing for their employees and the rise of housing cooperatives. The construction of private family homes was extended to towns and—like the housing cooperatives—was financially supported by the state through subsidies and soft loans.

The government introduced the legal regulation of rents. Rent levels took into account floorage, the quality and amenities of the flat, and the size and structure of the households of tenants with substantial rebates of as much as 50 percent for handicapped tenants or families with children (Government Regulation No. 60/1964 Coll. on Payments for Use of Flats and Services Related to the Use of Flat). The level of rent in state-owned housing did not change between 1964 and 1991, although in cooperative housing the rent and service fee reflected the real cost growth; for example, between 1980 and 1990 the payments in those flats increased by almost 71 percent (Jankovichová 2003, 63). The regulated rent and service fees did not cover the input costs, and the maintenance of housing and the housing stock consequently declined in condition.

Housing became one of the highest priorities in the regime's welfare system, and construction peaked in the late 1960s and in the 1970s. The planned housing construction focused on the development of urban areas with the construction of various forms of habitation and civic amenities (schools, hospitals, social services, recreational and cultural facilities) based on complex planning and scientific research. However, quantity mattered over quality, and systemic construction defects ultimately increased maintenance costs later on. Despite extensive production, the regime faced a constant housing deficit. Net growth of the housing stock was continuously undermined by the deterioration of old, unmaintained flats, and the concept of low-cost housing unceasingly stimulated a level of demand that could never be saturated (Havelková and Valentová 1998, 234). In the 1980s construction started to decrease as the country's economy declined and faced budget shortages, and the government began to promote housing development with the financial participation of users (in the form of cooperative and individual construction).

Between 1948 and 1990 as many as 1,352,843 new dwellings were built, of which 524,512 (39 percent) were private; 347,415 (26 percent) were state-owned; 376,797 (28 percent) were cooperative flats; and 104,119 (7 percent) were flats owned by other subjects (e.g., state enterprises, the armed forces). The number of dwellings increased from 823,158 (or 239 per one thousand inhabitants) in 1950 to 1,768,833 (or

335 per one thousand inhabitants) in 1991. The public housing system represented almost half of all housing in Slovakia.

A policy of full employment and wage setting translated into an extremely egalitarian distribution of income (Munich et al. 1999, 9). Rent and housing-related service fees regulated by the state, on the other hand, excluded, at least formally, existence of any social group that would have a problem with financial affordability of housing. The possibility of acquiring housing was thus only limited by deformations (unlimited demand), its inflexibility (bureaucratic burdens), ineffective management (nontransparency), and political bias during housing allocation (the favoritism of certain social groups and the exclusion of other, politically persecuted individuals).

With the exception of some urban areas dominated by detached housing and inhabited mostly by the establishment's nomenclature, and the historical town centers with flats inhabited largely by Roma (Gypsy) families,[4] the communist housing policy succeeded at creating a social mix in housing (occupational stratification was not reflected in residential distribution).

THE TRANSFORMATION OF HOUSING POLICY

After the collapse of communism, the new regime faced several challenges related to transforming the crumbling centrally planned economy into a market economy based on private ownership, establishing democracy, and repairing past injustices.[5] However, these objectives were sometimes conflicting, and their pursuit was sometimes held back by concerns about the presumed impact on the social situation of the population. Consequently, legal reforms proceeded at diverse speeds and some of them were postponed.

Within the Czechoslovak federation, housing policy was the responsibility of the two republics, although the federal government retained control over some 'sensitive' issues, such as rent regulation (Havelková and Valentová 1998, 238). In 1991 the central housing construction program was terminated and state subsidies for all forms of housing development were sharply reduced. Construction declined radically; between 1991 and 2000 only 78,319 new dwellings were built, most of them by private investors (50 percent) and cooperatives (31 percent); construction by the state/municipality decreased to one-fifth of what it had been in the previous decade.

As the Slovak government lacked the necessary funds to maintain public housing, it was transferred to the newly established local self-governments.[6] By an amendment to the Civil Code in 1992, sitting inhabitants' right of use of flats was converted into open-term rental contracts with strong tenant protections. For example, an owner could only terminate a lease for reasons defined in the law and only with the consent of a court; even in the case of termination of a lease the owner had to provide the tenant with substitute housing or accommodation (Act No. 509/1991 Coll. on Amendment of the Civil Code).

After the split of Czechoslovakia, Slovak law granted tenants of flats in buildings owned by the state, the municipalities, joint-stock companies with public share, and privatized companies the right to buy their housing at a favorable price and at the same time prohibited the transfer of the flat ownership to any other person than the flat's current tenant. The maximum purchase price was set by law in reference to the size of the flat and the age of the building (acquisition costs were reduced by 2 percent for every year of a building's existence up to 80 percent, and as a result flat prices in historical buildings in urban centers were much cheaper than flats in prefab building in new neighborhoods). Additional discounts and ten-year interest-free payment plans were provided (Act No. 182/1993 Coll. on Ownership of Residential and Non-Residential Premises). These prices were fifteen to twenty times lower than market prices for comparable dwellings (Suchalová and Staroňová 2010, 12), but the flats were generally in poor condition and the new owners had to refurbish and modernize them on their own.

Most of the housing stock developed by the state during the communist regime was privatized (Table 16.1); only 6.2 percent of flats were still the property of the municipalities in 2000, and these could conceivably be used for the purpose of social housing (although the real number of available dwellings would be much lower, as some would still be occupied by original tenants who did not use the opportunity to buy their flats and instead kept the open-term rental contracts). The process of privatization has continued. According to a survey conducted by the Ministry of Construction and Regional Development, as many as 639,329 dwellings have been transferred, and by the end of 2008 the available stock of rental housing owned by the municipalities had shrunk to 2.8 percent of all permanently occupied dwellings (Ministry of Construction and Regional Development of the Slovak Republic 2009).

Table 16.1 Changes in Tenure Structure during the Transformation

	[%]	
	1991	2000
Homeownership	0.24	0.32
Dwellings owned by housing cooperatives	0.23	0.34
Dwellings owned by municipalities	0.28	0.33
State-owned (state-owned companies) dwellings	0.23	0.3
	[Number]	
	1991	200
Total number of permanently occupied apartments	1,617,828	1,884,846
Total number of vacant apartments	151,000	209,316
Population of Slovakia	5,274,335	5,379,455

Source: Zapletalová et al. (2003, 303).

The restitution of property nationalized after 1948 to its owners or their heirs was not just a matter of reparative justice; the new political elite considered restitution a helpful means of speeding up privatization and developing the market economy (Kuti 2009, 78–79). Restitution also affected real estate and residential buildings with occupied flats. Currently rents in these flats are regulated at a level set by the Ministry of Finance of the Slovak Republic. They do not cover the costs of the secure operation and maintenance of the buildings (Grman 2011, 13). This situation will be changed by the new act adopted in 2011 (Act No. 260/2011 Coll. on the Termination Process and Structure of Certain Lease Agreements), which allows a gradual increase in rent and the termination of a lease by the dwelling's owner. Until 2017 municipalities are required to provide tenants in restituted housing in so-called 'housing need' (tenants who do not own another flat in the same municipality or do not have material resources to acquire proper housing) with adequate substitute housing with regulated rent and an open-term contract. If the municipality is not able to provide substitute housing, it has to pay the person or family in 'housing need' a monthly contribution to cover the difference between regulated rent and commercial rent usually at the local market.

According to estimates based on the 2001 Census, the total number of restituted dwellings may be as high as five thousand to seven thousand (Ministry of Construction and Regional Development of the Slovak Republic 2008, Annex 1). Although this amounts to less than 0.5 percent of the country's total housing stock, we can assume that the number of restituted dwellings is higher in certain municipalities, which will have thus exhausted their local housing resources.

THE RESPONSIBILITIES OF HOUSING POLICY

As part of the process of public policy reform and decentralization after 2000, housing policy became the responsibility of the local authorities (it is included among their 'original competencies', which are exercised independently from the central government and financed by the municipal budget, as opposed to 'transferred competencies', which are performed on behalf of the state, regulated by law, and funded by financial transfers from the central government). The law stipulates that the municipalities alone are responsible for the provision and approval of settlement zoning and the municipal strategies of economic and social development (Act No. 453/2001 Coll. on Amendment of Act No. 369/1990 Coll. on Municipalities and Other Acts). With this objective, municipalities can make their own investments or participate in commercial activities related to the planning, construction, and management of housing, technical infrastructure, and housing-related services.

The central government retained only normative powers over the technical, safety, and sanitary conditions of housing. The state also creates and partially manages the financial instruments that support the development of housing. Municipalities are eligible to apply through various grants and credit schemes for financial support to exercise their competency in the field of housing. However, whether the funding is actually provided depends on the state's economic means and budgetary allocations and the quality of the project applying for funding. At the central level the body responsible for housing policy is the Ministry of Transport, Construction, and Regional Development (MTCRD),[7] which since 1994 has formulated several national housing strategies (1994, 1995, 2000, 2005, 2010) and in 2005 prepared a specialized strategy focusing on housing for marginalized populations (Government of the Slovak Republic 2005).

All these documents emphasize the primary responsibility of citizens for their housing; on the other hand, they recognize the need to support the development of public rental housing and access to such housing for inhabitants who are unable to obtain housing on their own. The 2005 strategy introduced the term *social housing* aimed at vulnerable groups such as unemployed persons, the physically or mentally disabled, youth leaving institutional or protective care, elderly persons, lone-parent families, and large families. Special attention was given to socially excluded groups such as homeless people, long-term unemployed people, people in addiction recovery, and members of marginalized Roma communities (Government of the Slovak Republic 2005).

Their housing needs are to be addressed by providing them with affordable rental flats, developed and managed by the municipalities or not-for-profit organizations established by the local authorities with the financial support of the state, or by providing social care facilities, operated by municipalities, regional authorities, and private entities (profit or nonprofit) as part of the state's overall social policy (for example, pensioners' homes, charity shelters, emergency accommodation for victims of domestic violence, halfway housing for children leaving institutional care). The recent 2010 strategy states that rent in social housing should cover the costs of procuring, operating, and maintaining the housing, but should not generate a profit (Government of the Slovak Republic 2010). However, these strategies and new legislation on social housing adopted in 2010 do not introduce any new tools; they just confirm the financial instruments supporting rental housing development that have been in place, with slight modifications, since 1999 (see details in the following).

Besides supporting the supply side of housing, the state also provides poor inhabitants with a housing allowance as part of the social assistance policy implemented by the Ministry of Labor, Social Affairs, and Family. Since the restrictive welfare reforms introduced in 2003–2004, the housing allowance has been included among benefits of material need assistance paid to eligible individuals and families.[8] The amount of the housing allowance in 2011 is 68.5 U.S. dollars for individuals and 109.5 U.S. dollars for a household with more than one member (Order No. 324/2009 Coll.). Only persons or

Table 16.2 Housing Allowance Beneficiaries

Year	2006	2007	2008	2009	2010
Population	5,391,184	5,397,766	5,406,972	5,418,374	5,431,024
Registered unemployed population (job-seekers)*	299,181	250,938	230,433	340,243	380,791
Registered unemployment rate (%)*	10.4	8.4	7.7	11.4	12.5
Material need aid recipients (monthly average)	181,200	197,206	165,713	164,707	189,653
Housing allowance recipients (monthly average)	80,017	114,673	98,300	88,121	96,546
Housing allowance amount for a person (USD)**	58.23	62.51	63.80	67.23	71.98
Housing allowance amount for a family (USD)**	94.65	98.49	100.62	107.48	115.07
Average monthly nominal wage (USD)	803.35	862.65	932.71	960.41	992.01

Notes: Data marked with (*) are from the labor offices (and are lower than data gathered by the Statistical Office); data marked with (**) are valid as of January 1 of the given year.
Source: Statistical Office of the Slovak Republic; Central Office of Labor, Social Affairs and Family.

households with a legal housing tenancy or ownership or those permanently accommodated in a social care facility are entitled to the housing allowance. An additional condition is that an applicant cannot have debts on rent or services related to housing, or must have an installment plan to settle the existing debt. These entitlement conditions exclude inhabitants of informal Roma settlements (because their housing does not legally exist) and heavily indebted and low-income households (Table 16.2).[9] Moreover, as the amount of the housing allowance is fixed and does not reflect the real regional differentiation of housing costs, it restricts the spatial and social mobility of recipients of the benefit. They tend to remain or move to regions where there are lower housing costs, but also typically fewer employment opportunities.

SOCIAL HOUSING

The Social Housing Act (passed in 2010) defines social housing as any "housing procured with participation of public finances for adequate and dignified housing of natural persons who are not able to ensure housing by their own endeavor" (§ 20). Social housing is to be provided by the municipalities, regional self-governments, or not-for-profits established by them, who can apply for financial support from the state. State support is provided through subsidies from the MTCRD and the State Housing Development Fund (SHDF) for the construction of social rental flats with floorage up to 80 or 60 square meters, depending on the housing standard. Social housing can be allocated among households whose income is less than three times the amount of the subsistence minimum.[10] However, according to data from EU-SILC 2010, as many as 71 percent of households in Slovakia have a net income below this threshold, which indicates that the allocation of social housing to the most needy groups of housing seekers is not necessarily guaranteed.

In the case of lone-parent families; households with a handicapped person; or households with a member providing health, educational, cultural, or security services for inhabitants of the municipality, the income eligibility threshold is even higher—four times the subsistence minimum. Also eligible are people under the age of thirty who have left institutional care. The subsidies can also be used for the development of substitute housing for tenants of flats in restituted or privatized buildings where rent is being deregulated. The Ministry of Finance regulates the level of rent in social housing, and it can be no higher than 5 percent of the acquisition costs annually.

FINANCING SOCIAL HOUSING

Municipalities use soft loans (from SFHD) and grants (from MTCRD) to finance major part of the construction costs of social housing. In some cases of social housing construction in Roma communities, some municipal co-funding is provided in the form of work of future tenants (Hojsík and Perić 2009).

The MTCRD provides grants for the development of social rental housing (Table 16.3). Between 2001 and 2010, the MTCRD spent a total of 490 million U.S. dollars in subsidies for the construction of more than thirty thousand new dwellings through this scheme. Grant recipients must guarantee that only eligible tenants will use the housing, and 10 percent of the flats are allocated to households with a disabled member (if no eligible person applies for the housing, it can be rented to other applicants, but only with a one-year lease). Subsidized social housing must serve the purpose of social rental housing for at least thirty years, during which time the flats cannot be sold to their tenants or other persons. The municipality signs a lease with tenants for a three-year term (or ten-year term if the tenant is disabled), and the lease can be repeatedly extended.

The government supports the development of two categories of housing. One is a 'common standard' flat, in which the floorage may reach up to 60

Table 16.3 Subsidies for Construction of Social Rental Housing

Standard	Maximal floorage(m2)	Eligible costs per m2 (USD)	Maximal subsidy from the overall procurement costs	Maximal monthly rent calculated from eligible costs (USD)
	New construction and purchase			
	50	1,161	30%	243
Common Standard	56	1,148	25%	268
	60	1,135	20%	284
Lower Standard	45	677	75%	126
	55	658	70%	151
	Rehabilitation			
	50	839	30%	174
Common Standard	56	826	25%	192
	60	813	20%	204
Lower Standard	45	484	75%	90
	55	471	70%	108

Source: Act No. 443/2010 Coll. on grants for the development of housing and on social housing.

square meters and the grant ranges between 20 percent and 30 percent of the construction costs. The other provides a greater degree of assistance, where 70 percent to 75 percent of costs are covered, and use is made of 'lower-standard' flats, which are smaller in space (up to 55 square meters) and have fewer amenities, below the standard otherwise required for residential buildings.[11] Such low standards probably do not qualify as adequate housing according to the definition of the International Covenant on Economic, Social, and Cultural Rights (CESCR). Its concept of adequate housing requires the availability of facilities essential for health, security, comfort, nutrition, and the habitability of the housing, which must provide the inhabitants with adequate space and protect them from cold, damp, heat, rain, wind, and other threats to health (UN Committee on Economic, Social, and Cultural Rights 1991). The minimal requirements set by the MTCRD for amenities in lower-standard housing would probably not satisfy these requirements.

The SHDF additionally provides municipalities with soft loans that are intended for the construction or rehabilitation of housing (which can either be kept as rental housing or sold to its tenants) and for the construction, reconstruction, or rehabilitation of social care facilities that provide accommodation. Not-for-profit organizations can receive loans only for the construction of rental housing and the regional authorities only for the construction, reconstruction, or rehabilitation of social care facilities that provide accommodation. Typically, these soft loans cover the acquisition costs not covered by the grant. Loans are repayable, according to Order No. 432/2007 Coll., over a term of twenty to thirty years, and the interest rate is set at 1 percent or 5 percent per year, depending on the applicant and the investment project.[12]

A loan can cover up to 80 percent of the construction costs (a maximum 50,000 to 59,000 U.S. dollars). If the housing is for a disabled person, an additional nonrefundable subsidy is provided. The SHDF offers similar soft loans to individual applicants whose household income is no higher than three and a half times the subsistence minimum (81.8 percent of households). Loans up to 67,500 U.S. dollars can cover 80 percent of the costs of acquiring housing, and applicants must prove they have funding for the remaining 20 percent of the acquisition costs and the capacity to repay the loan within twenty to thirty years at an interest rate of 3.5 percent per year. More favorable conditions are set up for persons under thirty-five years of age (a longer repayment period and interest rate of 2 percent per year) and persons leaving institutional childcare (a loan covering up to 100 percent of the procurement costs with thirty-year repayment period and 1 percent per year interest rate).

Subsidized, low-standard housing is the usual scheme utilized for the construction of housing in marginalized Roma communities. The reason for the reduction of the minimal compulsory amenities by the subsidy provider is connected with anti-Roma prejudices and the widespread stereotype that the Roma destroy their housing. However, independent monitoring in 2008 showed that the poor technical condition of social housing in many Roma settlements is more the result of poor-quality construction and undelivered materials or equipment than to the behavior of the tenants. Furthermore, the monitoring revealed that almost 90 percent of social housing projects that target Roma conserve or even deepen the existing ethnic residential

Table 16.4 Completed Public and Private Dwellings between 2001 and 2010

Year	2001	2002	2003	2004	2005	2006	2007	2008	2009	2010	Total
Completed dwellings	10,321	14,213	13,980	12,592	14,863	14,444	16,473	17,184	18,834	17,076	149,980
Public	1,201	2,429	3,993	1,546	2,103	2,143	2,632	2,632	2,356	2,519	24,077
Private	9,120	11,784	9,987	11,046	12,443	12,301	14,552	14,552	16,478	14,557	125,586
Share of public (%)	11.64	17.09	28.56	12.28	14.15	14.84	15.32	15.32	12.51	14.75	16.05

Source: Statistical Office of the Slovak Republic.

segregation and virtually none of them have helped to foster an ethnic and social mix (Hojsík 2008).

In smaller municipalities, housing management is usually exercised by the municipal office itself, in larger towns by not-for-profit or for-profit companies established or contracted by the municipal authorities. The monitoring findings indicate that auditing for the proper use of public funds and the effective management of housing by municipalities is not sufficient. With the decentralization of public administration most housing governance powers were transferred to the municipalities from the central government, which retained for itself few if any control instruments for implementing or actively influencing housing policy at the local level.

In order to be eligible for any financial assistance from the central government, the municipal authority must have elaborated a local housing strategy or social and economic development plan. However, the actual content of these documents is not subject to scrutiny or evaluation by the MTCRD or any other authority independent of the municipality. A study into the transparency of social housing management showed that only about a quarter of district towns have official ex ante rules for the allocation of social housing; half of the municipalities allocate social housing upon 'individual examination' of the applications (Suchalová and Staroňová 2010, 50–54). We can conclude that neither vertical effectiveness (the extent to which the subsidies are actually allocated to those who really need help), nor horizontal effectiveness (whether any of the needy are excluded) of housing policies is fully achieved;[13] they depend entirely on the practices in individual municipalities.

CONCLUSION

Most of the existing dwelling stock in Slovakia was built during the communist regime with the strong financial support of the state. Public housing was supposed to be administratively allocated on the basis of applicants' needs (in reality, however, this system suffered from nontransparency and protectionism), and the rents were regulated and subsidized. In the first decade after the change of regime there was a dramatic decrease in the construction of new housing. It has started to increase again, but the volume of construction between 2001 and 2010 equaled only half that in the period 1981–1990. The amount of habitable residential stock in Slovakia (approximately 350 per one thousand inhabitants) is still lower than the standard in the EU (four hundred to five hundred per one thousand inhabitants).

After the division of Czechoslovakia, almost the whole public housing sector was privatized and sold to tenants, restituted to pre-1948 owners, or sold together with other state property to new private owners. Occupants exercising their right to buy got a comparative advantage, which reproduced inequalities from the communist period. On the other hand, they usually acquired poorly maintained property that required large investments in repairs and rehabilitation.

Privatization led to a substantial reduction in the amount of available public rental housing, and strong tenant protections and tenants' right to buy have served to restrict new housing development. Today, the share of public rental housing is only less than 3 percent of the whole habitable housing stock; private rental housing is moreover financially inaccessible to many. A lack of affordable rental housing in areas of economic growth and employment opportunities (Bratislava, Trnava region, and the largest towns of other regions) is an important barrier to labor mobility and a source of the high unemployment rate in Slovakia. A survey from 2007 indicated that private rental housing is four times (in Bratislava ten times) more expensive than public rentals.

Most new rental housing is provided through the construction of state-subsidized social housing. However, since the decentralization of public administration, the design and implementation of housing policy, including social housing, is in the hands of municipal self-governments. The central government does not have control over the effectiveness and efficiency of housing management.

The vertical effectiveness of social housing is limited due to the wide eligibility criteria; social housing is not reserved for the neediest groups of inhabitants, but is also open to the middle class (more than 70 percent of households satisfy the income criterion for access to social housing). Moreover, the allocation of social housing by the municipalities is not always transparent.

For certain social groups these circumstances create a barrier in access to housing. Low-income employees (the lower-middle class) are not eligible for restricted housing allowances, but at the same time they do not have enough income to afford their own housing even when they use the existing supports (soft loans, state premiums on building savings). Access to municipal social housing is limited by its shortage and unclear allocation procedures. Marginalized social groups, especially the Roma, are victims of persistent discrimination and residential segregation, often intentionally promoted by the municipal authorities.

NOTES

1. In the centralized communist polity, no local self-government existed. Public administration was exercised through a vertical system of local, district, and regional National Committees subordinated to the Communist Party of Czechoslovakia.
2. However, the lands remained *de iure* in the state's ownership and were only 'rented' to private investors, usually for a period of ninety-nine years.
3. "Between 1975 and 1989, as many as 97 percent of the multiple apartment buildings were constructed using the prefab technology . . . [and] made up

almost 42 percent of the total housing stock in Slovakia in 1990" (Zapletalová et al. 2003, 298).

4. The regime's policy of assimilation of the Roma focused on elimination of traditional rural settlements and their relocation into towns, often into historical buildings, which were seen as inferior because of a lack of modern amenities, poor maintenance, or old-fashioned architecture. However, after 1989 these flats became a matter of restitution to former (pre-1948) owners and commercially attractive (within the overall rehabilitation of central zones of towns); subsequently, their Roma tenants were among the first to lose their housing (see Hojsík and Perić 2009).
5. This reestablishment of justice was, however, selective. The right to restitution was conditional upon a claimant having Slovak citizenship and being a permanent resident in the country. The law also excluded restitutions to Sudeten Germans (in the Czech Republic) and Hungarians (in Slovakia) whose property was expropriated under the Beneš Decrees enacted in the aftermath of the Second World War and the restitution of national cultural sites (Kuti 2009).
6. Local self-governments were introduced in Czechoslovakia at the federal level by Constitutional Act No. 294/1990 Coll. and subsequently arranged separately on the national level by laws on municipalities adopted respectively by the Slovak National Council (Act No. 369/1990 Coll.) and the Czech National Council (Act No. 367/1990 Coll.).
7. Established in 1994 as the Ministry of Construction and Public Works, it was the Ministry of Construction and Regional Development between 1999 and 2010, and since 2010 has been MTCRD.
8. According to the Act No. 599/2003 on aid in material need, the amount of aid is calculated as the difference between different benefit entitlements (basic benefit, housing allowance, activation allowance, protection allowance, and others) and actual income of the household. The aid never reaches the level of the subsistence minimum.
9. According to sociographic mapping of Romany settlements in 2003–2004, 40 percent out of approximately 320,000 Roma in Slovakia live in rural and urban marginalized communities (including segregated settlements). About one-third of households in marginalized communities live in informal housing, including standard brick family houses, wooden houses, nonresidential buildings, shanties, caravans, tents, or other nonstandard housing (Jurásková, et al. 2004).
10. In 2011 the subsistence minimum is 257 U.S. dollars for one person, 172 U.S. dollars for each additional adult person, and 112 U.S. dollars for each child.
11. Decree of the Ministry of Health of the Slovak Republic No. 259/2008 Coll. on Details on Requirements for Interior of Buildings and on Minimum Requirements for Lower Standard Housing and for Accommodation Facilities. Order of the Government of the Slovak Republic No. 353/2006 Coll. on Details on Requirements for Interior of Buildings and on Minimum Requirements for Lower Standard Housing and for Accommodation Facilities.
12. The 5 percent per year rate applies for the construction of new dwelling in a residential building or in a family house (the municipality can sell them). A 1 percent per year rate is offered for the rehabilitation of an existing building, the construction of a new dwelling, or the purchase of an existing dwelling, which will be used as rental housing, and all investments into social care facilities.
13. Definitions from Lux (2003, 1).

REFERENCES

B. Č. and others v. Town of Sabinov and Ministry of Construction and Regional Development of the Slovak Republic, District Court Prešov, 25 C 192/2007 (2009). http://www.oad.sk/sites/default/files/downloads/Telek_rozsudok_EN.pdf accessed October 30, 2011.

Government of the Slovak Republic. 2005. *2005 Strategy of State Housing Policy by 2010*. Governmental Resolution No. 636/2005.

———. 2010. *2010 Strategy of State Housing Policy by 2015*. Governmental Resolution No. 96/2010.

Grman, J. 2011. "Problematika regulácie nájomného v podmienkach SR (The Issue of Rent Regulation in Slovakia)." *Bulletin slovenskej advokácie* 4 (17).

Havelková, E. and Valentová, B. 1998. "Komparatívna analýza bytovej politiky v Slovenskej a Českej republike v rokoch 1990–1996 (Comparative Analysis of Housing Policy in the Slovak and the Czech Republic in 1990–1996)." *Sociální politika v Čechách a na Slovensku po roce 1989*. Praha: Karolinum.

Hojsík, M. 2008. *Evalvácia programu obecných nájomných bytov v rómskych osídleniach (Evaluation of Municipal Rental Housing Program in Roma Settlements)*. Bratislava: Nadácia Milana Šimečku.

Hojsík, M. and Perić, T. 2009. *Case Study: Roma Housing Projects in Small Communities, Slovakia*. Vienna: European Union Agency for Fundamental Rights.

Ivanička, K., Zúbková, M., and Špirková, D. 2003. *Bytová politika (Housing Policy)*. Bratislava: Slovenská technická univerzita.

Jankovichová, E. 2003. *Nájomné bývanie (Rental Housing)*. Bratislava: Slovenská technická univerzita.

Jurásková, M., Kriglerová, E., and Rybová, J. 2004. *Atlas rómskych komunít na Slovensku 2004 (Atlas of Roma Communities in Slovakia)*. Bratislava: Úrad vlády SR.

Kuti, C. 2009. *Post-Communist Restitution and the Rule of Law*. Budapest: Central European University Press.

Long-Term Strategy of Housing for Marginalized Groups of Population. Governmental resolution No. 63/2005.

Lux, M. 2003. "Efficiency and Effectiveness of Housing Policies in the Central and Eastern Europe Countries." *International Journal of Housing Policy* 3 (3): 243–65.

Ministry of Construction and Regional Development of the Slovak Republic. 2008. Draft Act on Termination of Some Tenancies—New Version. Annex 1. Document from meeting of the Government of the Slovak Republic No. UV-3323/2008. February 14.

———. 2009. *Informácia o stave vlastníckej štruktúry bytového fondu v Slovenskej republike k 31. decembru 2008 (Information on the Status of the Ownership Structure of the Housing Stock in the Slovak Republic, 31 December 2008)*. http://www.build.gov.sk/mvrrsr/index.php?id=10&cat=&news=3867 accessed November 14, 2011.

Munich, D., Svejnar, J., and Terrell, K. 1999. *Returns to Human Capital under the Communist Wage Grid and during the Transition to a Market Economy*. Working Paper, no. 272. http://deepblue.lib.umich.edu/bitstream/2027.42/39656/3/wp272.pdf accessed October 30, 2011.

Šmídová, O. 1993. "Byty za (post)totality: osudy hrstky českých sociologů skrze jejich byty (Apartments during the [Post]Totalitarianism: The Fate of a Handful of Czech Sociologists through Their Apartments)." *Sociológia* 6 (25): 573–583.

Suchalová, A. and Staronová, K. 2010. *Mapovanie sociálneho bývania v mestách Slovenska (Mapping of Social Housing in the Cities of Slovakia)*. Bratislava: Ústav verejnej politiky a ekonómie FSEV UK.

UN Committee on Economic, Social, and Cultural Rights. 1991. *CESCR General Comment 4: The Right to Adequate Housing (Art. 11 [1])*. Geneva: Office of the United Nations High Commissioner for Human Rights.

Zapletalová, J., Antalíková, M., and Smatanová, E. 2003. "The Role of Self-Government in Housing Development in Slovakia: Local Government and Housing in Slovakia." *Housing Policy: An End or a New Beginning?* Budapest: OSI/LGI.

17 Slovenia

The Social Housing Sector in Search of an Identity

Andreja Cirman and Srna Mandič

INTRODUCTION

In the debates that accompanied the transition from socialism in Central and Eastern European (CEE) societies, *housing privatization* has been one of the key buzzwords. In Slovenia it has been a topical issue for more than a decade. Moreover, it represented a 'grand opening' to the process of transition, as the privatization of social housing was one of the earliest and most tangible 'transition' acts, directly affecting a massive population. However, having performed its role in this 'initiation rite' into the market economy, and after the grand story of transition lost its initial thrust, social housing has almost disappeared from the Slovenian political and research agendas. Its subsequent development has been slow and erratic.

In this chapter we observe the developments in Slovenia's social housing, understood in the traditional sense of the provision of affordable rental housing. In particular, we examine the specific dynamics of social housing in Slovenia. Seeing it as a significant social institution, we aim to explore its continuity—and discontinuity—within a historical framework and consider its organizational features. We intend to argue that there are a number of points of continuity and discontinuity between different historical periods, but that there seems to be more organizational continuity between pre-socialist and socialist social housing than between socialist and post-socialist social housing. Pre-socialist and socialist housing was firmly grounded in employer-owned rental housing, whereas during the post-socialist transition social housing was cut loose from this organizational base, thereafter remaining without an equivalent substitute.

To demonstrate the historical continuities and discontinuities in social housing in Slovenia, we will discuss its dynamics and social and historical contingencies in three historical periods: the pre-transition period, which goes as far back as the years before the Second World War; the transition reform period; and post-transition developments. Particular attention is paid to the institutional framework of social housing and to the question of the extent to which the changes in social housing after the transition can be seen as social housing strategies or, alternatively, as unintended consequences of other major economic changes. The current consequences of these changes are also discussed with regard to the new quality of social housing from the perspective of tenants. Finally, we conclude the account of Slovenian social housing by summarizing the factors that help explain its erratic course in post-transition development.

THE HISTORICAL AND GENERAL CONTEXT

The housing arrangements in place during the socialist era have often been regarded as specific (to that time) and inspired by socialist ideology. But it is possible to find a considerable degree of path dependence in Slovenian socialist housing policy in relation to prewar housing; specifically, there was continuity between two significant housing approaches in the first half of the twentieth century. The first approach was grounded in self-help housing provision, which dates back to the rural feudal tradition; self-help housing construction was also present during the early industrialization and urbanization periods, mainly on the outskirts of cities. The second approach was employer-owned housing provision, observed among the trades and in mining and industries like textile manufacturing; in the 1920s and 1930s this practice was also found in a number of public services, most notably in education, and railway employees were able to take advantage of rental housing provided by their employers and employee organizations. In contrast, two other major types of housing provision—private rental and cooperative housing—appeared in Slovenia on a very limited scale. Self-help construction and employer-owned housing provision thus had strong prewar roots.

The early postwar period typically saw heavy involvement by the state, which not only nationalized most of the housing stock, but was also the only actor in housing that could acquire and allocate new housing. Yet, already during the 1950s the provision of housing was decentralized and transferred from the central (at that time based in Belgrade) to the national (based in Ljubljana) governments and then to the municipalities. However, following the introduction of the self-management model of socialism, large-scale housing reform in 1965 even further decentralized the responsibility for the provision of housing and transferred it to each and every enterprise in social property, which thus became responsible for providing housing to its employees. The core of the self-management model of socialism was that enterprises in social property, organized and managed according to self-management principles, were able to make independent decisions about their economic activity, but they were legally and organizationally obliged to devote a certain proportion of their income to a housing fund. This housing fund was used for two purposes: to acquire new housing to be rented out to employees and to provide housing loans for employees to acquire their housing either by purchases on market terms or through self-help construction.

Thus, in the mid-1960s the form of housing provision adopted, developed to correspond to Yugoslavia's specific self-management model of socialism, was actually a continuation of the two dominant housing practices from the prewar period—employer-owned renting and support for self-help construction. Self-help construction also included a very popular practice of 'in-place housing adjustments', whereby people reconstructed their own residence or that of their relatives and did not move (Mandic 2001). Both types could be considered forms of social housing because when it came to their allocation the criteria of individual housing need and income were significant; in addition, both the rents to be paid and the loans to be repaid were provided at below-market prices. However, it was social rental housing that embodied the recognition of the social function of housing and the responsibility of employers for it. Two additional points should be made to complete the picture of social housing of that period. There were always long waiting lists for and shortages of available rental housing and available housing loans; in the allocation of both, other criteria besides need were applied, so often the members of the elite were prioritized. There were also municipal programs of 'solidarity and reciprocity', implemented in the 1970s to substitute employers' provision of housing in the case of people who were not employed. In 1990 social rental housing made up 33 percent of the total housing stock; its composition according to the type of owner was as follows: 68 percent enterprises; 30 percent municipalities; and 2 percent state agencies (Ministry for Environment Protection and Physical Planning 1991).

This self-management model of housing provision was formally abolished in 1991 (for more details, see Stanovnik 1994; Mandic 1994; Sendi 1995; Cirman 2006), but it was already on the decline throughout the 1980s. It had gradually been losing energy, and by the end of 1980s it was exhausted both financially and in terms of political support. The financial exhaustion had to do with inflation, which had eroded the lending capital that had accumulated in enterprise housing funds. Although the inflation rate reached 30 percent in 1982 and had risen to 132 percent in 1986, long-term housing loans were being repaid at a fixed interest rate below 10 percent. According to anecdotal sources from those times, a heavy long-term loan burden taken on for twenty years could in that period be easily paid off within a single year by a lucky homeowner. As a result of the difference between the inflation rate and the interest rate on loans, the lending capital in housing funds and banks lost one-half of its real value between 1982 and 1986; in terms of the share of GDP the amount of total lending capital fell from 4.8 percent of GDP to 2.4 percent of GDP (Yugoslav Institute for Urbanism and Housing 1987). Thus, through inflation and housing loans, 2.4 percent of GDP was transformed from 'social property' to 'private property'. This was actually a 'silent privatization', without any explicit reference to ideological issues.

Besides its shrinking financial base, the self-management model of housing provision also lost political and public support. During the 1980s it was often criticized, and the main target of this criticism was social rental housing. There were two main arguments. The first was economic and pointed out the inefficient management of social housing and the fact that it was 'dead capital' for their owners, for example, social enterprises. Enterprises could not freely dispose of their housing equity as it had been rented out on a permanent basis. The second was the 'social justice' argument, which highlighted the fact that elites had privileged access to social housing, a point frequently made by critical analysts. Paradoxically, empirical evidence in 1991 regarding this last point did not support this argument, as the share of social housing tenants among both the top and bottom educational categories was 22 percent (Mandic 1992, 7). It is quite likely that the small share of elites in social housing was the outcome of the reorientation of elites from rental housing to housing loans for homeownership that occurred in the last decade of socialism. However, in the public discourse, social housing became a symbol of social inequality and of how socialism failed to eradicate it.

From a historical distance, the critical arguments concerning the self-management model of housing provision may seem to contradict the social function of housing. According to the economic argument, the model was blamed for having too strong a social function, thus repressing the entrepreneurial instinct of owners; by contrast, the egalitarian criticism blamed the system for not fully realizing the social function of housing. However, by the end of the 1980s the self-management model of housing provision was exhausted: its first pillar—the system of social rental housing—came to be recognized as economically inefficient and socially unjust; its second pillar—the system of housing loans—lost most of its financial base. The system was thus ideologically and financially exhausted. The time for a new radical reform had come.

SOCIAL HOUSING STRATEGIES DURING THE TRANSITION

What attracted most attention and best embodied the 'transition to a market economy' was the sale of social rental housing to sitting tenants, that is, housing privatization. Some of the fundamental changes, however, barely even entered public debate. The transition era housing changes and the varied measures and activities that emerged in that period can be divided into two phases: the initial phase, aimed at abolishing the previous system and its state-dominated financial base, and the second phase, which involved the creation of new social safety-net provisions (Hegedüs et al. 1996). These two phases can be distinguished not so much in terms of their timing as much as in functional terms.

Three key measures were introduced during the initial phase of housing transition in Slovenia, only one of which was housing specific. The first measure already formed part of the 1989 Constitutional Amendments and eliminated the self-management model generally; in the domain of housing provision this meant that the 'solidarity and reciprocity' housing programs (together with rent subsidization and city renewal) were shut down and the responsibility for housing was transferred to the executive councils of the municipalities, which did not start dealing with the issue of housing until many years later. Some of them have yet to do so. The second measure came in 1991, when general financial legislation was amended so as to put an end to the legal duty of enterprises to invest a certain share of their revenue into housing funds. This eliminated the key national source of housing financing, and the search for a substitute source was deferred to a later date. The third measure was the privatization of social rental housing, as already described and analyzed elsewhere (see Stanovnik 1992; Sendi 1995; Mandic 1996; Cirman 2002), the bulk of social rental housing was sold to sitting tenants at below-market prices. Exempted from these sales was that part of social housing that had to be restituted to prewar owners and their heirs; in spite of the formal legal protection granted to sitting tenants, this arrangement caused many problems and conflicts (see Mandic 2000), which were ultimately brought before the European Court for Human Rights. Out of the three measures, only the third one seems to correspond to the notion of a 'social housing strategy', whereas the other two reflected other, nonhousing strategies.

The second phase, following on the collapse of the previous system, formally started in 1991 with the introduction of a governmental policy document called "Starting Points for the National Housing Program" and the subsequent 1991 Housing Act. The policy document introduced a new model of housing provision, in which the responsibilities for housing were redefined, with new actors, institutions, programs, and rules. As shown in Table 17.1, the implementation of this strategy was extremely modest. In 1991 the Housing Fund of the Republic of Slovenia was established to provide housing loans, some of the fund dedicated as lending capital created by collecting 20 percent of the purchase value of the social rental housing on sale.

The new housing model was based on the principle that each person is responsible for his/her housing, whereas the state supports those individuals who, due to inadequate means, are unable to do so by themselves and who are thus the target of social rental housing. In this way the state's responsibility changed from 'providing' to 'enabling'. In this phase, the 'enabling' function was defined in a very limited way and implied the strict targeting of social rental housing to the neediest part of the population with the lowest incomes. In addition to 'social rental housing' targeting the needy, lowest-income population and being supported by the state, 'nonprofit rental housing' was also introduced, envisioned as an independent and self-sustaining housing sector earmarked for the middle-income part of the population and serving as a substitute for the previous employer-owned housing. This sector was supposed to make use of the unsold enterprise-owned housing and even restituted housing.

EVALUATION OF SOCIAL HOUSING STRATEGIES DURING THE TRANSITION

However, the expectation that 'nonprofit rental housing' would develop out of private initiatives, generally without much state or municipal role in its implementation, turned out to be too optimistic. As Table 17.1 shows, the outcomes of the sector and of the whole system of housing provision followed a quite different logic than what was expected according to the policy document. Only a small amount of nonprofit housing was developed/built and it was not by independent, private nonprofit organizations, as anticipated, but mostly emerged within the municipal organizational framework. For this reason the categories of 'social' and 'nonprofit' rental housing were later merged into a single category.

Nonprofit rental housing takes a variety of forms. The nonprofit rental sector comprises housing units that were previously part of 'socially owned housing', some of which were privatized in/after 1991 and some of which were turned into 'dwellings leased for nonprofit rent'. This status guaranteed sitting tenants an open-ended rental lease and nonprofit rent. The landlords of these units are denationalized companies or individuals who got their property back in the restitution process, public agencies, and municipalities (for those dwellings with sitting tenants who decided not to participate in privatization and buy their housing unit). It also comprises post-privatization additions to the nonprofit housing stock that were constructed or acquired in the market by nonprofit housing organizations.

To sum up, the first decade after the transition saw the implementation of social housing measures that were almost microscopic in scale and extremely slow. For instance, Ljubljana, which had the country's most

Table 17.1 Housing Stock in Slovenia: Expected Structure and Resulting Structure after Privatization

	Initial structure prior to privatization according to Housing Census 1991	Expected structure for 2000	Resulting structure according to Housing Census 2002
Owner-occupied	67	75	90
Privately rented housing	0	5	2
Social housing	33	20	7
Other	–	–	1
Total	100	100	100

Source: Starting points for the preparation of the National Housing Programme, Ministry of Environment and Spatial Planning, Ljubljana (1991).

innovative city administration, only managed to create its first social housing program and allocate social housing in 1995, and many municipalities have yet to create any program.

THE INSTITUTIONAL FRAMEWORK FOR SOCIAL HOUSING SINCE THE YEAR 2000

With the introduction of the National Housing Program in 2000, the development of provisions to support the social function of housing started to make progress. Further, the responsibility for housing provision began to be perceived more broadly in the sense of promoting the efficient functioning of the entire system of housing provision. This was reflected in the emergence of a widening range of financial instruments, such as the subsidizing of housing loans, the provision of housing loans for nonprofit housing, or the subsidizing of rents in private rental housing. There were also some important innovations on the municipal level, particularly in Ljubljana; besides emergency housing, a number of new programs were implemented for specific groups, such as the disabled, the elderly, victims of violence, homeless people, people with mental health problems, other groups in need of supported housing, and artists (studios). In addition, social housing began to adopt and apply innovative environmental and energy-efficient

Table 17.2 Implementation of the National Housing Program in Slovenia: Additions to the Nonprofit Housing Stock

Year	Nonprofit housing (actual construction in housing units)	National Housing Program (housing units)	Index
2000	580	650	89
2001	444	850	52
2002	538	1,100	49
2003	411	1,400	29
2004	264	1,800	15
2005	524	2,250	23
2006	442	2,700	16
2007	439	3,200	14
2008	498	3,800	13
2009	*400	4,500	9
Total	**4,540**	**22,250**	**20**

* *Data for 2009 are estimates from the Ministry of Environment and Spatial Planning.*
Source: National Housing Program (2000); the Ministry of Environment and Spatial Planning (2010).

measures. Social housing is now changing somewhat in terms of its scope and target groups. It is shifting between two ideal types of social housing. On the one hand, it focuses especially on providing the minimum to the most marginalized groups; on the other hand, it supports innovation in quality housing and energy saving.

Although the National Housing Program set ambitious targets for the development of the social housing sector, its real results lagged far behind. In the transition process the system of social housing was adapted to the economy's new market orientation and brought more in line with comparable developed European countries. However, even with the National Housing Program of 2000 and with the amendments to the Housing Act after 2000, most of the changes remained on a declaratory level, as the institutional setting was far from supportive of the development of a modern social housing sector.

There are several reasons for this failure. At the national and municipal levels housing was too often regarded as a low-priority issue. This attitude also led to the program not being adequately financially supported for it to be put into practice. Established by the Housing Act, the Housing Fund of the Republic of Slovenia is a central institution for supporting the implementation of the National Housing Program in the field of social housing. Under the program the government was supposed to increase the capital in the national housing fund in the 2000–2009 period by 334 million U.S. dollars. In reality, however, capital was increased by just 39 million U.S. dollars (11.6 percent of the amount planned). The situation at the municipal level was similar.

Social housing in Slovenia is regulated by legislation at the national level. The Housing Act defines the status of social housing, stipulates that leases must be open-term, outlines rental provisions and eligibility, and sets the level of rent and rent subsidization. Nonprofit rent is set according to a regulated methodology for determining rent in nonprofit housing, defining rent as a percentage of the value of the housing unit, and according to a methodology for determining the value of housing units. Nonprofit rent is set at a maximum of 4.68 percent of the value of the housing unit and covers the following elements: upkeep and maintenance (up to 1.18 percent);[1] the cost of management (up to 0.4 percent); unit depreciation for the life period of sixty years (up to 1.67 percent); and the capital cost of investment (up to 1.5). Tenants below a certain means-tested income level can apply for a subsidy of up to 80 percent of the nonprofit rent. The subsidy is paid from the municipal budget.

A large drawback to investment in and the financial viability of social housing in Slovenia lies in the methodology used to valuate housing units. The value of a housing unit is determined with the use of a legally prescribed administrative valuation procedure. The valuation methodology assumes that the land and the infrastructure are acquired free of charge from the local authority, and therefore the assessed value only takes the construction costs into account. Because this is rarely the case in practice, rents do not cover all the costs of providing housing. This has a negative impact on the interest of (especially private) nonprofit housing organizations in contributing to the existing stock of nonprofit dwellings (Cirman 2004) and detracts from financial viability of such an investment. The result of the administrative valuation model is a value established in points, which is then multiplied by the attributed value of the point. Before entering the Eurozone the value of a point was indexed first to the German mark and later to the euro. However, once the country adopted the euro this indexation stopped and the value of a point has stayed nominally the same since 2006.

Given the very few additions to the nonprofit housing stock in the last two decades, the bias of privatization towards housing units in better condition (Stanovnik 1994) and the conversion of restituted dwellings with sitting tenants to nonprofit housing status, the nonprofit housing stock is quite unbalanced in terms of its age structure and quality. Nonprofit housing organizations face another obstacle in the fact that the rent-pooling mechanism does not work properly.

On the regulatory level, the provision of nonprofit rental housing is defined as a 'service of general interest, realized through benefits targeted at registered nonprofit housing organizations'. They are established for the acquisition of housing units, management, rental, administration, and sale of housing. In practice, they operate as departments of the municipalities (municipal budget funds), municipal housing funds (independent legal entities), or as nonprofit housing organizations that operate as private companies. Nonprofit housing organizations come in different sizes, ranging from less than one hundred to about three thousand nonprofit dwellings, with most being geographically limited to operations within a specific municipality.

The Ministry of Environment and Spatial Planning supervises nonprofit organizations and their operations and maintains a register of nonprofit housing organizations. It was last updated in 2004. At that time there were fifty-nine nonprofit housing organizations, of which 42 percent had private or private/public ownership and 52 percent were owned by municipal housing funds. However, it is impossible to find out how many of them are still active today. According to an estimate by the Director of the Housing Chamber of Slovenia, the public and municipal housing funds are still active, but very few others still exist. The demise of a significant share of nonprofit housing organizations established as private companies can be attributed to the institutional setting, which has been unfavorable towards private initiatives, in particular the nonprofit rental policy and the existing institutional arrangements for nonprofit organizations.

Nonprofit housing organizations operate under specific conditions. In addition to the development, acquisition, renovation, rental, management, and administration of nonprofit housing they can also engage in commercial activities. The net profit earned by a nonprofit housing organization must be used for the acquisition of housing units, renovation, reconstruction, and maintenance, with a minimum of 70 percent of the net profit earmarked for additions to the stock.

Nonprofit housing organizations can also enter into private–public partnerships (PPPs) with the public sector and are eligible for subsidies from the government and local authorities or for specific tax exemptions; they can receive grants in the form of building land, with or without infrastructure, reductions in communal taxes, and so on. The Housing Fund of the Republic of Slovenia provides favorable loans to nonprofit housing providers (up to 50 percent of an investment if the Housing Fund also participates with equity stakes), forms joint ventures with municipalities, and enters into PPPs with nonprofit housing organizations, again participating with equity stakes. Yet, in practice, the public housing funds are limited in the use of financial leverage to 10 percent of its assets. This very much reduces their ability to embark on new investments. On the other hand, the rent-setting regime and widespread liquidity problems stemming from the limited effectiveness of the rent-pooling mechanism also deter private companies from making such investments.

There is no effective supervision of nonprofit housing organizations. According to the Housing Act, supervision is exercised by the Housing Inspection (Office) within the Ministry of Environment and Spatial Planning, which can remove a company from the register of nonprofit housing organizations if it has acted in breach of the regulation. The last inspection of nonprofit housing organizations, however, was performed in 2002. That inspection also revealed that most of the organizations were operating at a loss. Those nonprofit organizations that also engaged in other commercial activities had better results, but only a few of them operated with any profit (Stanovnik et al. 2003). The collected rents are not enough to permit them to purchase new housing stock or sometimes to renovation of the existing stock. Many nonprofit organizations have also suffered from liquidity problems, the exception being those organizations that manage older housing stock and no longer pay off loans for its purchase.

Not only has the institutional setting of the nonprofit housing sector resulted in only small additions being made to the non-profit housing stock; it has even contributed to a decrease in housing stock. According to the Ministry of Environment and Spatial Planning, the municipalities owned 21,260 housing units in 2000. Despite some additions to the stock, however, by 2009 they owned just 15,728 housing units. The difference can be attributed to the sale of social housing, mostly units that were previously socially owned housing. Some tenants made late use of their right-to-buy option, established in the Housing Act of 1991, and some nonprofit housing organizations decided to sell their housing units to their sitting tenants. It was especially the right-to-buy option from 1991 that enabled sitting tenants to buy their housing on almost absurd terms. In the early privatization period tenants had the right to buy their dwellings at a heavy discount (e.g., in Ljubljana at about 10 percent of the unit's market value). But two decades later the same nominal terms still applied. For example, in Ljubljana, where market prices in 2008 and 2009 ranged between 3,250 and 4,550 U.S. dollars per square meter, the Housing Fund of the Municipality of Ljubljana had to sell its housing units for prices ranging from 10–185 U.S. dollars per square meter. The proceeds from the sale of nonprofit housing could therefore never make up for the reduction of the housing stock.

OUTCOMES FROM THE PERSPECTIVE OF TENANTS

The high demand for nonprofit rental housing and its very limited supply led to the introduction of subsidies for private rental housing in 2008. For example, in Ljubljana only 10–15 percent of applicants for nonprofit rental housing could be granted such housing. Unsuccessful yet eligible applicants for nonprofit housing were consequently forced to find a market solution to their housing problems; hence, the government decided on a subsidy scheme. The housing allowance is paid to landlords and the funds are provided by local authorities. The allowance is calculated as the difference between the maximum accepted market rent, set in conformity with the regulation, and the nonprofit rent level, set at U.S. dollars 3.8 per square meter. However, tenants in market rental housing are only eligible for an allowance equal to the difference between market and nonprofit rent, but not for an allowance for the full rent, like tenants in nonprofit rental housing are. Moreover, the maximum eligible rent varies by region, in Ljubljana

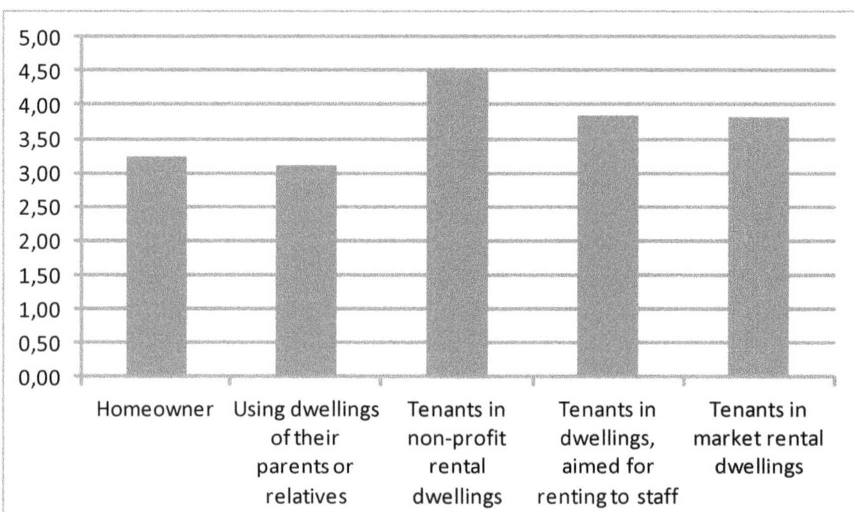

Figure 17.1 Average monthly operating costs in U.S. dollars per square meter.
Source: Cirman (2005)

it is set at 9 U.S. dollars per square meter—a price far below actual market rents. As a consequence, only 210 U.S. dollars in allowances for households in the profit rental sector were paid to 333 households in 2009 in Slovenia, which illustrates the significant limitations to this scheme.

Another problem facing nonprofit housing is maintaining the housing and especially upgrading it in terms of energy efficiency. As noted earlier, the nonprofit rental sector is unbalanced in its structure and it has a large amount of relatively old housing, which suffers from liquidity problems and whose maintenance was put off in the past. The Housing Fund of the Republic of Slovenia tries to stimulate energy-efficient refurbishment in the nonprofit housing sector by offering favorable loans for this purpose; however, there is no effective demand for them. This is largely attributable to the fact that the methodology for determining the value of housing units used as a basis for calculating nonprofit rent does not account for the impact of energy-efficient refurbishment and consequently blocks investors' motivation because they are unable to recoup their investment by increasing the rent.

As a result, the operating costs of housing for tenants in nonprofit housing are high, especially in the colder part of the year. The Housing Survey conducted in 2005 revealed that operating costs in the nonprofit rental sector were higher than the operating costs in all the other housing sectors. Some of these high costs can be attributed to the poor energy performance of housing in this nonprofit housing sector owing to its age, the lack of interest in and conditions for energy-efficient refurbishment of nonprofit housing, and the lack of financial resources. Despite the strong need for investment, the shortage of funding and institutional barriers is effectively blocking the renovation and especially the energy-efficient upgrading of the nonprofit housing sector.

Yet another problem is the quality of service in nonprofit housing. Issues relating to the availability and financial sustainability and the quality of dwellings and of housing services are much less debated. Moreover, the quality of service in nonprofit housing has not yet been systematically monitored or evaluated. No official data are available for such an assessment, so we can use data from the Housing Survey 2005 (Mandić and Cirman 2006) based on a representative sample of four thousand households. To observe and identify the quality features that are specific to nonprofit housing, it was compared to three other tenures: owner-occupied housing, private for-profit rental housing, and the use of housing without paying rent (e.g., mostly people residing in a dwelling owned by a relative other than a household member) (Mandić and Cirman 2006, 29–37).[2] The results indicate that nonprofit tenants gave the same negative assessment of their situation as private tenants and reported a much worse situation than owner-occupiers. Moreover, 66.5 percent of nonprofit tenants complained of excessively high rents and 74.4 percent of too high operating costs; these figures are even higher than the number of private tenants who made similar complaints—64.7 percent and 71.9 percent, respectively.

CONCLUSION

In Slovenia, social housing experienced a tremendous shock during the transition, a shock from which it is still gradually recovering. In a certain sense it seems to have served as 'a wealth reservoir' from which the 'social costs' of the transition were paid. Although the housing reform aimed to enhance market and economic rationality, it was taken for granted that the social protection of tenants would remain more or less the same, as though such protection was guaranteed by the general level of social democratic achievements in Europe. It was also taken for granted that the housing reform was based on the rational decision making model (aims, instruments, implementation, monitoring, evaluating, fine-tuning). From today's perspective, both of these assumptions are quite questionable.

The pursuit of market and economic rationality interrupted the development of social rental housing. The case of Slovenian housing reforms reveals a tremendous discrepancy between what was planned and what was realized in the area of social housing. More than expected, social housing has proven to be an extremely vulnerable and unstable institution. Although it was easy to retrench, its recovery has turned out to be very difficult and demanding. Although acknowledged as one of the top priorities of the National Housing Program, the program's application to social housing has revealed a clear lack of commitment and an operational inconsistency between words and actions. The program's results in terms of the size and quality of the social sector suggest that social housing will soon be a marginalized safety net available to only the neediest part of society.

The new, post-transition social environment seems to lack a number of elements that are essential to the social function of housing. The institutional framework of operations in the nonprofit housing sector is negatively affecting the financial stability of existing providers of nonprofit housing. It exposes tenants to potential energy poverty and effectively blocks new investment into the stock, especially from the private sector. What is also still missing is a well-developed and responsive legal environment, which would define and defend the boundary between housing and property rights in order to address conflicting interests between tenants and landlords. It also seems that normative or ideological arguments that would support redistributive justice in housing (defining what is decent, affordable housing) and defend collective provision in times of individualization and privatization are too weak or remain unarticulated. As the social democratic discourse fades into the background, these issues remain difficult to articulate, and even more so because, given that vulnerable groups are numerous, fragmented, and in competition with each other, the power of interest organizations and coalitions, which could make relevant policy demands, is weak and dispersed.

NOTES

1. Rent without the cost of heating (cold rent).
2. A shortage of space was reported by 47.5 percent of tenants in nonprofit housing and 52 percent of profit-housing tenants, whereas owner-occupiers suffered from a shortage of space to a much smaller extent, only 23 percent. The average floor space per person was estimated at 24 square meters for nonprofit tenants, 25 square meters for private tenants, and 34 square meters for owner-occupiers. The lack of an indoor flushing toilet and/or bath or shower was reported by 30.5 percent of nonprofit tenants, 35.3 percent of private tenants, and 22.9 percent of owner-occupiers. Similar results were found with regard to rot in windows and floors, damp or leaks in walls or roof, and a lack of daylight.

REFERENCES

Cirman, A. 2004. *Modeli finančne spodbude za delovanje neprofitnih stanovanjskih organizacij v bodoče (Financial Stimulation Models for the Future Operation of Nonprofit Housing Organizations).* Ljubljana: Faculty of Economics.

———. 2005. "Uspešnost stanovanjske politike v luči rezultatov Stanovanjske ankete (Effectiveness of Housing Policy in Slovenia in Light of the Housing Survey Results)." *Proceedings from the Conference: Država, državjani, stanovanja.* Portoroz: Slovenian Chamber of Commerce and Industry.

———. 2006. "Housing Tenure Preferences in the Post-Privatization Period: The Case of Slovenia." *Housing Studies* 21:113–34.

Hegedüs, J., Mayo, E., and Tosics, I. 1996. *Transition of the Housing Sector in the East-Central European Countries.* Budapest: USAID, Metropolitan Research Institute.

Mandic, S. 1992. "Stanovanjska preskrba: trend 1984–1991 (Housing Supply: Trend 1984–1991)." *IB revija za planiranje,* 25:3–9.

———. 1994. "Housing Tenures in Times of Change: Conversion Debates in Slovenia." *Housing Studies* 9:27–38.

———. 2000. "Trends in Central Eastern European Rented Sectors." *Journal of Housing and the Built Environment* 15:217–31.

———. 2001. "Residential Mobility versus 'In-Place' Adjustments in Slovenia: Viewpoint from a Society 'in Transition'." *Housing Studies* 16:53–73.

Mandic, S. and Cirman, A., eds. 2006. *Stanovanje v Sloveniji 2005 (Housing in Slovenia 2005).* Ljubljana: Faculty of Social Sciences.

Ministry for Environment Protection and Physical Planning. 1991. *Izhodišča za Nacionalni stanovanjski program (Starting Points for Preparation of the National Housing Program).* Ljubljana: Ministry for Environment Protection and Physical Planning.

Sendi, R. 1995. "Housing Reform and Housing Conflict: The Privatization and Denationalization of Public Housing in the Republic of Slovenia in Practice." *International Journal for Urban and Regional Research* 19:435–46.

Stanovnik, T. 1994. "The Sale of the Social Housing Stock in Slovenia: What Happened and Why." *Urban Studies* 31:1559–70.

Stanovnik, T., Zupancic, D., Blaganje, D., Cirman, A., Nagode, P., Srdic, A., and Cebul, S. 2003. *Elementi neprofitne najemnine in njihovi deleži glede na vrednost stanovanja (Elements of Nonprofit Rent and Their Relationship to the Value of Housing Units).* Ljubljana: Faculty of Economics.

Yugoslav Institute for Urbanism and Housing. 1987. *Finansiranje stambene izgradnje (Financing of Housing Construction).* Belgrade: Yugoslav Institute for Urbanism and Housing.

18 The Ukraine

Waiting Lists without Housing

Irina Zapatrina

INTRODUCTION

This chapter briefly describes how approaches to social housing in Ukraine emerged, and it analyzes several challenges that have accompanied the introduction of the concept of 'social housing' and that have influenced the direction of development of social housing policy. The Soviet legacy has an important role in this. For several reasons that will be discussed in the following, the 'new system' of public housing has essentially involved the creation of several new waiting lists, but as there is no housing to be allocated, this remains more of an idealized than a practical strategy.

The term *social housing* is used in the chapter in its traditional sense. It is rental housing at below-market rent allocated to those in need. Given that Ukraine makes almost no use of interest rate subsidy schemes, capital grants, tax exemptions, and similar measures aimed at helping households to afford a socially acceptable level of housing consumption, we will necessarily focus on rental solutions.

THE HISTORICAL CONTEXT OF UKRAINE'S SOCIAL HOUSING STRATEGY

In Ukraine, the provision of housing, in particular social housing, reflects influences from the Soviet era, when public policies were based on the theory of social homogeneity and it was the state's obligation to ensure that everyone, regardless of income, had housing, and to maintain the housing stock with minimal financial participation from the population. Until 1992, when the privatization of housing began, only detached housing units were privately owned. Apartments in multifamily buildings were rented through local authorities. Members of the public could register on a waiting list to obtain housing free of charge. To qualify to register a person's living conditions had to be poor (they were residing in a living space smaller than the minimum standard). At the same time, the rights attached to the allocated rental housing were pretty much the same as in private housing: tenants enjoyed indefinite occupancy rights and the right to bequeath, sublet, or exchange their housing unit for another one. Clearly, at that time the term *social housing* meant something very different than what it does today, or what it did even then in Western Europe (Marcuse 1994).

The situation changed when housing privatization began and market conditions were created. More than 92 percent of apartments are now privately owned, and housing privatization is still an ongoing process.

In past decades, approximately 2 percent of the state budget was spent on public housing construction. This has changed in recent years; financial constraints have brought the construction of state and municipal housing to a halt. As a result, the waiting list for housing never gets any shorter and it now contains 1.3 million families. Social housing is still awaiting conceptual reforms that would respond to the need to operate in conditions of a shrinking social housing sector and growing demand (Tsenkova and Turner 2004). Under such circumstances, the continued (giveaway) sale of housing (in privatization) constitutes a loss of resources.

There is a great demand for housing, especially among the poorer strata. In 2007, almost one-quarter of all households were unsatisfied with their living conditions and another one-third (34.1 percent) were not very satisfied (Zapatrina 2010). A survey carried out by the Institute of Sociology of the National Academy of Sciences of Ukraine (2008) found that 51.2 percent of the Ukrainian population were living in conditions that require improvement, and 3.1 percent were living in conditions considered unsuitable.

Housing affordability is a critical issue for large numbers of families in Ukraine. For 80 percent of the population, the possibility of refurbishing their homes or improving their living conditions remains remote. The remaining 20 percent could change or improve their housing either on their own or with the help of credit.

Still, over the years the number of families and singles on the waiting list for housing has barely declined, primarily because it can in theory take as long as sixty-five to sixty-seven years to obtain a flat through the 'regular' housing allocation system, that is, from the waiting list. Many households have now been on the waiting list for more than ten years, and their numbers are growing (see Table 18.1).

Table 18.1 Structure of Housing Waiting List (%)

	1990	2006	2007
Percentage of people on the housing waiting list for less than ten years	89.0	32.4	31.4
Percentage of people on the housing waiting list for more than ten years	11	67.6	68.6

Source: Institute of Sociology of the National Academy of Sciences of Ukraine (2008).

There are a few structural reasons for this attitude of relying on the state for the allocation of housing rather than on the market for a solution to one's housing needs. Estimates indicate that no more than 15 percent of the population is in a position where they might be able to purchase a dwelling, and only 3 percent of the population (1.4 million people) might be able to do so within the next five years. In response to this, certain policy steps have been taken to develop the 'social housing' sector, targeting those most vulnerable.

As noted earlier, the term *social housing* did not exist in the former Soviet Union and it is still incomprehensible for the majority of the Ukrainian population. Nevertheless, Articles 47 and 48 of the Constitution acknowledge the principle of inviolability of housing and guarantee the citizens of Ukraine the right to housing. This is to be done by ensuring the creation of conditions in which every citizen is able to build a dwelling or to purchase or rent one in order to maintain a decent standard of living. By law, citizens who need social housing are entitled to receive housing from the state or municipal government free of charge or at an affordable price.

The legacy of the Soviet era influences not just how the term *social housing* is understood, but also the public's expectations as to what it means in everyday life. We could argue that there is a historically shaped public attitude towards housing that it is something that the (paternalistic) state is obliged to support. For this reason most of the population still believes that the state should provide free housing that, in conformity with the post-Soviet context, could eventually be privatized. Further evidence of this is that even though the current housing waiting list in Ukraine barely budges, citizens keep registering on it in the hope of obtaining housing.

Because waiting list eligibility is based exclusively on 'housing norms' for a family (i.e., the floor space and number of rooms the applicant currently lives in), whereas financial status and income levels are not considered, the information on the public need for state assistance to obtain housing is biased and insufficient. Thus, the waiting list system in its current setup in Ukraine is just an administrative tool that has been of little practical use to families waiting for housing and to policymakers.

In sum, the model of social housing that exists in Ukraine evolved out of the Soviet approach of providing housing for broad groups of the population, but refined with the following qualifications:

- Housing is provided free of charge, but tenants must pay for maintenance costs.
- Disposal rights on the housing are limited: the housing cannot be privatized, given away, or inherited.
- Allocation of housing is based on a waiting list made up of eligible candidates and containing privileged categories (people given special priority in allocation).[1]

The only changes since the Soviet past are that social housing now quasi targets the poor and is provided for a defined period and that there is a limited number of dwellings. Social housing is only to be provided to the population with low income (those who need social protection), on a temporary basis (for a certain period of time), by granting access to rental housing that conforms to certain physical parameters (normative requirements of floor space, planning and quality). But given the very limited number of dwellings available for allocation—for example, in the case of families and singles no more than fifty dwellings have been allocated each year in the last decade—the system has more of a shop-window function than a practical impact on improving the situation (Institute of Sociology of the National Academy of Sciences of Ukraine 2008).

THE REGULATION OF SOCIAL HOUSING IN UKRAINE

The current Housing Act dates back to 1983 and to the times of the Ukrainian Soviet Socialist Republic. It defines social housing as that part of the housing stock, in particular, apartments in multifamily buildings, detached houses, and other forms of housing tenure that is to be provided to citizens who need social protection in accordance with the law.

It was not until 2005 that a model of public housing support for socially vulnerable citizens was formulated in the form of the concept of the State Program for Social Housing(i.e., in the fourteenth year of Ukrainian independence).[2] In just ten years it was supposed to ensure social housing for all persons who were registered on the waiting list as of January 1, 2005 (the costs were to be covered by the state and local budgets or other sources). This can be seen as an attempt to reform the housing waiting list system and replace it with a waiting list for 'social housing', which would not be privatized and would be provided for a certain period of time.

A year later, however, development took a different turn: the Act on Housing Stock for Social Purposes, adopted on January 12, 2006, defined 'housing for social purposes' as all social housing provided to the citizens of Ukraine who need social protection. Based on this legislation, social housing is housing, of various ownership forms, provided free of charge on the basis of a rental agreement for a certain period to the citizens of Ukraine who need social protection. Shelters, halfway houses, temporary housing for the homeless, special housing for veterans, the disabled, the elderly, the poor, and so on, are all forms of social housing.

The legal framework, however, does not clearly and coherently define all the conditions attached to social housing, which hinders the sector's further development. This problem is caused by the contradictory framework that exists for rent setting, which states, on the one hand, that social housing should be provided free of charge and, on the other, that the management of the housing stock should be covered by a user fee, composed of a fee paid directly by the tenant and a state assistance contribution provided for the household in need. Another example is that, despite the fact that all kinds of tenure forms can serve as social housing, the housing has to be provided by the local authorities, which necessarily limits the source of social housing provision to public housing.

Besides local authorities, there are other players in the social housing policy arena: the Cabinet of Ministers of Ukraine is in charge of policy development and control, and local offices of public administration implement state policies and manage the housing stock (Zaslavets 2003). Nevertheless, the most important role is played by the local authorities, who have the greatest powers over social housing, including the power to create new social housing, covered by the local budget and other financing sources; they are also responsible for the management, maintenance, repair, and control of social housing and for defining and collecting the housing fee. Waiting list registration and the allocation of housing are other key competences of local authorities. Moreover, local governments must annually monitor the eligibility of households registered on the waiting list for social housing and monitor existing social tenants and, in cases where eligibility can no longer be demonstrated, delete people from the waiting list or terminate the relevant individuals' social housing contracts.

However, the devolution of so many of the responsibilities connected with social housing provision to the local level is unrealistic, because new construction, reconstruction, the refurbishing of run-down buildings, and restitution in kind cannot be performed without financial resources. In order to implement these tasks, local governments need funds that they do not have.

Despite all these challenges, the new law has one important merit: for the first time since the transition it introduced the term *social housing register*, which is the waiting list of people entitled to social housing. This register is a list of people in very poor living conditions, with low income, who are unable to cover housing expenses and have few assets. People living in shelters or halfway houses, the disabled, the unemployed, and the elderly can also be included in the register. Allocation is carried out by the local government. Rental agreements for allocated social housing are effective until the social tenant's situation improves considerably and the tenant loses eligibility to such housing. After a period of three years, however, people can be reentered on the list.

The 'regular' waiting list for housing also still exists, despite the introduction of the aforementioned more targeted social housing register, which means that citizens may simultaneously be on both waiting lists. There are also twelve household categories that take priority and are entitled to receive housing first on the regular waiting list or to come first in line on the waiting list. They include, for instance, war veterans with disability, victims of the Chernobyl nuclear disaster, orphans and children leaving foster care, disabled children without parents and in specialized foster care arrangements, and families with five or more children. Various circumstances can allow a person to jump to the top of the waiting list, such as having been involved in a military operation or a war resulting in disability or having received an award (Heroes of Ukraine, Heroes of the Soviet Union, Heroes of Socialist Labor). Young families and single parents with three or four children are also given priority. This results in a lack of transparency to the allocation of social housing.

In principle, civil society can play an important role in social housing provision, as in conformity with their charters civil (both for profit, and nonprofit) organizations may take part in providing housing for specific target groups under the supervision of local governments.

Social housing is not provided free of charge (in contravention of one of the regulations set out in the Housing Act), but it is provided at low rent. Rent levels are set based on the tenants' income and assets, household composition, and the physical characteristics of the dwelling. In theory, the sum paid should cover the rent and fees for building maintenance and communal services. Because the amount the tenant should be required to pay is capped (at 20 percent of the monthly household income),[3] the state supplements the remaining amount in the form of a benefit. The local authorities transfer the funds to pay for the capital repair of social housing to the entity/person who manages the building the housing is in, because social housing units are normally located in buildings with mixed ownership and the management of these buildings is not run by public authorities. In the case where social housing is run by a private landlord, the private owner and local authorities make an agreement on the amount of this payment.

The financial burden put on local governments (and potentially on any other types of organizations that would engage in social housing development) for both the development and management of the social housing makes running this service for the poor very unappealing, which is reflected in the small size of the sector. Despite efforts to increase state funding and introduce incentives, for instance, through the National Program for Social Housing Development drafted in 2008, no concrete steps towards improvement have been taken and no funds have been allocated for implementation of the program.

THE CHALLENGES OF SOCIAL HOUSING REFORM

To date the social housing program has not started working in Ukraine. This is caused, on the one hand, by the choice of an inadequate social-economic model for the sector's operation and, on the other hand, by the timing of its planned implementation in 2008.

Firstly, even pessimistic calculations of the state funds necessary to starting the program proved that there was no chance of these funds becoming available in a medium-term perspective. According to the forecasting calculations of the Institute of Economy and Forecasting of the National Academy of Sciences of Ukraine (2008), a minimum of approximately 6 percent of the existing housing stock as of 2006 would be required to meet the demand for social housing until 2025. This means that even if calculated at a price of 1,000 U.S. dollars per square meter, the total cost of the program would be 30 billion U.S. dollars (assuming housing would be provided free of charge and utilities would be paid for out of the local budgets and not taking into account inflation forecasts), which amounts to almost 50 percent of nominal GDP of Ukraine and is 1.55 times higher than the expenditures of the consolidated budget in 2007. Moreover, if we take into account costs related to infrastructure, the total costs of the program increase considerably.

Secondly, the time when the National Program for Social Housing Development was to be prepared by the Cabinet of Ministers of the Ukraine and submitted for review to the Ukrainian Parliament (January 1, 2008) coincided with the beginning of the financial-economic crisis in the Ukraine. As a result not only this document, but also the Concept of the National Program of Social Housing Development have not yet been approved.

Luckily, however, social housing was able to reenter the general housing policy agenda a year later. Social housing options were addressed in the "National Program of Reform and Development of Housing and the Local Economy for the years 2010–2014," adopted in July 2009, and in a draft law 'on the main principles of the state housing policy', which envisaged a comprehensive and systematic approach to solving the housing problem. These documents were intended to develop a unified, nationwide housing program for Ukraine, and one of the components of this program would be a mechanism for 'ensuring social housing for citizens'.

Unfortunately, the draft law 'on the main principles of state housing policy' has not yet been adopted as legislation by the Parliament of Ukraine—for political reasons. Consequently, social housing issues have been left to be dealt with in the National Program of Reform and Development of Housing and the Local Economy.

The program articulated several goals:

- organizing registration on the waiting list for those Ukrainian citizens entitled to social housing, and the provision of state support for the purchase of housing—2009–2010
- monitoring housing needs in relation to supply in a medium- and long-term perspective—2010–2012

Independently of developments surrounding the National Program for Social Housing' that ultimately led to its rejection by Parliament and the incorporation of some of its goals in the National "Program of Reform and Development of Housing and the Local Economy", some regions have adopted programs for social housing development. However, these programs have not yet begun to operate owing to a lack of financial recourses. For example, a social housing program was approved in Kiev for the years 2010–2015. It planned to provide housing for 1,450 families (the 'average' dwelling size would have been 51 square meters). But as of January 2011, the program has still not been launched.

There is another challenge to the creation of social housing policy in Ukraine and it has to do with competing institutions in the field. In 2009, the term *affordable housing* appeared in Ukraine, and it basically knocked the concept of social (rental) housing off the agenda and drew attention away from the urgent need to develop social housing stock. According to the law of Ukraine 'on ensuring affordable housing for citizens' adopted by Parliament in 2009, thus, around the same time as the National Program of Reform and Development of Housing and the Local Economy, *affordable housing* means residential buildings (complexes) and apartments already built or in the process of construction with the assistance of the state. Unlike social housing, affordable housing could be built or purchased by citizens who are eligible (their living conditions need improvement) and have the financial resources for this (supplemented by state funding).

With the adoption of this law, a third 'state register of citizens eligible for affordable housing' was established. This register was constructed the same way as the regular waiting list and the social housing register, so it consists of three categories: a general waiting list for affordable housing, supplementary allocation procedures for people who can be given priority on the list, and those who belong to groups who automatically come first on the list.

According to the regulations, any citizens living in bad conditions whose income exceeds the eligibility threshold for social housing, but at the same time is no more than four times the average monthly wage in their region, are eligible to register on this list. Thus, in theory, this register may contain better-off households than the social housing waiting list. Households on this list can receive state support for the construction or purchase of affordable housing, but only once. Households that receive such support are then the full owners of the dwelling they built or buy. State support can be provided in the form of:

- payment to cover a portion of the construction (purchase) costs of affordable housing, and/or the receipt of a subsidized mortgage loan from an authorized bank
- payment of premiums to citizens who have a contract savings scheme and to members of housing-construction cooperatives who have accumulated enough housing savings to partially pay for the construction of affordable housing

Housing support works with a concept of housing size equal to 21 square meters per person and for every additional family member 10.5 square meters. For dwellings beyond these parameters the additional costs are paid for by the eligible household.

Since the adoption of the law 'on ensuring affordable housing for Ukrainian citizens', the social housing program had lost the attention of the state, and public money has been steered towards running the program for affordable housing construction or purchase.

We could argue that this development can largely be ascribed to the housing construction lobby's successful representation of its interests. Even more so when we observe that when housing construction halted as a result of the financial crisis and a number of buildings were left unfinished in many Ukrainian cities, construction companies began looking for opportunities to attract funds from the state and local budgets in order to complete their construction projects, so they suggested to the state that it stimulate housing demand by providing the public with a financial contribution to the cost of purchasing housing. The state, in fact, did this and helped the construction sector overcome the crisis.

Nevertheless, the introduction of the category 'affordable housing' caused a crack in the reform process, halted the preparation and implementation of the National Program for Social Housing Development, and resulted in the definitive loss of the population's trust in the ability of the state to solve the current housing problems.

THE SOCIAL HOUSING MODEL IN UKRAINE: EFFECTIVENESS AND EFFICIENCY

In Ukraine, the right to housing is guaranteed in the Constitution, so the state must assist those citizens who are unable to solve their housing problems themselves. The most effective way for the state to do so is by designing a comprehensive social housing model based on the realistic financial involvement of the state and good targeting of state assistance.

However, the model set up by the Act on Housing Stock for Social Purposes does not satisfy either of these criteria. Moreover, since its adoption in 2006, no steps have been undertaken to create a housing sector for citizens at risk of poverty. The reasons are manifold: a lack of mid- and long-term funding, exacerbated by the fact that the state lacks resources to cover all the obligations laid out in the current legislation. Without additional resources, the social housing program will remain just a piece of paper. Recent discussions about introducing a real estate tax (starting from 2011) raise some hope that this new source of state revenue form could be used to help cover the costs of taking measures to increase the supply of social housing.

Moreover, currently the housing registers and waiting lists are not fulfilling their function, which is not surprising considering that without the development of new social or affordable housing the composition of the waiting lists will remain unchanged for years. Also, the introduction of an additional two separate registers contradicts the logic of targeting: one list exists for ordinary 'affordable housing' that may be privatized later, and the other exists for social housing. In recent years only approximately 1–1.5 percent of the people registered on the waiting list for 'ordinary affordable housing' have been allocated a dwelling, and no new social housing was even built. If eligibility for these lists were narrowed—which was intended by the draft aforementioned law in the case of the targeting of social housing—the waiting lists would become more functional. The system of prioritizing certain categories also needs to be revised.

As of 2007 there were 1.4 million families and singles on the waiting list for ordinary affordable housing, 21 percent of them entitled to be "first on the waiting list"; 7.5 percent were people from priority categories that automatically puts one on the top of the list, even if the person did not register yet. At the same time, annually only 1–1.5 percent of people on the waiting list receive a dwelling (Institute for Sociology of the National Academy of Sciences of Ukraine 2008). This example proves the inexpediency of maintaining such a waiting list for housing, or even a register for social housing with three categories of regular applicants, priority groups, and those who without having registered are automatically eligible for social housing.

The current model of social housing grants local authorities wide powers for dealing with housing issues. But these powers are not backed with financial support. It is the local governments that are obliged to develop and manage the (social) housing stock, but they lack financial resources for the construction or reconstruction of housing or the conversion of nonresidential dwellings into residential ones. Since the adoption of the 'Law on ensuring affordable housing for Ukrainian citizens' several years ago, no state budget funding or local resources have been earmarked for these purposes. Moreover, local governments have to bear the administrative burden of the nonfunctioning register system, maintaining the housing registers and monitoring the income of applicants on the waiting list for social housing, even though there is almost no turnover in the social housing stock, so there are rarely any new allocations.

In sum, the Ukrainian social housing model is exceptionally declarative, ineffective, and inefficient. It needs to be reformed as part of the development of an entirely new housing policy in Ukraine.

CONCLUSION

Creating and implementing comprehensive social housing reforms and meeting the demand for social housing remain challenging issues in Ukraine. Constraints on access to affordable and secure housing in general impact the public's work productivity, health, quality of life, and sense of security about the future. According to research conducted by the Ukrainian Centre for Social Reforms and Social Monitoring in 2008 (Libanova et al.

2009), the unresolved housing problem ranks second after financial problems as the reasons people cite for postponing the birth of their first or next child. In order to solve the housing problem for socially vulnerable citizens the state developed and approved a social housing concept. Attempts at its implementation failed, and it is only a new and nonfunctional waiting list that has been put in operation.

In order to formulate a housing policy based on new principles, in particular, that of ensuring social housing for citizens in need, in 2009 the state launched a program of housing and communal sector reform.[5] The draft law on this program was very ambitious: it outlined a new state housing program, including new models of housing development that would meet the demand for housing of various standards and would offer a number of loan guarantee schemes. The draft law proposed created a single state housing program that would ensure everyone's constitutional right to housing and the provision of social housing to certain categories of the population.

Unlike the current social housing model, the draft law stipulated that the social housing stock would comprise various tenures, for example, halfway or supported housing, but also, more generally, housing in public ownership, allocation of which would be based on a waiting list established by law or by a decision of the local government. All long-term social housing would be owned by the local governments.

The new housing policy strategy was to have been backed with financial support from the state via the introduction of a real estate tax to cover social housing construction and the development of housing-communal infrastructure, but was to have been accompanied by demand-side programs promoting homeownership with grants for the purchase of building plots, dwellings, or for capital repair and improving housing affordability (allowance schemes for communal services fees).

Unfortunately, the draft law was not adopted in 2009. Its main provisions were, however, included in the draft of the new Housing Code of Ukraine, which is under consideration in the Ukrainian Parliament and is being prepared for a second reading in early 2011.

To conclude, there are several obstacles to the creation of an efficient and effective model of social housing in Ukraine. The biggest challenges are the shortage of necessary funds in the state and local budgets and the absence of instruments other than social housing to ensure the right of socially vulnerable citizens to housing. Reforms should include the creation of criterion for targeting social housing and a basis for effective social housing management.

Other challenges are the general lack of political support to revise the housing waiting lists and to focus on more vulnerable households instead of the production of owner-occupied housing, which is at odds with objectives of the construction lobby, and the need to change the general public's understanding of what social housing is. The public still expects the state to privatize dwellings and provide housing for free to 'eligible' households 'in need'. Under the current financial constraints, the state is only able to and should only support vulnerable citizens by ensuring decent living conditions so that scarce public funds are not wasted.

NOTES

1. Ukraine has retained since Soviet times a general housing waiting list on which households can register based on their housing needs. However, there are two prioritized categories of 'eligible households': households that automatically get on the top of the list (due to some special merits, for example) and families who do not even have to register on any waiting list and still have the highest priority for obtaining housing. Such an approach was useful when these two categories represented a very small share of families registered on the general waiting list. At the moment such differentiation seems to be irrelevant.
2. On September 3, 2005, the concept of the State Program for 'Social Housing' was approved by the Order of the Cabinet of Ministers of Ukraine (No.384–p).
3. Since 2010—15 percent.
4. The Ministry of Housing and Communal Services (2008) of Ukraine has developed the draft law of Ukraine, "On Main Principles of State Housing Policy", and registered it in the Ukrainian Parliament on 18.06.2009 N4676.

REFERENCES

Institute of Sociology of the National Academy of Sciences of Ukraine. 2008. *Report on the Performance of the Social Research of Population's Vision Regarding how to Solve Housing Problems.* Kiev: The Ministry of Housing and Communal Services of Ukraine.

Libanova, E., Makarova, O., Cherenko, L., Tkachenko, L., and Palii, O. 2009. *Social Protection and Social Inclusion in Ukraine.* http://ec.europa.eu/social/BlobServlet?docId=5757&langId=en accessed May 10, 2012.

Marcuse, P. 1994. "Privatization, Tenure, and Property Rights: Towards Clarity in Concepts." *Social Rented Housing in Europe: Policy, Tenure and Design.* Amsterdam: Delft University Press.

Ministry of Housing and Communal Services of Ukraine. 2008. *Strategic Plan of Work of the Ministry of Housing and Communal Services of Ukraine.* Kiev. The Ministry of Housing and Communal Services of Ukraine.

Tsenkova, Sasha and Turner, Bengt. 2004. "The Future of Social Housing in Eastern Europe: Reforms in Latvia and the Ukraine." *International Journal of Housing Policy* 4 (2): 133–49.

Zapatrina, I. 2010. *Living Conditions and Communal Infrastructure: Reforms and Their Financial Conditions (Жилищно-коммунальная инфраструктура: реформы и система их финансового обеспечения).* Kiev. Institute of economics and forecasting of the National Academy of Science.

Zaslavets, T. 2003. "Prerequisites for the Formation of the Concept for the Construction of Social Housing in Ukraine—Architectural and Typological Aspect." Presented at Proceedings of the UNECE Workshop on Social Housing, Environment and Quality, Prague, May 19–20.

Part IV

19 New Social Housing Strategies in Post-Socialist States

Effectiveness, Efficiency, and Sustainability

Martin Lux and Petr Sunega

INTRODUCTION: THE CHANGING ROLE OF PUBLIC HOUSING

From a Society of Official Tenants and de facto Quasi Homeowners . . .

As mentioned in Part I of this book, before 1990, most of the economy in socialist states was in state ownership and was subject to central planning. Despite some differences (especially the reemergence of market logic in some parts of the economy in the former Yugoslavia and in Hungary), in the field of housing, this meant extensive public (state) interventions directed at decommodifying housing, such as housing subsidies, property expropriations, and rent/price regulations. These interventions created a segment of mass public (semipublic) rental housing, where rent-setting systems ensured that rents were kept at extremely low levels.

No definition of *social housing* existed under socialism (with some exceptions such as the former Yugoslavia). Nor can this term simply be applied to the mass public housing stock created during socialism. The key principle of socialist housing policy was to allot flats for free 'according to people's needs': *need* was defined technically as the right to occupy a specified amount of housing space (housing need). Defining needs and standards was basically the task of social engineers, planners, and architects.

In income leveled societies the allocation of public housing on the basis of income was officially unnecessary. Similarly, in reality there was no income-targeted social policy whatsoever: the term *social policy* disappeared from official vocabulary for some time (1950s), as it implied the existence of social problems that had officially been taken care of. The role of nonstate actors (church, charity, nongovernment organizations) in the social field was suspended, and the whole system of 'social policy' was centralized under the umbrella of the omnipotent state (Krebs et al. 2005).

As labor income varied only marginally (Hamilton and Hirszowicz 1993; Breen and Rottman 1995; Crompton 1998), the main source of stratification in socialist society centered on access to social security and 'privileges'. Social paternalism was an instrument of both social security and political control (Večerník and Matějů 1999, 198). Those who were not loyal to the prevailing political ideology had difficulty finding work corresponding to their education and skills.

The same applied for housing (Kornai 1992; Lux 2003). As in the case of access to a decent job, public housing became a tool of the regime to distribute socialist 'privileges': as the country chapters in this book show, the people who obtained public housing the fastest and/or with the highest implicit value tended to be members of the Communist Party, people loyal to the socialist regime (*nomenklatura*), or people who effectively used their clientele networks or employed corrupt means to acquire public housing.

In Hungary, Szelényi (1983) and Dániel (1985, 408) demonstrated that despite the declared intentions of communists, the allocation of public dwellings "didn't reduce but, on the contrary, increased inequality within the Hungarian society". The official egalitarianism (incorporating ideology of 'housing for all') led to artificial housing scarcity and ineffective consumption, and this in turn led to the politically based distribution of housing 'privileges'.

Tenants who were allotted dwellings by the state/municipality/public enterprise obtained unlimited occupancy rights in the form of a so-called 'deed' to the flat. In many countries the officials do not speak about 'renting', but about the 'personal use' of a flat. 'Personal use' became an institution separate from that of rental tenure—it could be inherited or transferred to relatives, or exchanged with some other holders of user rights—all this was later called quasi-homeownership (Lux 2009; Hegedüs and Tosics 1996). Consequently, socialist state rental housing more resembled homeownership than a typical tenancy (Marcuse 1996).

. . . To a Society of Official Homeowners and de facto Quasi Tenants . . .

After 1990, the new democratic governments wanted to reintroduce private property and establish a market economy. Governments in most post-socialist countries shared the view that part of public rental housing should be transferred to private hands. However, the transfer of public housing into private hands ultimately took the form of a mass giveaway sale to sitting tenants, who obtained housing wealth almost or wholly free of charge (see more details in Chapter 2, this volume). Other forms of privatization (such as the sale of public flats to professional private investors or to not-for-profit private housing associations or cooperatives, or the selective privatization of public flats for market prices to sitting tenants) were barely discussed. Public housing, as well as rental housing generally, in most post-socialist states almost disappeared—within a few years it diminished to a residual share of just marginal significance.

There were a few exceptions, and this policy differentiation led several scholars to speculate about a possible divergence of social housing models in the future (Tsenkova and Turner 2004; Lux 2003). For example, in Poland and the Czech Republic right-to-buy legislation was not passed and public housing privatization was left to the municipalities as an open option. The decision of these governments not to apply right to buy policy preserved public rental housing for some time. However, were the policies in these two countries really different? From the perspective of their ultimate effect on recent housing tenure structure (2011) it seems that they were not.

Municipalities in these two countries, although not obliged to sell their newly acquired housing, were unable to introduce any effective way of managing public housing stock that could save them from subsidizing it. With their hands tied by rent control and the quasi-homeownership entitlements of public tenants, municipalities often saw the sale of public housing as a good way of getting rid of this unwanted gift from the state. The giveaway privatization of public housing to sitting tenants was delayed but ultimately did happen. For example, in the Czech Republic 70–75 percent of originally public housing had been sold to sitting tenants under advantageous price terms by 2009 and the share of public housing had decreased from 35 percent in 1990 to an estimated 10 percent in 2009.

. . . Where the Equity Consequences of 'Reform' Were Simply Ignored . . .

As mentioned in Chapter 2 of this volume, there are several papers in which the giveaway privatization of public housing to sitting tenants is justified. Some arguments in support have been very strong: "The surest and most efficient way to restore housing market equilibrium without creating additional distortions during the transition is to unwind totally the socialist housing legacy by eliminating all housing subsidies and the taxes that finance them and giving away the existing stock . . . equity concerns are not a legitimate obstacle to rapid market reforms" (Buckley et al. 1995, 74–75). "Managing the transition toward markets requires the simultaneous pursuit of two very distinct sets of policies which should match the dualistic structure of the housing system. One set of policies is needed to privatize the large inefficient stock of public housing, and the other to encourage the rapid growth of the very small new private sector" (Renaud 1995, 39).

However, the discussion surrounding the equity consequences of the mass giveaway privatization of public housing was neglected or biased. The regressive character of wealth redistribution resulting from privatization has been shown only recently by Lux (2009) (for the Czech Republic), Pichler-Milanovich (2001), and in more detail by Yemtsov (2007) (for Russia, Serbia, Poland, and to some extent other post-socialist states). It is a fact that all former public tenants were made 'richer', thanks to housing transfers, but the former *nomenklatura* became even 'richer' due to the higher property values of their dwellings.

"It is obvious that housing privatization programs created winners and losers depending on where people happened to be living at the beginning of transition . . . privatization universally, in all three countries favored the rich . . . It therefore contributed to the increase of inequality" (Yemtsov 2007, 10, 23). In this respect it is surprising that advocates of public housing privatization often talk about 'reform'. Marcuse (1996, 143) writes that the recommendation favoring giveaway privatization, "whether appropriate or not, is a question not of property rights development, but of the reallocation of already existing rights that have been lodged elsewhere in the past . . . with substantial and differential impacts on different groups in society."

. . . And Where New Social Housing Programs Showed to Be Unsustainable in the Long Term

As will be shown in the following section, giveaway public housing privatization, originally intended as a temporary, *ad hoc* public intervention at the beginning of transition, proved to have strong staying power and had a long-term impact on post-socialist housing systems: it not only changed 'countries of tenants' into 'countries of homeowners', but because of its giveaway approach it also extended the socialist legacy in housing policies well beyond 1990 and, indirectly, became one of the barriers to the introduction of a new, sustainable social housing policy after 1990. We call this situation the 'privatization trap', which simply means:

1. Once politicians started to privatize public housing originally allocated with no real needs assessment (and, therefore, occupied by many affluent and politically influential people) for giveaway prices they would face serious political troubles if they wanted to limit it only to part of the total stock and/or stop at a particular time point.

↓

2. As public housing privatization is politically difficult to stop or limit in scope, an unintended consequence of the original action is the establishment of a social norm stipulating that all public tenants have the right to buy the public dwelling that they occupy for a giveaway price.

↓

3. As this norm reflecting the institutional arrangements inherited from the socialist period (quasi-homeownership) acquires legitimacy in the new democratic and market environment, any new social housing program will be challenged by it, and, consequently, even new social flats often become the subject of a giveaway sale to tenants.

↓

4. As the housing system remains predominantly based on homeownership tenure and state interventions are too weak to change it, the character of rental housing becomes more and more skewed, so that it serves as just a residual and temporary form of housing, and the

inequality between housing tenures deepens; this leads to the further, irreversible residualization of social/public housing.

↓

5. Divergence in early transformation policies concerning the application of right to buy and/or new forms of social/public housing support surprisingly ends in the convergence of all post-socialist housing systems due to the 'privatization trap': the residualization of social/public housing (as well as rental housing in general) and growing social/spatial segregation.

As discussed in Part I of this book, another important motto of the economic reforms, next to privatization, was the decentralization of power (dismantling central planning and the weakening of the state power in favor of more power to local governments). Therefore, the second aspect of general reform strategies that had an important effect on future social housing policy in this region was the decentralization of decision making because housing played a prominent role in this process.

Despite the many positive aspects of decentralization, such as bringing decision making closer to the local population, when it came to the introduction of a new social housing strategy the large-scale decentralization of power proved to be more of an obstacle than an impetus to the creation of sustainable policies. This could be called the 'paradox of decentralization' referred to in behavioral economics: decision making is decentralized to a large number of small entities that are financially and politically so weak that they refuse to make financially (costly) and politically (unpopular) risky decisions.

The social housing strategy is an example of such a risky decision: it is not politically popular to help the poor, it is a very expensive activity (as housing is an expensive good generally), and there is a danger that the actors involved will be punished for their efforts if other actors do not do the same. In other words, the creation of an effective social housing strategy in one small municipality can lead to immigration of poor people from neighboring municipalities and intensify the problem there instead of solving it.

The third important contextual aspect concerns the nature of the economic reforms themselves. If the legal system undergoes a radical change there is always a danger of legal gaps emerging, thus weakening the power of law—at least for a transitional period of time. This situation creates incentives for illegal economic activities (non-declared income, clientelism, corruption, and the growth of organized crime), and a substantial part of the economy starts to perform in a shadow zone. Under such circumstances it is hard to target social assistance to poor (needy) households on the basis of income. Official income and wealth declarations are not reliable and, consequently, any means-tested policy holds a risk of abuse.

Finally, the post-socialist economies, especially the small ones, entered what was already a global economy in the 1990s. In the global economy, the price of energy, raw materials, and consequently of many building materials were set globally, determined by supply from supranational (global) firms and the nature of global demand. This often led to a situation where new housing construction was extremely expensive because building costs did not reflect the purchasing power of the local population. The market segment of newly built housing could not effectively compete with the market segment of existing housing because the price gap for dwellings in similar locations and of a similar size was too deep.

Public investment in new social housing construction therefore faced a dilemma: whether to spend public money to build a small amount of social/public housing with low rent targeting those in real need, or whether to build more housing with less affordable rents (or prices) that could not be targeted to those most in need. When faced with such a dilemma, most governments opted for the second option. There are basically four explanations for this: (a) the first option held the political and financial risks mentioned in the preceding; (b) the first option would have led to a marginal number of newly built dwellings that would not meet the expectations of people accustomed to the kind of mass housing construction they saw in the past; (c) the second option would have benefited the middle classes, which were important for the sustainability of economic transformation; and (d) the second option was much closer to the socialist legacy surviving in the minds and behavioral patterns of the population, such as the practice of allocating housing to everyone.

The overall connotation of the term *social housing* was also not very positive during the early transition period given past experiences in western countries and especially given the spatial segregation of social housing estates. Social housing in western countries was undergoing a reform. It is logical that governments in post-socialist states did not want to follow policies that were being critically revised even in the West. The danger of the ghettoization of poor people has often been used as an effective argument by opponents to social housing.

The main contextual and ideological factors were therefore far from ideal for social housing growth in post-socialist states: the trap of privatization, the paradox of decentralization, the informal economy, the rules of the global economy affecting the costs of new housing, and a re-evaluation of the idea of social housing in the West.

CONTEXTUAL AND BASIC INDICATORS ON SOCIAL/PUBLIC RENTAL HOUSING

Table 19.1 shows further contextual information (economic and demographic data) for each country in our sample. GDP per capita in purchasing power parity (PPPs) indicates the relative strength of the countries' economies (average GDP per capita in PPP was set as 100 percent). The real GDP growth (decline) rate in 2009 should demonstrate how deeply the countries were hit by the recent global economic crisis. The real GDP growth rate in 2010 shows whether the countries reported an economic recovery or showed further economic decline in 2010. Ukraine and Estonia in particular were countries severely hit by the recession (the decline in real GDP in 2009 was by more than 14 percent). Some other countries (Slovenia, Russia) heavily impacted by the recession in 2009 showed positive real GDP growth in 2010. Poland was the only exception among the sample countries, as it saw real GDP growth both in 2009 and in 2010 and the impact of the crisis was thus relatively mild.

The Gini coefficient shows how equally incomes are distributed in each country. The more equal a country's income distribution, the lower the Gini coefficient and *vice versa*. Incomes are distributed less equally in Russia, Bosnia and Herzegovina, Romania, Estonia, Poland, and Ukraine than in the other countries. The at-risk-of-poverty rate around 2010 shows the share of population that after social transfers had an income below the poverty threshold.[1] The highest at-risk-of-poverty rate was recorded in Russia, Romania, Croatia, Bosnia and Herzegovina, and Poland. The lowest at-risk-of-poverty rate was found in the Czech Republic. The last columns in Table 19.1 show the population size in 2010 and the number of occupied dwellings per one thousand inhabitants around 2001. The highest number of occupied dwellings per one thousand inhabitants was found in Estonia, Ukraine, Croatia, and the Czech Republic; the lowest ratio was in Poland, Slovakia, and Romania.

Table 19.2 confirms that the decline in public housing, which started with the giveaway privatization in the early 1990s, has not yet been reversed even today, and new social housing strategies have proved to be weak, unstable, and unsustainable in the long term. Table 19.2 shows the basic characteristics of social/public housing for all the countries in our sample: the size of the sector, the existence of an official definition of social housing, central regulations on rents and central rules on the allocation of social/public housing, and the relative evaluation of new social/public housing output (between 1995 and 2010) and its trend. The evaluation of new output was based on the relative value of share of estimated number of new social/public dwellings built between 1995 and 2010 on the number of permanently occupied dwellings in each country.

The highest share of public/not-for-profit/social housing in total housing stock is recently (2011) observed in Russia (16 percent), Poland (12 percent), and the Czech Republic (10 percent); in Ukraine it makes up 5 percent of the total; in Estonia, Hungary, and Slovenia 4 percent; in Slovakia 3 percent; in Croatia, Bosnia and Herzegovina, and Romania 2 percent; and in Serbia 0.5 percent.

Although the municipalities emerged as the main social housing landlords, they did not receive enough public funds to allow them to seriously take up this new role. Moreover, in most countries old rental contracts are still bound by relatively strict rent regulation regimes (Czech Republic, Romania, Russia, Ukraine, Slovakia, Slovenia, Croatia, Bosnia and Herzegovina, Serbia), and this may prevent municipalities from preparing and realizing their own social housing policies. In sum, the municipalities

Table 19.1 Selected Economic and Demographic Information on Sample Post-Socialist States

Country	GDP in PPP in 2010[a]	Real GDP growth rate in 2009 (%)	Real GDP growth rate in 2010 (%)	Gini coef-ficient around 2010	At-risk-of-poverty rate around 2010	Population size in 2010	Occupied dwell-ings per 1,000 inhabit-ants around 2001
Bosnia and Herzegovina	75.9	-2.8	1.0	34.1	18.4	3,843,126	342
Croatia	105.1	-6.0	-1.2	27.0	17.9	4,425,747	374
Czech Republic	136.6	-4.7	2.7	24.9	9.0	10,506,813	373
Estonia	107.9	-14.3	2.3	31.3	15.8	1,340,127	394
Hungary	109.4	-6.8	1.3	24.1	12.3	10,014,324	365
Poland	106.5	1.6	3.9	31.1	17.6	38,167,329	304
Romania	76.9	-6.6	-1.9	33.3	21.1	21,462,186	319
Russia	106.1	-7.9	4.0	42.0	26.0	142,905,200	338
Serbia	61.8	-3.5	1.0	29.5	17.7	7,306,677	366
Slovakia	129.0	-4.9	4.2	25.9	12.0	5,424,925	307
Slovenia	148.9	-8.0	1.4	23.8	12.7	2,046,976	334
Ukraine	35.9	-14.8	-4.2	31.0	13.0	45,870,700	391

Note: a GDP per capita in PPP as a percentage of average GDP per capita in PPP for compared countries.
Source: World Bank (GDP in PPP), Eurostat, national statistical offices, expert estimates.

became the main heir of the former stock of public rental housing. However, their rights to dispose of this heritage were largely restricted by the state: either by central right to buy legislation and/or by central rent regulations.

Not-for-profit housing is a new phenomenon, having only appeared since the collapse of socialism. However, there are only two post-socialist countries in our sample where not-for-profit housing now makes up a visible share of the housing stock: Poland and Slovenia (2 percent of the housing stock in both of them). Moreover, the growth of this sector has probably ceased in both of them: Slovenia recently turned from supply-side subsidies towards housing allowances and Poland stopped its support for not-for-profit housing development. In Poland, it is expected that not-for-profit dwellings will be offered for sale to tenants and thus the sector is predicted to decline sharply. Not-for-profit housing programs have therefore so far been unsuccessful in the region. Additionally, not-for-profit (formally) often means municipal (in fact) because most not-for-profit organizations in Poland and Slovenia are municipally owned.

Formally, the new social housing models in many post-socialist states bear many similar features to social housing models in the West. Official

Table 19.2 Characteristics of Public/Social Housing on Sample Post-Socialist States, 2010

Country	Public / not-for-profit housing as % of total housing stock	Not-for-profit housing as % of total housing stock	Central rent control for existing SH/PH	Central rent control for new SH/PH	Central (official) definition of SH	Central allocation rules for SH/PH	New SH/PH output (1995–2010)	Trend for SH/PH output	Central (state) funding of SH/PH	Local (municipal) funding of SH/PH
BA	2.0	0.02	Yes, AVP	No	No	No	Marginal	No trend	Yes	No
HR	2.0	–	Yes, AVP	No	No	No	Marginal	Slight increase	Yes, marginal	Yes
CZ	10.0	–	Yes, since 2012 SG	Yes, CP	No	Yes, but till 2002 no targeting	**Substantial**	**Sharp decrease**	Yes	No
EE	4.0	–	No	No	No	No	Low	Slight increase	No	Yes
HU	4.0	–	No	Yes, CP	No	No	Marginal	Decrease	Yes	No
PL	12.0	2.00	Yes, SG	Yes, CP	Yes, since 1995	Yes, but TBS is finishing	**Medium**	**Sharp decrease**	Yes	No
RO	2.0	–	Yes, IR	Yes, IR	Yes, since 1996	Yes, general list of target groups	Low	No trend	Yes	No
RU	16.0	0.20	Yes, ST	Yes, ST	Yes, since 2005	Yes, but till 2005 no targeting	Marginal	Slight increase	Yes, matginal	Yes
RS	0.5	–	Yes, ST	Yes, ST	Yes, since 2009	Yes, general list of target groups	Medium	**Sharp decrease**	Yes	Yes, capital
SK	3.0	–	Yes, but planned deregulation	Yes, CP	No	Yes, income limits	**Substantial**	Slight increase	Yes	No
SI	4.0	2.00	Yes, AVP	Yes, AVP	Yes, since 1991	Yes, general statement	**Substantial**	**Sharp decrease**	Yes	Yes, in capital
UA	5.0	–	Yes, ST	Yes, ST	Yes, since 2006	Yes, income limits	Marginal	No trend	Yes	No

Note: SH - social housing, PH - public housing. APV – appraised value principle; SG – second generation; IR – income related; ST – strict tariffs; CP – cost principle. BA - Bosnia and Herzegovina; CZ - Czech Republic; HR – Croatia; EE – Estonia; HU – Hungary; PL – Poland; RO – Romania; RU – Russia; SK – Slovakia; SI – Slovenia; RS – Serbia; UA – Ukraine.
Source: Country chapters and expert estimates.

definitions of social housing have already been formulated in half of countries analyzed here (Poland, Romania, Russia, Serbia, Slovenia, Ukraine), rents in existing social/public housing are centrally regulated at below-market levels in ten of them (with the exception of Estonia and Hungary) and rents and allocation rules (targeting) for newly built social/public housing are centrally set in all the countries with any central social/public housing subsidies. However, the actual performance of new social/public housing strategies, especially in terms of their sustainability, has been poor.

As Table 19.2 (column 8) shows, there are three countries where new social/public housing output built between 1995 and 2010 can be considered substantial (when related to the size of the country's housing stock and the situation in other countries in the sample), and these are the Czech Republic, Slovakia, and Slovenia. By rough estimates obtained from the authors of the country chapters, between 1995 and 2010 eighty-five thousand to ninety thousand public dwellings were built in the Czech Republic; twenty-four thousand public dwellings in Slovakia; and twenty-three thousand public and not-for-profit dwellings in Slovenia. When divided by the total number of permanently occupied dwellings the ratio is especially high for Slovenia (3.5) and the Czech Republic (2.1).

However, in the Czech Republic most new public housing output had *de facto* status of homeownership, because the original state support for municipal housing was in fact converted into support for co-op housing: 'tenants' paid large contributions from their own pockets; became co-op members rather than pure tenants; and, as co-op members, had relatively extensive disposal rights similar to the rights of homeowners. Moreover, the program ended up with the state subsidizing the construction of luxurious dwellings, secondary homes, and flats acquired purely for speculation. When the program was amended in response to its deficits (co-op form was banned and income targeting was introduced), the scale of output substantially decreased and in recent years has become of marginal significance. In Slovenia, the former relatively generous social housing programs were recently scrapped and replaced by a housing allowance scheme, which is expected to be better targeted and make more efficient use of scarce public sources; this led to a substantial decrease in new social housing output.

A medium level of social/public housing output after 1995 was also observed in Serbia and Poland. However, the Serbian program ended up applying right-to-buy for tenants, and the stock became part of the owner-occupied housing stock (that is why Serbia now has the lowest share of public housing in the total housing stock out of all the countries in the sample). In Poland, the only country with a substantial not-for-profit social housing scheme (TBS) in the region, subsidization of new social housing output recently stopped, and flats built during the program's existence will probably be privatized to sitting tenants.

Social/public housing output is stable (or variable but with no clearly decreasing trend) only in countries with low or marginal new output

(Bosnia and Herzegovina, Croatia, Estonia, Romania, Russia, Ukraine) and in Slovakia. Slovakia is the exception in our sample: the construction of new social/public housing can be considered to be substantial and the trend is stable or even slightly increasing. This, however, is the only such example in our sample of post-socialist states.

The systems vary not only according to the amount of output but also according to the background ideology and the role of central institutions. Whereas some new social housing strategies strongly resemble the centralized systems under socialism (this is especially the case of Ukraine where three different waiting lists coexist, one of which is universal, just like under socialism), other systems rely explicitly on a free housing market and perceive social housing as a local and residual measure (such as in Estonia, Croatia, or to some extent in Hungary).

Table 19.2 shows that in nine out of twelve countries the new social/public/not-for-profit housing programs were funded mainly from the central (state) budget between 1995 and 2010 (Czech Republic, Poland, Romania, Hungary, Slovakia, Slovenia, Bosnia and Herzegovina, Serbia and Ukraine), whereas in three sample countries there were no significant state subsidies and new social housing output was exclusively or mainly funded from the local budgets of the municipalities (Croatia, Estonia, Russia). Hungary and the Czech Republic are important outliers in this respect: despite the fact that central rent regulation and central allocation rules for social/public housing were abolished (or will soon be abolished) and no central legal definition of social housing has been adopted, the main source of finance for new social/public housing output has come from the state. This is yet further evidence of the financial weakness of the municipalities in these largely decentralized countries.

CATEGORIZATION OF SOCIAL/PUBLIC HOUSING STRATEGIES APPLIED BETWEEN 1995 AND 2010

The social/public housing strategies applied in the period of 1995–2010 could be categorized from different perspectives. One way they can be categorized is by the volume of new social/public housing output built between 1995 and 2010 and the ideology framing it: *conservative strategy* (Ukraine, Russia); *emergency strategy* (Croatia, Serbia, Bosnia and Herzegovina); *market complement strategy* (Poland, Czech Republic, Slovenia, Slovakia); and *market residual strategy* (Estonia, Hungary, Romania). The conservative strategy is characterized by the survival of many features of socialist system: preservation of central waiting lists, application of the ideology of 'public housing for all', quasi-ownership rights of tenants, very strict rent regulation, and extremely low rents.

In countries affected by political instability and war the emergency strategy to social/public housing mainly addressed the housing needs of victims of war or forced migration. Its main goal was to meet emergency housing needs. In some of these countries there have recently been signs of a move towards the market strategy (Croatia). The market strategy attempts to define the role of social/public housing under free housing market conditions and is typical for advanced post-socialist states with a developed market-based housing finance system, a suitable legislative framework in place for housing market institutions, and some history of a functioning housing market. It contains both the role of social/public housing as important complement to the market (market complement strategy) and the role of a residual addition to the housing market (market residual strategy).

Another categorization combines the characteristics of social/public housing and the general economic performance of a country: *declined strategy* (Ukraine); *rational strategy* (Poland, Russia); *decentralized strategy* (Estonia, Hungary, Croatia); *central underdeveloped strategy* (Bosnia and Herzegovina, Romania, Serbia); and *central advanced strategy* (Czech Republic, Slovakia, Slovenia). In the declined strategy a country has a poor general economic performance; high at-risk-of-poverty rate; deep income inequalities; and, at the same time, a small share of social/public housing; very strict rent regulation; long and ineffective waiting lists; and marginal new social/public housing output. In the rational strategy to social/public housing also there is relatively unequal income distribution and a high at-risk-of-poverty rate in the country, but there is relatively significant share of social/public housing in the housing stock and even new output is not insignificant.

The decentralized strategy, like the declined strategy, is typically characterized by a small share of social/public housing in the total housing stock. However, thanks to the country's better economic performance, it is not, in fact, in decline and there is a stable volume of new social/public housing construction, mostly funded by local budgets; there are no central allocation rules and no official definition of social housing. For the central underdeveloped strategy the economy (in general) performs weakly; there are significant inequalities in society; and, at the same time, there is a marginal share of social/public housing in the housing stock. There is, however, an official definition of social housing; central rent control; and new social housing construction is mostly funded by state programs. In contrast to the declined strategy, the level of new output is stable (though marginal) and there is some funding from the state; in contrast to the rational strategy the overall share of social/public housing in the total housing stock is low.

The central advanced strategy is typically found in a country with above-average economic performance; higher income equality; a lower at-risk-of-poverty rate; significant share of social/public housing on total housing stock; and a relatively large volume of new social/public housing output; rent is regulated at the state level, and new social/public housing construction is funded mainly by central programs.

One would expect that new social/public housing output (measured as the share of new output built between 1995 and 2010 out of the total number of permanently occupied dwellings) would be greater in countries with a high at-risk-of-poverty rate (i.e., in countries where a relatively significant part of the population is considered to live in poverty). As Figure 19.1 shows, the opposite is true. The largest relative volume of construction was in Slovenia, the Czech Republic, and Slovakia, that is, countries with the lowest at-risk-of-poverty rates in our sample. The countries with the highest at-risk-of-poverty rates (Russia, Romania) reported only a 'middle' volume of social/public housing output.

If we take into account equality of income distribution (measured by Gini coefficient) and relative social/public housing output in the period 1995–2010, we get a picture similar to Figure 19.1 (only the differences among countries are smaller). Similarly, countries with relatively the lowest income inequality (Slovenia, Czech Republic, Slovakia) have the highest relative social/public housing output. Hungary and Croatia represent 'outliers' to some extent: despite their relatively equal income distribution, social/public housing output is rather low.

Another hypothesis is that higher economic performance (measured as GDP per capita in PPP) should be connected with higher public budget expenditures (i.e., also higher public expenditures on housing) and therefore higher relative social/public housing output. Figure 19.2 shows that this hypothesis is robustly confirmed for our sample of post-socialist countries.

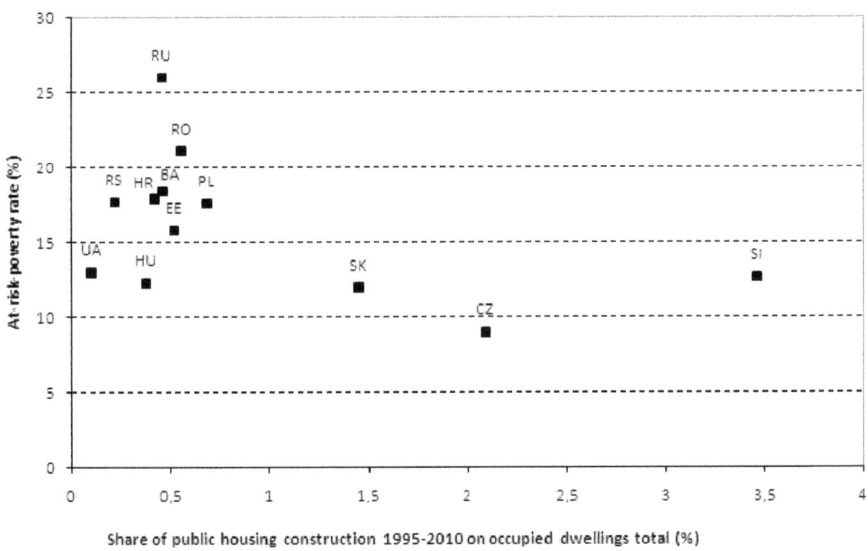

Figure 19.1 At-risk-of-poverty rate and public housing construction, 1995–2010.
Note: BA - Bosnia and Herzegovina; CZ - Czech Republic; HR – Croatia; EE – Estonia; HU – Hungary; PL – Poland; RO – Romania; RU – Russia; SK – Slovakia; SI – Slovenia; RS – Serbia; UA – Ukraine.
Source: Country chapters, expert estimates, Eurostat, national statistical offices.

The relative size of new social/public housing output grew with the level of GDP per capita at a rapid (logarithmic) rate, that is, a marginal increase in relative GDP above a certain level is followed by a significant increase in social/public housing output.

We might expect that countries hit hard by the economic recession (i.e., with strong decline of real GDP in 2009) would have been forced to cut their budget expenditures, including social/public housing subsidies. Consequently, the economic recession would have an impact on the trend in social/public housing construction in the future. However, there doesn't seem to be any connection. The countries hit hardest by the economic recession (Ukraine and Estonia) show stable (Estonia) or variable (Ukraine) trends in social/public housing construction. Conversely, Poland as the only country with a positive real GDP growth rate in 2009 shows a decreasing trend in new social housing construction.

Another important question is whether the existence of an official definition of social housing is positively connected with the level of new social/public housing output. However, this doesn't seem to be the case. Slovakia and the Czech Republic have no definition of social housing at the central level, but in spite of this they have a much higher level of social/public housing output than most of the countries that have adopted a legal definition of social housing.

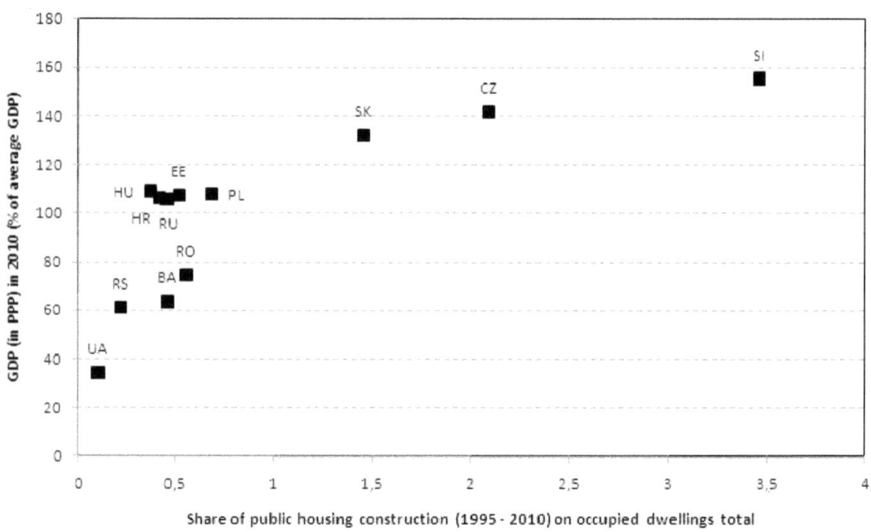

Figure 19.2 GDP (in PPP) in 2010 (as a percentage of average GDP in the sample) and public housing construction output, 1995–2010.

Note: BA - Bosnia and Herzegovina; CZ - Czech Republic; HR – Croatia; EE – Estonia; HU – Hungary; PL – Poland; RO – Romania; RU – Russia; SK – Slovakia; SI – Slovenia; RS – Serbia; UA – Ukraine.

Source: Country chapters, expert estimates, World Bank, national statistical offices.

THE EFFECTIVENESS AND EFFICIENCY OF NEW SOCIAL/PUBLIC HOUSING STRATEGIES

There may be a whole range of possible evaluation tools to assess new social housing policies in our sample of post-socialist states, but welfare economics is gradually becoming the standard approach for such analysis in policy studies. It is a branch of economics that simultaneously determine allocative efficiency within an economy and the income distribution associated with it.

The concept of efficiency originated in neoclassical economics as a social welfare function (the work of F. Y. Edgeworth, H. Sidwick, and A. Marshall described, e.g., in Ng 1983). However, this early approach produced rather different conclusions about 'efficient' social welfare, including such distributions that would lead to deep income and wealth inequalities in a society. The New Welfare Economics (studies by W. Pareto, J. Hicks, and others) distinguished between the *efficiency* and *equity (effectiveness)* parts of theory: the former is analyzed using the Pareto criteria of economic efficiency, and the latter (equity, effectiveness) can be analyzed only in close conjunction with particular social norms and values. In this way the concept of efficiency has been 'freed' from the influence of varied normative statements and/or social justice theorizing. In contrast, the concept of equity (effectiveness) has become fragmented into various theories of social justice and consequently into many types of particular welfare state regimes.

Efficiency is therefore defined through the Pareto lens: if any alternative allocation of goods increases utility from consumption for at least one actor on the market and at the same time does not decrease utility from consumption for other actors then we say such allocation is inefficient and there is room for improvement in market performance. For housing markets, particular examples of market failure may be the existence of oligopoly or monopoly in housing finance or production, asymmetric information access, externalities during housing production, or consumption. An example, which points to our main interest, is the situation where the state spends taxpayers' money for the production and allocation of goods or services that could be allocated by private entities, or where the social/public housing strategy is set up in a way that makes it financially unsustainable (unrealistic).

Effectiveness is closely associated with the idea of social justice and the welfare state;[2] it relates to the 'fair' distribution part of social welfare studies. As such, it is closely connected with particular welfare state regimes, social norms, and redistributive policies. Effectiveness may be understood as the degree to which the originally defined redistributive goals of state intervention are met, that is, whether public funds are actually spent where they were allocated and whether those for whom they were intended actually benefited from them.

However, the concept of effectiveness is not open to an infinite variety of definitions; the concept was thus, at least partially, generalized into the assumption that whatever state redistribution of wealth is finally applied, it should decrease social inequality in society. Policies should help the worse-off with the means of the better-off. The scale of wealth redistribution may be small (residual welfare state regime) or large (social-democratic welfare state regime), but in either case, all modern concepts of social justice share the assumption of the direction of wealth redistribution from less needy to more needy members of society.

Welfare economics also distinguishes between 'vertical' and 'horizontal' effectiveness (Barr 1993). Vertical effectiveness measures the degree of redistribution of income, consumption, and wealth from affluent (rich) to disadvantaged (poor). In the case of a particular housing subsidy it measures the extent to which such subsidy is actually allocated to those who really need help. Horizontal effectiveness is connected with the idea of setting a minimum standard of consumption that would be ensured for all members of society and with the assumption that all needy (poor) households have equal and unrestricted access to subsidies. In the case of a particular housing subsidy it measures whether any needy (poor) household is not eligible to apply for the subsidy (whether it is implicitly or explicitly excluded from state assistance).

We drew on the following assumptions (inspired by Lux 2009) to assess new (after-1990) social/public housing strategies in the sample of post-socialist states. For effectiveness the assumptions are:

Assumption 1: An effective social/public housing strategy assists lower-income (needy) households more than higher-income (less needy) households (vertical effectiveness).

Assumption 2: An effective social/public housing strategy does not exclude any lower-income (needy) households (horizontal effectiveness).

For efficiency, the main assumption was:

Assumption: A social/public housing strategy is efficient when it is not possible to find another strategy meeting the same goal that would be less costly to public budgets, and when it is financially sustainable in the long term.

Assessing effectiveness basically involves the measurement of the distribution of a particular subsidy in a society: in the case of social housing, this means whether it serves really vulnerable/needy households and whether all needy household are eligible for it. Measuring and evaluating the efficiency of subsidies is far more difficult. For example, housing policy reforms (alternative subsidy settings) could lower public expenditures and increase the efficiency of public spending in the short term, but many side effects, caused by the speed of reform and the application of a 'black-and-white' perspective in practical policies, may create substantial problems in the long term. Policy changes often create the need for unexpected additional public expenditures after their implementation. Such expenditures may offset a substantial amount of the public savings achieved.

All the authors of the country chapters made a partial assessment of the efficiency and effectiveness of new social/public housing strategies. It must be acknowledged that in every case they had to deal with a lack of the necessary statistical data and therefore they could make only a partial and often subjective (i.e., not substantiated by quantitative data analysis) assessment. Following is a summary of the main conclusions for each country drawn from the country chapters in this volume.

Slovenia

The main barrier to the sustainability of the social housing strategy in Slovenia is, according to the authors, the methodology used to valuate the housing units for rent regulation. Owing to this inappropriate rent control regime, rents do not cover the costs of housing provision and discourage nonprofit housing organizations from becoming more deeply involved in the provision of social housing (their housing facilities were operating at a loss). The lack of supervision of nonprofit organizations has been also mentioned as a problem. Because of the ineffective targeting of newly built social housing to those most in need and the efficiency problems, Slovenia recently stopped supply-side subsidization and turned to housing allowances. Moreover, there is ongoing privatization of both existing and new social housing at advantageous prices to sitting tenants, and this decreases the amount of stock available for needy households.

Estonia

The authors of the Estonian chapter mentioned the following drawbacks: extremely low rents in the residual social housing segment (equal to about one-third of the costs of the housing), which is the main efficiency deficit, and poor targeting in the allocation of new social dwellings, which is the main effectiveness deficit (many new allocations went to young families, key workers, former tenants of restituted housing with no test of their need). Various PPP projects with private developers have not functioned well, from either the effectiveness or efficiency perspectives: local governments pay developers unreasonably high rents and the rent/subsidy conditions are not flexible enough to reflect recent changes in the market resulting from the economic crisis. Moreover, social housing has increased segregation levels and the spatial pattern of new social housing output has reinforced differences inherited from the past.

Hungary

Hungary had the lowest new (weighted) social housing output of all the countries in our sample after 1995. Its only serious social housing program, the so-called Szecheny program, had several weaknesses: costs were very high (as well as relating cost rent) and allocation criteria for new tenancies were not regulated; the higher rents (when compared to existing public housing) and unregulated allocation allowed local governments to distribute it mainly among key workers and middle-class families, whereas the needs of only some vulnerable households were met. The program finished after three years of operation and was replaced with a means-tested housing allowance scheme. The authors identify the shadow economy incomes as one of reasons for ineffective targeting.

Croatia

Croatia was an example of an emergency strategy to social/public housing (aiming to satisfy the acute housing needs that arose after the Balkan War), but there have recently been signs of the system moving towards a residual market strategy. The country's first central program had had too many drawbacks: supply of newly built housing failed to meet the demand; some new buildings were of low quality; conversely, higher-quality dwellings were allocated using political rather than social criteria—some newly built dwellings were also purchased on speculation. The local program introduced in the capital of Zagreb was targeted more at key workers than needy households; poor targeting here is again explained as being due to the existence of a large informal incomes from shadow economy. Outsiders, mostly very vulnerable households, generally do not receive any effective help from the state in this field.

Romania

In Romania new social housing output is directed by the centrally based National Housing Agency, which acts both as a funding entity and a developer. The authors give this model a positive evaluation, but they note that the allocation of newly built social housing is nontransparent and most dwellings are allocated to young families (and young does not necessarily mean the most needy). Moreover, the rents are so low that they do not cover the costs and create a barrier to migration and a higher turnover of tenants. Due to the low rents, local authorities are obliged to cover the gap with an additional allowance scheme (the system is over-subsidized) and this decreases its financial sustainability. Despite the low rents, the number of people with rent arrears is high—it was estimated that one-third of social/public tenants are in rent arrears in bigger cities. Evictions for rent arrears are rare and politically unpopular.

Slovakia

Slovakia is an example of a country with relatively stable and large (when weighted to the size of the housing stock) new social/public housing output. Social/public housing, financed through preferential loans from state funds and grants from the responsible ministry, has enjoyed long-term political support. However, the allocation of new social/public housing again is not transparent. Moreover, more than 70 percent of households are eligible for new social/public housing under the central criteria. As a result, allocation rules may change quickly and preferential treatment may be given to groups of households that do not belong among vulnerable households. Marginalized social groups, especially the Roma, are victims of persistent discrimination and residential segregation.

Russia

The Russian social/public housing strategy is still similar in many ways to the socialist model of public housing: quasi-ownership entitlements of tenants; very low rents insufficient to cover housing costs; and a long waiting list based on a universal housing need assessment, which has included income among its criteria only since 2005 (registrations made before 2005 remained valid). Inefficiencies and gaps in the legal framework for condominiums create a somewhat paradoxical incentive for dwelling occupants to remain public tenants despite a generous right to buy offer. The plan to use a waiting list system to provide housing for low-income citizens was never put into practice: the financial resources of the municipalities are not sufficient to meet this demand (the average waiting time on the list is more than twenty years).

Poland

For a long time, the Polish model of not-for-profit housing provided by housing associations (TBSs) served as a unique example of well-functioning, financially sustainable, and economically efficient market strategy to social housing in the post-socialist region. There were allocation (effectiveness) deficiencies in the TBS system because, despite the income ceilings set by law and restricting access to less than half of the population, it was still targeted more towards the lower-middle classes than towards the poorest part of society. However, this fact was explained by high construction costs and, consequently, the higher rents in the newly built TBS dwellings than in existing social/public housing. However, owing to the growing fiscal deficit and successful pressure from tenants to buy their flats, which they paid for in part with a refundable deposit, the TBS system came to an end. The application of a right to buy policy will probably lead to the decline of this social housing segment in the future. In public housing, there is still a serious rent arrears problem: it is estimated that more than 40 percent of public tenants are in arrears.

Ukraine

Ukraine, like Russia, applied conservative strategy to social housing, retaining many of the institutional features that existed under socialism. Unlike

Russia, most tenants did use their right to buy option, but the remaining tenants as well as tenants of newly built public housing continue to have large quasi-homeownership rights and pay rents that are well below cost levels. The allocation procedures are still based on a waiting list system, which is nontransparent and badly targeted: there are now three different waiting lists and very little public housing available for allocations. The waiting period is extremely and unsustainably long: annually only 1–1.5 percent of people registered on the waiting list for 'ordinary' housing obtain a dwelling, and no housing stock for households registered on the 'social housing' waiting list has even been created.

Czech Republic

The Czech Republic is the country with the largest (weighted) new public housing output in the period of 1995–2010. However, official public housing support turned into *de facto* support for co-op (basically owner-occupied) housing and, owing to the absence of any limits on construction costs or the income of eligible households, the program was largely abused for the construction of luxurious dwellings, secondary housing, and housing for affluent households. Consequently, this system had serious deficits in terms of both effectiveness and efficiency. After a necessary amendment to the program, new public housing production sharply decreased and since the second half of the 2000s there has been very little new public housing construction. One positive development is that rents in existing public housing were deregulated and increased to cost levels.

Serbia

Serbia had a medium amount of new social housing output after 1995: new public housing was mainly used for emergency purposes to cover the acute needs of forced migration and it has been financed for a long time by the system of Solidarity Housing Funds that existed under socialism. However, all the tenants in both existing and newly built public housing were given a generous right to buy option and therefore the support *de facto* ended up going to highly subsidized owner-occupied housing. The allocation criteria, next to emergency requirements, were targeted more towards key workers and the middle class rather than poor households. The share of social/public housing in Serbia in recent years is the lowest of all the countries in our sample.

Bosnia and Herzegovina

Housing reconstruction after the war and the provision of housing for returnees were the strategic goals of the government in this country, and these required enormous housing investments. However, these investments managed to address only housing problems in rural areas and mostly took the form of support for owner-occupied housing. The emergency strategy to social housing appeared in this country only thanks to international donor financing involving both municipalities and NGOs. However, it also primarily targeted the victims of the war, irrespective of their income levels: families of war victims, individuals disabled by the war, civilian war victims, families with four or more children, inhabitants of undeveloped municipalities, and key workers. These housing programs applied immediate crisis solutions but did not take into account a targeting perspective (effectiveness) or long-term sustainability (efficiency).

CONCLUSION

An evaluation of new social/public housing strategies shows that there are serious deficiencies in both the efficiency and effectiveness in all the post-socialist states in our sample. All the strategies, regardless of the ideology behind it and regardless of the amount of new social/public housing output between 1995 and 2010, proved to be unsustainable in the long term and did not lead to any decisive growth in social/public renting. Those countries where new social/public housing output was assessed as substantial are now undergoing reforms and, consequently, the future trends look negative (with the exception of Slovakia).

Both the vertical and the horizontal effectiveness of strategies have been found to be low: long waiting lists based on universal housing needs in the conservative strategies were only combined with middle class and key workers preference in new social/public housing allocation in the market strategies. The low level of effectiveness has sometimes resulted in social/public housing being used for speculative purposes, being allocated non-transparently, or being allocated according to political criteria. The factors that were identified as the main causes of the lack of sustainable, efficient, and effective social housing schemes in post-socialist region are as follows:

- *Trap of privatization*—when social rental housing is built, sooner or later there is a demand for its privatization to the new social/public tenants; or it is transformed in practice into *de facto* homeownership support (applies to Serbia, Bosnia and Herzegovina, Croatia, Estonia, Poland, Czech Republic, Ukraine, Russia).
- *Paradox of decentralization*—small and politically weak municipalities (the main social landlords in the region) do not have sufficient fiscal sources to maintain an active social housing policy and, moreover, often refuse to make financially (costly) and politically (unpopular) risky decisions (applies basically to all post-socialist states).
- *Informal (shadow) economy* (applies to all post-socialist states) and *illegal settlements* (applies especially to Bosnia and Herzegovina,

Serbia and Croatia) make it difficult to estimate the real social and housing need, and targeting social housing according to declared income holds a risk of abuse.

- *Global economy and high construction costs*—due to the high price of new housing (when compared to the price of existing stock) public investment faces a dilemma: whether to build less housing with low rents targeting those in need or whether to build more housing with less affordable rents that cannot be targeted to those in need. The second option is path dependent (more consistent with public expectations of extensive state intervention, known from the past) and wins the much needed support of the middle classes for economic reforms (applies basically to all post-socialist states).
- *Socialist legacy in allocation schemes*—the legacy of universal 'housing need' and waiting lists in the allocation schemes of the conservative strategies, and the key workers schemes ('young and perspective employees') in the allocation schemes of the modern strategies (applies to all post-socialist states).
- *Not-for-profit schemes (usually inspired by the French HLM system) and PPP projects face mistrust or are generating unreasonably high costs.* Not-for-profit and PPP schemes failed to gain long-term support and not-for-profit actors are financially and politically weak (applies to Estonia, Slovakia, Slovenia and Poland); sometimes such schemes have been abused owing to the weakness of the law in the post-socialist environment.
- *General lack of public finance* as a result of war, the banking crises, the economic transformation, budget deficits. Every program ends up being halted after several years of operation and there is a sharp discrepancy between original intentions and real outcomes (applies basically to all post-socialist states).
- *Rent in social/public housing is usually set far below the cost level* and therefore it is not financially sustainable in the long term; despite this fact, households living in social/public housing often have large rent arrears.
- *Limited information about the efficiency and effectiveness of different programs*, which makes it impossible to thoroughly evaluate them.

With some exceptions, the recent trends in new social/public housing construction are mostly negative: the Polish and Slovenian systems of support for not-for-profit housing have *de facto* ceased operating; the Hungarian social housing policy has turned into demand-side subsidies; the scale of new social/public rental housing construction substantially decreased in Serbia, Ukraine, Russia, and the Czech Republic. Stable or positive trends are found only in countries where there is little social/public housing output (such as Bosnia and Herzegovina, Croatia, and Estonia). The only exception to the aforementioned rule is Slovakia, but there the share of public housing in the total housing stock is still very low.

The generally negative trends in social housing production and the low level of effectiveness (targeting) of social housing policies raises an important question: how do poor (needy) people obtain housing? Firstly, many older low-income households received generous economic subsidies in the early part of the transformation period (the giveaway sale of public housing or low rent in public housing) and therefore do not need any more substantial assistance. However, in the future, new households will not be able to benefit from subsidies similar to those derived from giveaway privatization and rent regulation.

Secondly, many newly formed low-income households rely on the intergenerational transfer of housing wealth and housing 'privileges'. The intergenerational transfer of housing privileges was common under socialism and was a deeply rooted behavioral pattern in all post-socialist societies. It probably served as the main bulwark against the rise of serious social problems in the early stage of the transformation of these societies.

Finally, in some countries (Czech Republic, Hungary and Slovenia) new means-tested housing allowances have now started to play a crucial role in increasing housing affordability for low-income households. In all the countries in the sample, however, social segregation grew during the last decade and inequalities in housing consumption deepened. This shows that the current systems, based on old economic subsidies and their intergenerational transfer, and on the housing allowance, are not sufficient to tackle the problem of worsening housing access among vulnerable households in post-socialist countries. Policies that ignore the dynamics of emerging economies (new demographic trends, divorces, migration) and are more or less a reflection of the socialist legacy will prove to be ineffective at tackling new social problems. Social housing may get a new and original face. However, it is hard to imagine that post-socialist states can live entirely without it.

NOTES

1. The annual national at-risk-of-poverty threshold according to Eurostat methodology was set at 60 percent of the national median income per equivalent adult.
2. We use the term *effectiveness* rather than *equity* in the text of this chapter. The reason is that equity, which is closely related to income distribution, need not be equal to housing consumption distribution; income inequalities do not have to fully reflect particular housing inequalities. The broader meaning of the term *effectiveness* is therefore more appropriate for the purpose of housing policy assessment (see Lux 2009).

REFERENCES

Barr, N. 1993. *The Economics of the Welfare State.* Oxford: Oxford University Press.

Breen, R. and Rottman, D. B. 1995. *Class Stratification. A Comparative Perspective.* New York: Harvester.

Buckley, R., Hendershott, P., and Villani, K. 1995. "Rapid Housing Privatization in Reforming Economies: Pay the Special Dividend Now." *Journal of Real Estate Finance and Economics* 10:63–80.

Crompton, R. 1998. *Class and Stratification: An Introduction to Current Debates.* Cambridge: Policy Press.

Daniel, Z. 1985. "The Effect of Housing Allocation on Social Inequality in Hungary." *Journal of Comparative Economics* 9:391–409.

Hamilton, M. and Hirszowicz, M. 1993. *Class and Inequality: Comparative Perspective.* Hemel: Harvester.

Hegedüs, J. and Tosics, I. 1996. "Disintegration of East-European Housing Model." *Housing Privatization in Eastern Europe.* Westport, CT: Greenwood.

Kornai, J. 1992. *The Socialist System: The Political Economy of Communism.* Oxford: Oxford University Press.

Krebs, V.,, Durdisová, J., Kotýnková, M., Mertl, J., Poláková, O., Žižková, J., Vlček, M., Vychová, M. 2005. *Sociální politika (Social Policy).* Prague: ASPI.

Lux, M., ed. 2003. *Housing Policy: An End or a New Beginning?* Budapest: Open Society Institute.

———. 2009. *Housing Policy and Housing Finance in the Czech Republic during Transition.* Amsterdam: Delft University Press.

Marcuse, P. 1996. "Privatization and Its Discontents: Property Rights in Land and Housing in the Transition in Eastern Europe." *Cities after Socialism.* Cambridge: Blackwell Publishers.

Ng, Y-K. 1983. *Welfare Economics.* London: Macmillan.

Pichler-Milanovich, N. 2001. "Urban Housing Markets in Central and Eastern Europe: Convergence, Divergence or Policy 'Collapse'?" *European Journal of Housing Policy* 1:145–87.

Renaud, B. 1995. "Housing Finance in Transition Economies. The Early Years in Eastern Europe and the Former Soviet Union." *Housing Finance International.* http://www.housingfinance.org/uploads/Publicationsmanager/9512_Tra.pdf accessed May 5, 2011.

Szelényi, I. 1983. *Urban Inequalities under State Socialism.* Oxford, New York: Oxford University Press.

Tsenkova, S. and Turner, B. 2004. "The Future of Social Housing in Eastern Europe: Reforms in Latvia and Ukraine." *European Journal of Housing Policy* 4 (2): 133–49.

Večerník, J. and Matějů, P., eds. 1999. *Ten Years of Rebuilding Capitalism. Czech Society 1898–1998.* Prague: Academia.

Yemtsov, R. 2007. *Housing Privatization and Household Wealth in Transition.* Research Paper No. 2007/02, United Nations University UNU-WIDER.

Contributors

Wolfgang Amann, Austria—Wolfgang Amann is a leading international expert in housing finance, housing policy, and housing legislation. As director of IIBW, the Institute of Real Estate, Construction and Housing Ltd., Vienna/Austria, he has executed some three hundred research and consulting projects in Western Europe and many CEE countries. A main focus in his professional activities is the implementation of PPP models in housing in transition countries. In this context he has published studies and influential articles in international journals and has executed consultancy and implementation projects in countries such as Albania, Armenia, Bulgaria, Hungary, Kyrgyzstan, Montenegro, Romania, Russia, and the Ukraine. He is consultant to the United Nations (REM—Real Estate Market Advisory Group) and the World Bank. Dr. Amann is an Associate Professor, teaching real estate economics at several graduate programs in Austria and is active in the European Network for Housing Research (ENHR). He holds the Decoration of Merit in Silver to the Republic of Austria.

Ioan Bejan, Romania—Ioan Bejan is an independent consultant specializing in housing finance and housing policy and currently the acting head of the Cabinet in the Romanian Ministry for the Economy. Until recently he worked as a business development manager for RAIFFEISEN BANCA PENTRU LOCUINTE, the "bauspar" subsidiary of Raiffeisen Bank in Bucharest. Prior to that, he was on the staff of the National Housing Agency, a public institution under the authority of the Romanian Ministry of Transport, Construction, and Tourism. As senior adviser and, for some time, a member of the board of directors, Ioan Bejan has focused on housing market and housing finance research, improving Romanian housing policy and housing subsidy programs, and developing the new housing finance legal framework. He has provided market analyses and assessments on housing policy and housing finance topics for the World Bank, the OECD, the European Mortgage Federation, the UN-ECE, the UN-HABITAT, USAID, and the Romanian government and has particular research experience in this field for the Central and East European region. He is the editor of the book *The Mortgage Loan* (2008) and is the author of a number of articles published in local newspapers.

Catalin Berescu, Romania—Catalin Berescu, PhD, is a Bucharest-based architect working in the field of extreme poverty areas and improper living conditions. He has coordinated several research and intervention projects in poor neighborhoods for which the teams received prizes for urban planning, published a book (*Housing and Extreme Poverty*, 2006) and various articles on Roma housing issues, and led a team that in 2008 created a ministerial methodology for improving housing conditions in areas affected by exclusion. In the last years he has presented papers at numerous conferences and given speeches in public events organized by various civil and political institutions across Europe on the recent formation of new Roma ghettos and other housing discrimination issues. Besides his academic activity, formerly at the Theory Department of the University of Architecture in Bucharest (digital imaging, contemporary theory), now at Babes-Bolyai in Cluj, he was involved in various international artistic actions aimed at drawing attention to the situation of people living in poverty. He is also an adobe building enthusiast.

Gojko Bežovan, Croatia—Gojko Bežovan is a professor of social policy at the Faculty of Law, Department of Social Work, University of Zagreb. He is active in research in the field of housing and housing policy, social policy, civil society, and welfare mix development. He is head of the interdisciplinary postgraduate program of urban management at the University of Zagreb. Currently he is implementing a housing survey–housing needs assessment in Croatia. He is adviser to the mayor of the city of Zagreb on housing and housing policy. He has published several articles and books in the mentioned field, such as *Stambena politika i stambene potrebe* (Housing Policy and Housing Needs, 1987), *Stanovanje i stambena kriza* (Housing and Housing Crisis, 1987), *Alternativna stambena politika* (Alternative Housing Policy, 1990), *Europske stambene inicijative* (European Housing Initiatives, 1993), "Stambena politika" (Housing Policy, 2005), and "Stanovanje i stambena politika" (Housing and Housing Policy, 2008).

Andreja Cirman, Slovenia—Andreja Cirman, PhD, is Associate Professor at the Faculty of Economics, University of Ljubljana, serving as Vice Dean for Academic Affairs since 2007. In her research work her main fields of expertise are housing and real estate, reflected in a variety of published articles, contributions, research works, and consultancy projects in Slovenia and abroad. She is a member of European Network for Housing Research (ENHR), American Real Estate Society, Housing Council of the Republic of Slovenia, and other professional organizations. She is also serving as a president and member of advisory boards in companies in Bosnia and Herzegovina and Slovenia.

József Hegedüs, Hungary—József Hegedüs, PhD, is a founding member of the Metropolitan Research Institute, which was established in 1989 in Budapest, Hungary. He has been a co-organizer of the East European Working Group of the European Network for Housing Research since 1989 and a member of the Housing Policy Council, a high-level advisory group in housing policy matters since 1996 in Hungary. Since 1994 he has been a part-time Associate Professor at Corvinus University Budapest. In the past two decades he has written extensively on housing issues, and his two most recent publications are on social housing in Hungary and social housing in transition countries, published in *Social Housing in Europe*, edited by C. Whitehead and K. Scanlon (London School of Economics, 2007). He was the coeditor of *The Reform of Housing in Eastern Europe and the Soviet Union*, edited by B. Turner, J. Hegedüs, and I. Tosics (Routledge, 1992); *Housing Privatization in Eastern Europe*, edited by D. Clapham, J. Hegedüs, K. Kintrea, and I. Tosics (Greenwood, 1996); and *Housing Finance: New and Old Models in Central Europe, Russia and Kazakhstan*, edited by J. Hegedüs and R. J. Struyk (OSI/LGI, 2005).

Marek Hojsík, Slovakia—Marek Hojsík is a public policy analyst and consultant in the Field of Roma inclusion. He focuses on topics of housing, de/segregation, social policy and EU Structural Funds. From 2010 to 2012 he was head of Social Development Fund, national agency for social inclusion responsible also for the implementation of European Social Fund programs. He designed and launched two large-scale national projects of social field work and community centers in Romany settlements. Previously he was involved in implementation of Open Society Institute's initiative Making the Most EU Funds for Roma in Slovakia. Between 2004 and 2007 he worked as advisor to the Slovak Government Commissioner for Roma Communities and participated in development and monitoring of public policies, including a pilot Comprehensive Approach of Romany Settlement Development. He conducted several field researches including Evaluation of municipal rent housing program's implementation in Romani settlements (published in 2008 in Slovak).

Anneli Kährik, Estonia—Anneli Kährik, PhD, has been a researcher and lecturer in human geography at the Department of Geography, University of Tartu in Estonia since 1999. Her main research areas are residential mobility and segregation, urban and housing issues, and urban governance in post-socialist cities. She has participated in a number of international research projects as a country's team coordinator or researcher, for example, Open Society Institute LGI–funded project on Local Government and Housing in CEE Countries (2002); European Commission–funded project on Access to Housing for Vulnerable Groups in Estonia (2003); EU 5th Framework Program–funded project on Neighborhood Housing Models (NEHOM) (2000–2004); and she is active in COST project Cities Regrowing Smaller (TU0803) (2009–2013). She is currently holding a four-year (2009–2012) research grant of the Estonian Science Foundation. Anneli Kährik has published extensively on urban and housing issues in the main international journals in the field, such as *Urban Studies*, *Housing Studies*, *Cities*, and more.

Jüri Kõre, Estonia—Jüri Kõre, sociologist and social policy researcher, is an Associate Professor at the University of Tartu, and has been an adviser to the Estonian Ministry of the Interior (1996–1999), and deputy mayor of the City of Tartu (1996–1997, 1999–2001, and from 2011). He is a member of several international and national social welfare and housing research projects. He has been a consultant to the Estonian Parliament and the government, the Ministry of Social Affairs, the Statistics Office of Estonia, and the Association of Estonian Cities. He is the author or coauthor of six books, such as: *Housing Policy in Europe and Estonia* (Tallinn, PRAXIS, 2002), *Housing Policy—An End or a New Beginning?* (Budapest, LGI, 2003), *Housing Policy in Transition Countries* (Tallinn, PRAXIS, 2004), and *Support and Housing* (Tartu, 2006). He has also written several articles published in the *European Journal of Housing Policy*, the *Acta et commentationes Universitatis Tartuensis*, and the *Estonian Human Development Reports*. He is a researcher for FEANTSA (European Federation of National Organizations Working with the Homeless) (2004–2006). His main interests are comparative social policy and housing policy, social housing, social welfare and social services management, and local government issues.

Martin Lux, Czech Republic—Martin Lux, PhD, sociologist and economist, head of the Department of Socio-Economics of Housing at the Institute of Sociology, Academy of Sciences of the Czech Republic in Prague. He was the leader of several international and national housing research projects, a consultant for LGI, MOW, UN-ECE, the Czech government, and the Czech banking sector. He has edited ten books, such as *Housing—Res Publica* (Prague, SLON, 2002) and *Housing Policy—An End or a New Beginning?* (Budapest, LGI, 2003, translated into three other languages), and is the author or coauthor of articles published in *Urban Studies*, *Housing Studies*, *Journal of Housing and the Built Environment*, *European Journal of Housing Policy*, *European Sociological Review*, *Communist and Post-Communist Studies*, *Post-Communist Economies*, *Czech Journal of Economics and Finance*, *Czech Sociological Review*, and others. He is a member of the European Network for Housing Research, the Association for Housing Market Development, and the Advisory Board for the International Journal of Housing Policy. His main interests are comparative housing policies, social housing, housing finance, and housing economics.

Srna Mandič, Slovenia—Srna Mandič is an Associate Professor at the Faculty for Social Sciences at University of Ljubljana, and Head of the Centre for Welfare Studies. She has served as a member of the Group of Experts on Access to Housing at the Council of Europe, a member of the Coordination Committee of the European Network for Housing Research, one of the coordinators of the European Observatory on Homelessness at FEANTSA, and a member of the National Housing Council of the Ministry of the Environment of Slovenia. Her recent publications have covered the topics of homelessness, housing reforms, and housing mobility as well as cross-national comparisons in home-leaving, housing conditions, and the role of housing assets. Her publications include "Rental Housing in Central and Eastern Europe as No Man's Land" (cowritten with H. Priemus) in the *Journal of Housing and the Built Environment*; "Trends in Central Eastern European Rented Sectors" in the *Journal of Housing and the Built Environment*; "Residential Mobility versus 'In-Place' Adjustments in Slovenia: Viewpoint from a Society 'in Transition'" in *Housing Studies*; "Home-Leaving and Its Structural Determinants in Western and Eastern Europe: An Exploratory Study" in *Housing Studies*; "The Changing Role of Housing Assets in Post-Socialist Countries" in *Journal of Housing and the Built Environment*; and, with A. Cirman, "Housing Conditions and Their Structural Determinants: Comparisons within the Enlarged EU" in *Urban Studies*.

Alexis Mundt, Austria—Alexis Mundt, economist and historian, is a research associate at the Vienna-based IIBW—Institute for Real Estate, Construction and Housing Ltd. His areas of research include the history of the welfare state, social policy evaluation, comparative housing policy, and social housing. He has worked on a number of projects that have investigated and evaluated housing policy in Austria and Europe.

Alina Muzioł-Węcławowicz, Poland—Alina Muzioł-Węcławowicz, PhD, is senior lecturer at the Warsaw University of Technology and expert in National Economy Bank, Warsaw, Poland. She previously was working at the Institute of Geography and Spatial Organization of the Polish Academy of Sciences. Her research interests are housing policy and finance, regeneration policy, and urban development. Her research and consultancy activity concern local and national housing and urban regeneration issues. She wrote several articles on housing reforms in Poland, published in books on housing reforms in Central and Eastern Europe. Recently she published *Perspectives of Development of Social Rental Housing* in *Immovable Financing*, a quarterly of the Union of Polish

Banks; "The Regeneration of Central Districts of Polish Cities" in the book *Spatial Aspects of Urban Regeneration*; and edited *Examples of Urban Regeneration Programs* (both published in Polish by the Urban Research Institute, Cracow).

Mina Petrović, Serbia—Mina Petrović is an Associate Professor in sociology in the Department of Sociology at the Faculty of Philosophy of Belgrade, where she teaches urban sociology, the sociology of housing, social and residential segregation, the sociology of youth, and some courses in methodology. Her research interest is in socio-spatial mobility and exclusion, social housing, urban culture, and local governance. She has published five books and numerous articles in journals and edited volumes. Her book titled *Housing Policy: Challenges and Opportunities* (2004, in Serbian) covers the key issues of social housing in a comparative perspective, in particular the questions of its efficiency in relation to different welfare concepts and redistributive goals. Petrović's latest book, titled *Transformation of Cities: Towards the De-Politicization of the Urban Question* (2009, in Serbian), is devoted to an analysis of the rising socio-spatial inequalities in contemporary European cities. She wrote about the post-socialist housing transformation in Serbia for the *European Journal of Housing Policy* (2001). Her latest publications in English include: a chapter on Belgrade's post-socialist urban evolution in the book *The Post-Socialist City*, edited by Stanilov (Springer 2007, coauthor with S. Vujović); and two articles on Belgrade urban neighborhoods' development, published in *Children's Geographies* (2010, coauthor with S. Tomanović) and in *International Journal of Urban and Regional Research* (2011, coauthor with S. Hirt).

Alexandr Puzanov, Russia—Alexandr Puzanov is a research analyst in the fields of housing and social policy and regional, urban and community development. He is one of the six founders of the Institute for Urban Economics, a Russian think tank providing analysis and assistance in urban issues. In 2004 he was also appointed Chair of Urban Economics and Municipal Governance in the Department for State and Municipal Management of the Higher School of Economics. He is a member of the advisory boards of the journals *Urban Research and Practice* and the *Review of Urban & Regional Development Studies*. His main publications have dealt with the provision of affordable housing to moderate income households, social housing, housing legislation and real estate market development, rent reform and housing allowances, monitoring Russia's experience with housing allowances, and income adjustments owing to rent increases in post-Soviet economies.

Elisabeth Springler, Austria—Elisabeth Springler, economist, is deputy director of the program of studies European Economy and Business

Management and coordinator of Economics at the University of Applied Sciences bfi-Vienna, Austria. Previously she was appointed as Assistant Professor at the Vienna University of Economics; Visiting Professor at the University of Applied Sciences, Volda, Norway; and Marshallplan-Chair at the University of New Orleans, Louisiana. Besides of housing economics, her research interests include Post-Keynesian monetary economics and European Integration. She is editorial board member of the journal *Kurswechsel* as well as reviewer for many international journals. She has numerous publications in these fields including edited books, like *Heterodoxe Ökonomie*, together with colleagues from Vienna University of Economics (2009). She published, together with Nathalie Homlong, the book *Wirtschaftspartner Indien* as result of her research on the Indian subcontinent.

Petr Sunega, Czech Republic—Petr Sunega, an economist, is one of the founding members of the Department of Socio-Economics of Housing at the Institute of Sociology, Academy of Sciences of the Czech Republic. He has participated in most of the research projects undertaken by the department—projects supported by national grant agencies, ministries and by the European Commission's Fifth Framework research program (Sustainable Refurbishment Europe). His field of specialization is housing allowances in comparative perspective, housing economics, and simulation modeling. He is the coauthor of several books, such as four books published in the Housing Standards series (Prague, Institute of Sociology) and *Housing—Res Publica* (Prague, SLON, 2002). He is also the coauthor of one chapter in a book titled *Housing Allowances in Comparative Perspective* (Bristol, Policy Press, 2007), and the author or coauthor of articles published in the *European Sociological Review*, *Urban Studies*, *European (International) Journal of Housing Policy*, *Journal of Housing and the Built Environment*, *Sociologický časopis/Czech Sociological Review*, *Czech Journal of Economics and Finance*, and others.

Gorana Stjepanović, Bosnia and Herzegovina—Gorana Stjepanović is a PhD student at the Faculty of Architecture of Belgrade University. Her field of interest includes social housing, socio-spatial segregation, and the role of national policy in terms of social housing. She participates in conferences on social housing and in research on social housing concepts, which is linked to her PhD thesis.

Nóra Teller, Hungary—Nóra Teller, a sociologist, has worked on several international projects for the Council of Europe, the Friedrich Ebert Foundation, the European Commission's Fifth, Sixth and Seventh Framework research programs on various aspects of housing (OSIS, DEMHOW) and ESPON. She has conducted research on issues about social housing construction and housing allowances in Hungary, and has been involved in the development of local-level housing strategies in Hungary and in consultation on the development of some national-level housing programs. She was one of the housing experts and evaluators of the Roma settlement rehabilitation program in Hungary in 2005–2007 and 2010 and led the evaluation team assessing the impact of EU Funds for Roma integration in Hungary in 2011. In the framework of an OSI/LGI Fellowship, she conducted a research about the links of segregated urban areas and local development in 2007. In 2008, as part of an EU-funded project, she was advising the state government of Bosnia and Herzegovina on the development of a national-level social housing policy strategy. She has published several papers on social housing policy and decentralization and coedited a publication on security and insecurity issues of homeownership (M. G. Elsinga, P. De Decker, N. Teller, J. Toussaint, *Home Ownership beyond Asset and Security*, 2007). She is member of the European Network of Housing Research and the European Observatory on Homelessness of FEANTSA. She is one of the editors of the European Journal of Homelessness. Her ongoing PhD research focuses on Roma housing mobility in Hungary.

Irina Zapatrina, Ukraine—Irina Zapatrina used to be the Deputy Minister of Housing and Communal Services of Ukraine, which is responsible for strategic development, housing policy, international relations, and scientific development. She holds a doctorate in economic science and is the head of the State Finance Department of the Academy of Financial Management. She has published more than eighty scientific papers in the areas of finance, economic development, housing, and communal services. She is the author of the recently published monograph *Budget Mechanism of Economic Growth* and coauthor of the book *Social Housing in Ukraine: Problems and Perspectives*. She is working on the development of housing legislation in Ukraine.

Index

M

N

O

P

Q

R

S

www.ingramcontent.com/pod-product-compliance
Ingram Content Group UK Ltd.
Pitfield, Milton Keynes, MK11 3LW, UK
UKHW022004180926
475701UK00003B/186
* 9 7 8 1 1 3 8 8 0 9 5 6 7 *